MYCOBACTERIUM AVIUM–
COMPLEX INFECTION

LUNG BIOLOGY IN HEALTH AND DISEASE

Executive Editor

Claude Lenfant
Director, National Heart, Lung and Blood Institute
National Institutes of Health
Bethesda, Maryland

The opinions expressed in these volumes do not necessarily represent the views of the National Institutes of Health.

MYCOBACTERIUM AVIUM– COMPLEX INFECTION

PROGRESS IN RESEARCH AND TREATMENT

Edited by

Joyce A. Korvick

*National Institute of Allergy
and Infectious Disease
National Institutes of Health
Bethesda, Maryland*

Constance A. Benson

*Rush Medical College/Rush-Presbyterian–
St. Luke's Medical Center
Chicago, Illinois*

Marcel Dekker, Inc.　　　**New York • Basel • Hong Kong**

Library of Congress Cataloging-in-Publication Data

Mycobacterium avium–complex infection : progress in research and treatment / edited by Joyce A. Korvick, Constance A. Benson.
    p. cm. — (Lung biology in health and disease ; v. 87)
    Includes bibliographical references and index.
    ISBN 0-8247-9403-6 (hardcover : alk. paper)
    1. Mycobacterium avium. 2. Mycobacterial diseases. 3. AIDS (Disease)—Complications. 4. Opportunistic infections. I. Korvick, Joyce A. II. Benson, Constance A. III. Series.
    QR82.M8M94 1995
    616.2'4—dc20
                                                   95-31147
                                                  CIP

The publisher offers discounts on this book when ordered in bulk quantities. For more information, write to Special Sales/Professional Marketing at the address below.

This book is printed on acid-free paper.

MARCEL DEKKER, INC.
270 Madison Avenue, New York, New York 10016

Current printing (last digit):
10 9 8 7 6 5 4 3 2 1

PRINTED IN THE UNITED STATES OF AMERICA

INTRODUCTION

The perpetual enemies of the human race, apart from man's own nature, are ignorance and disease.

—Alan Gregg, 1941

Contemporary medical researchers often refer to "emerging infections." This term applies to diseases caused by newly discovered bacteria and viruses. However, sometimes it could also apply to the resurgence of conditions that have been forgotten, or were not considered of great public health importance.

Infections have been of concern for centuries. The existence of transmissible agents was first recognized by Marcus Varro in the first century B.C., who noted that it was unsafe to live close to swamps because of "certain minute creatures which cannot be seen by the eyes, which float in the air and enter the body through the mouth and nose and then cause disease."

Mycobacterium tuberculosis is by far the most famous—or infamous —of all the mycobacteria. Although it was identified only in 1882 by Koch, tuberculosis was described in 1500 B.C. and there is some evidence that it might have existed as early as 4000 B.C. (1). It is in the year 1950 that non-tuberculosis mycobacterial diseases began to be recognized; among these causing agents *Mycobacterium avium* complex may be the most common. Of course, the bacteria was active long before 1950, but its effect was often hidden by the condition with which it was associated. Since then, *Mycobacterium avium* complex has been reported to occur usually in patients with underlying chronic lung disease, particularly in elderly persons. Others have concluded that it can also affect individuals without predisposing conditions, particularly elderly women. Yet, it is the occurrence of the acquired immunologic lung syndrome that greatly contributed to the dissemination of *Mycobacterium avium* complex and heightened the interest in the resulting infection.

This volume edited by Drs. Joyce A. Korvick and Constance A. Benson presents the readership with state-of-the-art description —from epidemiology to treatment—of the infection caused by *Mycobacterium avium* complex. As we see no end to the AIDS epidemic, it is evident that we must not ignore the causes and consequences of one of its complications. This is why the series of monographs *Lung Biology in Health and Disease* includes two volumes on *Pneumocystis carinii*.

The editors have assembled experts in many disciplines to contribute to this volume. As the goal of the series is to present to the readers the most recent advances in lung biology or in related issues, this volume is an important addition. I am thankful to its editors and contributors for their participation.

Claude Lenfant, M.D.
Bethesda, Maryland

[1]Philip C. Hopewell. Mycobacterial Diseases in Textbook of Respiratory Medicine. J.F. Murray and J.A. Nadel, Editors. W.B. Saunders Co. 1988.

PREFACE

Until recently, generations of practicing clinicians have been reluctant to treat *Mycobacterium avium*–complex (MAC) infection. Therapeutic intervention required numerous agents, with considerable toxicity and limited proven efficacy. In the United States, disseminated MAC infection has emerged as the most common bacterial infection occurring in patients with AIDS, affecting up to 43% of HIV-seropositive persons. Limited therapeutic success with multidrug regimens, consisting of conventional antimycobacterial drugs, has led clinicians to approach the treatment of disseminated MAC infection with pessimism. New, more effective approaches to prevention and therapy are clearly needed.

The clinical presentation of MAC infection is dependent upon underlying host characteristics. The classical presentation of modestly symptomatic and indolent pulmonary disease was commonly seen in older adults with underlying parenchymal lung processes such as chronic obstructive pulmonary disease, prior cavitary tuberculosis, or pneumoconioses. MAC would be isolated from sputum specimens. Therapy, which consisted of multiple, conventional antimycobacterial agents, was not usually instituted unless the patient had significant pulmonary symptoms and/or pulmonary infiltration. Disseminated MAC disease is most commonly seen in HIV-seropositive individuals whose CD4+ T-cell counts are under 100 cells/mm^3. The symptoms of disseminated MAC include fevers, night sweats, weight loss or wasting, diarrhea, fatigue, and abdominal pain. Laboratory abnormalities include anemia (out of proportion to that expected of the underlying disease state) and elevated serum alkaline phosphatase (often indicative of liver infiltration). MAC is most frequently isolated from blood, but can be recovered from other sterile body sites in these patients. Studies suggest that HIV-seropositive individuals with disseminated MAC infection have a shorter duration of survival than those without MAC.

In contrast to most conventional antituberculosis drugs, the newer expanded-spectrum macrolides, clarithromycin and azithromycin, have been shown to have substantial in vitro and clinical activity against MAC. This discovery, coupled with the increasing numbers of HIV-infected persons coinfected with *Mycobacterium avium* complex, has resulted in expanded interest in developmental therapeutics for MAC disease. Recent clinical studies have demonstrated that clarithromycin and azithromycin can decrease the quantity of MAC in the blood; however, longer-term studies are needed to determine if there is a survival benefit when these agents are used for treatment. Even though the macrolides have great promise in the treatment of MAC, the development of resistance to them, also shown in recent clinical trials, remains a real threat to their continued usefulness.

In view of the largely bacteriostatic activity and potential for engendering resistance among these agents, the therapeutic armamentarium currently at hand for MAC remains suboptimal. Additionally, more potent agents are needed. However, barriers to early preclinical testing of potential new compounds exist including the slow growth rate of *Mycobacterium avium* complex, the lack of "standards" for in vitro susceptibility testing, the diversity of colony morphology and virulence, and the controversy regarding appropriate animal models and their relation to human disease. The recent application of new approaches in immunology and molecular biology to MAC promises to overcome some of these limitations.

This monograph reviews the current status of preclinical and clinical research on *Mycobacterium avium* complex in the 1990s. Emphasis will be placed on epidemiology, the clinical presentation of MAC disease, the results of clinical trials for treatment and prophylaxis of MAC disease, and the pharmacokinetics of newer anti-MAC agents. In order to bridge the gap between the clinic and the laboratory, the microbiology, pathogenesis, and immunopathology of *Mycobacterium avium* complex as they relate to developmental therapeutics are integrated with the clinical topics. In addition, this monograph briefly describes what is on the horizon and to what extent new techniques in molecular biology, genetics, and immunology can be applied to MAC research to further enlighten our current state of knowledge. Developmental therapeutics for MAC will not only include pharmacological agents but could ultimately involve immunological and gene therapy as well.

The primary audience for this monograph is the practicing clinician, AIDS researcher, and student of MAC infection. This monograph is intended to link preclinical and clinical knowledge of MAC disease in addition to identifying potential areas for scientific inquiry open to young investigators. Although scientific advances have been made in this field, significant research opportunities remain. This is an area of research that is expected to grow into the next decade.

Joyce A. Korvick
Constance A. Benson

CONTRIBUTORS

Constance A. Benson, M.D.   Associate Professor of Medicine and Infectious Disease, Department of Medicine, Section of Infectious Disease, Rush Medical College/Rush-Presbyterian–St. Luke's Medical Center, Chicago, Illinois

Luiz E. Bermudez, M.D.   Senior Scientist, Kuzell Institute for Arthritis and Infectious Diseases, California Pacific Medical Center Research Institute, San Francisco, California

William J. Burman, M.D.   Fellow, Division of Infectious Diseases, University of Colorado Health Sciences Center, Denver, Colorado

David L. Cohn, M.D.   Director, Denver Disease Control Service, Denver Health and Hospitals, and Division of Infectious Diseases, University of Colorado Health Sciences Center, Denver, Colorado

G. L. Drusano, M.D.   Professor and Director, Departments of Medicine and Pharmacology, Albany Medical College, Albany, New York

Jerrold J. Ellner, M.D.   Professor of Medicine and Pathology, Department of Medicine, Division of Infectious Diseases, Case Western Reserve University, Cleveland, Ohio

Joseph O. Falkinham, III, Ph.D.   Professor of Microbiology, Department of Biology, Virginia Polytechnic Institute and State University, Blacksburg, Virginia

C. Robert Horsburgh, Jr., M.D.   Professor of Medicine, Division of Infectious Diseases, Department of Medicine, Emory University School of Medicine, Atlanta, Georgia

Clark B. Inderlied, Ph.D.   Associate Professor, Department of Pathology and Laboratory Medicine, University of Southern California, Children's Hospital Los Angeles, Los Angeles, California

Michael D. Iseman, M.D.   Professor of Medicine, Division of Pulmonary Sciences and Infectious Diseases, University of Colorado School of Medicine, Denver, Colorado

John L. Johnson, M.D.   Assistant Professor of Medicine, Division of Infectious Diseases, Department of Medicine, Case Western Reserve University and University Hospitals of Cleveland, Cleveland, Ohio

Thomas P. Kanyok, Pharm.D.   Assistant Professor, Department of Pharmacy Practice, College of Pharmacy, University of Illinois at Chicago, Chicago, Illinois

Aaron D. Killian, Pharm.D.   Research Fellow, Department of Pharmacy Practice, College of Pharmacy, University of Illinois at Chicago, Chicago, Illinois

Joyce A. Korvick, M.D.   Medical Officer, Division of AIDS, National Institute of Allergy and Infectious Disease, The National Institutes of Health, Bethesda, Maryland

Michael McNeil, Ph.D.   Associate Professor, Department of Microbiology, Colorado State University, Fort Collins, Colorado

Kevin A. Nash, Ph.D. Research Associate, Department of Pathology and Laboratory Medicine, University of Southern California, Children's Hospital Los Angeles, Los Angeles, California

Hiroe Shiratsuchi, Ph.D. Instructor, Division of Infectious Disease, Department of Medicine, Case Western Reserve University, Cleveland, Ohio

Lowell S. Young Kuzell Institute for Arthritis and Infectious Diseases, California Pacific Medical Center Research Institute, San Francisco, California

CONTENTS

Contents

1

Epidemiology of *Mycobacterium avium* Complex

C. ROBERT HORSBURGH, JR.
Emory University School of Medicine
Atlanta, Georgia

I. *Mycobacterium avium* Complex in the Environment

A. Birds

Mycobacterium avium complex (MAC) was first isolated from birds in the nineteenth century; thus the organism was named *M. avium*. Although it was recognized at the time that the organism caused disease in both domestic and wild birds, acceptance of MAC as a human pathogen did not occur until the 1950s. Most MAC disease in birds is caused by the traditional "avium" serotypes; namely, serotypes 1–3 (1–4). In contrast, most human disease is caused by "intermediate" serotypes (serotypes 4–9, particularly 4, 6, and 8), although MAC pulmonary disease is frequently caused by "intracellulare" strains (serotypes 10 and higher). These observations suggest that birds are not a common source of human infection (1).

B. Water and Aerosols

In the 1970s, MAC organisms were isolated from water by a number of investigators. Ocean water, freshwater ponds, and piped water systems have

1

all been identified as reservoirs for MAC (5–8). MAC from ocean water and freshwater ponds are also generally different from human isolates by serotype, DNA typing, ability to grow at 43°C, antibiotic susceptibility pattern, plasmid profile, susceptibility to heavy metals, and ability to grow on specific media (9–17); this suggests that these sources are not common reservoirs for human disease. However, in some instances, isolates from freshwater ponds have been similar to patient isolates (18,19). MAC organisms appear to be present in water in all geographical areas, although prevalence may be less in developing countries (20,21).

MAC isolates similar to patient isolates are often found in piped water systems, particularly hot water systems with recirculating holding tanks that are kept at less than 140°F. MAC organisms isolated from such systems have been of the same serotype as those isolated from some patients in several studies (6,22–24); in one report, isolates recovered from institutional hot water systems were identical to patient isolates by pulsed-field gel electrophoresis (24).

Since pulmonary disease is a major manifestation of MAC infection, much interest has been directed to potential aerosol routes of MAC exposure. Since MAC is known to reside in many bodies of water, water aerosols have been proposed as a mechanism for MAC transmission (8,17,25,26). Supporting this are the similarity of MAC from aerosols to clinical isolates (10,26) and the concentration of MAC in water aerosols in a laboratory model of aerosolization (17).

C. Amphibians and Mammals Other than Humans

MAC organisms have been most commonly isolated from pigs and cattle, where they may cause disease or subclinical colonization. MAC serotypes from these animals resemble human serotypes, with serotypes 2, 6, and 8 predominating (1,4,27–34). However, this may merely reflect the widespread distribution of these serotypes of MAC in the environment, as MAC isolates have also been recovered from hares, cats, dogs, deer, wild boar, and monkeys (4,35). Kazda isolated MAC serotype 8 from frogs, suggesting this animal as a possible reservoir of infection (18).

D. Soil

Mycobacteria of all types are common in soil, and MAC organisms have been isolated from this site as well. MAC organisms have been found in loam, clay, mud, and sand, but these isolates were not further characterized (18,20,29,36). In other reports, MAC isolates from soil with serotypes similar to patient isolates were recovered (20,29,38) but no direct links to human infection were established.

E. Food

The presence of MAC in cattle, pigs, chickens, and turkeys indicates that undercooked beef, pork, chicken, and turkey are potential sources of MAC infection in humans. In addition, MAC isolates have been found in milk, both pasteurized and unpasteurized, and in raw oysters (39–41). Chapman has postulated that milk is the source of MAC cervical lymphadenitis in children (42), but this hypothesis has not been tested. Vegetables have not been identified as sources for MAC, although MAC has been recovered from dried plants (43).

F. Humans

Humans may have transient or prolonged carriage of MAC in oral or bronchial secretions (44,45). MAC was isolated from about 1% of asymptomatic persons in these studies; the duration of this carriage was not examined. Persons with chronic lung disease may have prolonged colonization with MAC, although separation of this entity from early invasive disease is a persistent diagnostic dilemma (46). Stools of control patients in studies of the role of mycobacteria in the etiology of Crohn's disease have shown that healthy persons may have MAC in the gastrointestinal (GI) tract (47,48), suggesting that ingestion of MAC and passage through the GI tract are common occurrences in the absence of disease.

G. Other Sites

Beerworth has reported recovering MAC from insects living in sawdust, on trees, and elsewhere as summarized by Meissner and Anz (4).

II. Human Exposure to MAC

A. Skin Test Reactivity

Interpretation of results of skin testing to determine exposure to MAC presents two difficulties. The first is the fact that testing has been done with two preparations, one of which, purified protein derivative Battey (PPD-B) is no longer available. This preparation, made from an *M. intracellulare* strain, was used from 1956 to about 1976, when supplies were exhausted (49–51). A new batch was prepared by the Public Health Service but has not been standardized and is not currently available (52). A second preparation, "*M. avium* sensitin'' (Statens Seruminstitut, Copenhagen, Denmark), made from an *M. avium* strain, is available in Europe but is only available for investigational use in the United States at the present time (53–59). Although the two preparations are not made from the same MAC strain, they have produced similar results in the one area where both have been studied (59), and for the purposes of this review, they will be considered together.

The second difficulty in evaluating the results of skin testing for MAC is the cross reactivity of the antigen. In areas where tuberculosis (TB) is prevalent, persons with TB infection or disease will have a positive skin test to MAC as well. This problem necessitates dual skin testing with tuberculin purified protein derivative (PPD) as well as the MAC reagent; individuals are characterized by which of the two reactions is larger (i.e., MAC dominant or TB dominant) (49,50,58,59). Therefore, there is some degree of imprecision when neither reaction is dominant. However, in areas of low TB prevalence, such as the United States, a positive MAC skin test has a useful predictive value (59). Exposure to other nontuberculous mycobacteria may also lead to a positive skin test. In particular, the similarity between distribution of skin test reactivity to MAC and to a skin test preparation of *M. scrofulaceum* (PPD-G) suggested that a positive MAC skin test might more truly be considered to represent exposure to either MAC or *M. scrofulaceum* (50). Nonetheless, skin testing has revealed important features of environmental exposure to MAC.

In a study in North Carolina in 1965, MAC skin test positivity was first seen at age 2 years, and it increased in a linear fashion up to age 20, at which age 60–80% of the population had a positive test (Fig. 1) (51). After age 20, rates were relatively stable. Whites were less likely to be positive than blacks, and women were less likely to be positive than men. This increase in reactivity with age in children was also seen in a study of Swedish schoolchildren in 1985–1988 (54,55).

A large national study done in military recruits by Edwards and Palmer in 1958 showed considerable geographical variability in reactivity to PPD-B (49,50). In the northern United States, generally less than 20% of recruits had a positive test (Fig. 2). Reactivity increased as the home county of the recruit moved south, to greater than 60% positivity in recruits from the gulf or south Atlantic coasts. Recruits from rural areas were more likely to have a positive test than recruits from urban counties.

MAC skin test positivity occurs in many geographical areas, although the rates of positivity vary and cannot be directly compared because of demographical differences among the groups studied. Swedish schoolchildren aged 4–5 years from an urban area had a positivity rate of 8%, whereas by

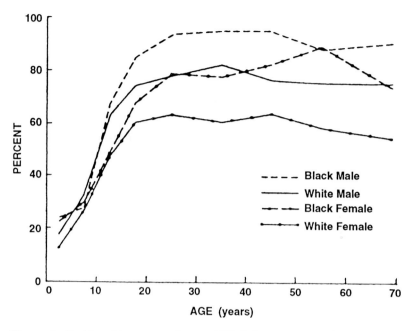

Figure 1 Positive skin test reactions to PPD-B by age, sex, and race in North Carolina, 1956–1960. (From Ref. 51.)

age 8–9 years the rate was 25% (54,55). In contrast, in rural Swedish school-children aged 8–9 years, the rate was 9.7% (56). In Saudi Arabia, 16% of BCG unvaccinated schoolchildren had a positive MAC skin test (57). A study of British recruits aged 18–20 years (using a different PPD-B preparation) in 1961 showed 24–30% positivity (60). In a study of adults in Finland, Kenya, Trinidad, and the United States in 1992–1993, MAC skin test positivity was 7–12% at all sites (58).

These data indicate that environmental exposure to MAC is common in all geographical areas and increases with age at least to age 20. MAC skin test positivity is considerably more frequent than clinical MAC disease, indicating either widespread subclinical MAC infection resulting in sensitization or cross-reactive sensitization to MAC by other environmental mycobacteria.

B. Anti-MAC Antibodies

Studies of antibody to MAC also are plagued by the nonspecific nature of such antibodies. The most immunogenic mycobacterial epitopes, such as li-

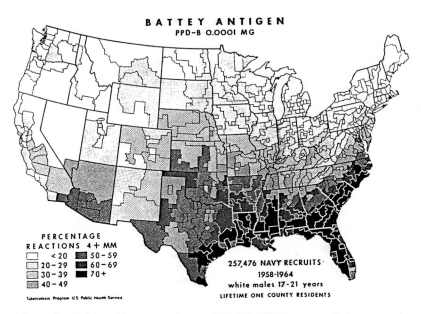

Figure 2 Positive skin test reactions to PPD-B in US Navy recruits by geographical area, 1958–64. (From Ref. 50.)

poarabinomannan (LAM), are shared by all mycobacteria. Low levels of such antibodies are common in the general population and may result from exposure to MAC as well as environmental mycobacteria other than MAC (61,62). On the other hand, patients with MAC pulmonary disease (with presumed normal humoral immunity) have distinctly elevated titers. In contrast, patients with acquired immunodeficiency syndrome (AIDS), with or without MAC disease, have undetectable antibody titers, presumably reflecting an immunological inability to respond to antigenic stimulation (63–65).

Assays for antibody to MAC type-specific glycopeptidolipid antigens or recombinant mycobacterial protein antigens have also been evaluated (62,66). Such studies also show high levels of antibody to MAC in immunologically normal patients with MAC disease but low levels of antibody in the general population and in patients with AIDS. Thus, although such antibodies may be useful in the diagnosis of disease in the normal host, they do not appear to be useful in diagnosis of MAC disease in the immunologically compromised host.

The presence of antimycobacterial antibodies in much of the general population raises the question of the proper interpretation of a "positive" test result. Several of the reported studies have defined a "normal" range on a population basis that results in a large number of persons being "positive." A more realistic breakpoint is obtained by choosing a value that separates patients with MAC pulmonary disease from those without. When this is done, it is seen that the prevalence of such antibodies is much less common than MAC skin test reactivity. The utility of such antibody assays to evaluate exposure to MAC appears limited.

C. Epidemiological Studies of Exposure to MAC

Studies of MAC pulmonary disease and disseminated MAC disease in patients with AIDS have shown that person-to-person spread of MAC is unlikely (46,67). This is supported by detailed analyses of patient isolates which show that such isolates from individual patients are unrelated (68). The one exception to this finding is the report by Hamson et al. that some patients with AIDS may have genetically similar isolates by DNA fragment analysis (69). However, that report analyzed only a single genomic fragment; more detailed analyses (by pulsed field gel electrophorasis [PFGE] or multifocal enzyme electrophoresis) do not show such clonality among patient isolates (unpublished observations).

Several studies of the relationship of MAC skin test positivity or disease to potential environmental reservoirs have been performed. Lind et al. showed an association between the presence of birds in the home and a positive MAC skin test in Swedish schoolchildren, but they were unable to address whether there was an association with MAC lymphadenopathy because of the rarity of this disease (54). We investigated environmental risk factors for MAC in patients with advanced human immunodeficiency virus (HIV) disease and showed an increased risk for disease associated with consumption of hard cheeses (cheddar, Swiss, jack), but we were unable to recover MAC from such cheeses (67). No association was found between MAC disease and exposures to birds, water, water aerosols, animals, soil, or other foods. In contrast, von Reyn et al., in a similar study, have reported a preliminary finding that MAC disease in HIV-infected persons was associated with exposure to water in spas, and that lifetime soil exposure was protective (70). Taken together, these data suggest that there are multiple environmental reservoirs for MAC infection in humans, and that geographical variability in these reservoirs may play a part in determining the risk of specific exposures.

III. MAC Lymphadenitis

A. Demographics

Cervical lymphadenitis due to MAC is an uncommon disease. In 1981–1983, about 300 cases annually were reported in the United States (71). Since many cases do not achieve a definitive diagnosis because culture is not performed or is negative, the actual number of cases is likely closer to 500. Patients are almost always less than 5 years old, with the majority being less than 3 years of age. Girls may be affected slightly more often than boys, and most patients are white (72). Some investigators have noted a predominance of cases in the winter and spring (42,73), whereas others have not (74).

B. Trends Over Time

More cases of MAC lymphadenitis are reported now than were reported in the past, but this may reflect improved detection. From 1950 to 1970, the predominant cause of cervical lymphadenitis in the United States was *M. scrofulaceum*; case series from that period showed a predominance of *M. scrofulaceum* over MAC (2,74–75). However, the CDC survey revealed that by 1981–1983, MAC had become the predominant cause of this condition (71). Recent case series have substantiated this finding (76–79,80). Lymphadenitis due to MAC has also been reported from Canada, Australia, Sweden, and England (83–86). In Sweden, as in the United States, the disease appears to be increasing in frequency (79,85).

IV. MAC Pulmonary Disease

A. Demographics

MAC pulmonary disease, unlike tuberculosis, is not a reportable condition in most states. However, a national survey performed by the CDC from 1981 to 1983 estimated that approximately 3000 cases of MAC pulmonary disease occurred annually in the United States (71). Most patients were over 40 years of age, and there was a slight male predominance (Table 1). The majority of cases were in whites. In the United States, the disease was originally recognized in the Southeast, and a 1979 survey showed high rates of disease in southern states; however, equally high rates were seen in many other states, so that the disease does not appear to have a particular geographical localization in the United States (86). Similarly, the rate of 1.3 cases per 100,000 seen in the United States is similar to the rates of 1.3 cases/100,000 reported from Japan (87) and of 0.9 cases/100,000 reported from Switzerland (88).

Table 1 Age and Sex Distribution of Patients with Pulmonary MAC Disease

Age (years)	Male (%)	Female (%)	Total
0–9	13 (46)	15 (54)	28
15–29	10 (45)	12 (55)	22
30–44	52 (70)	22 (30)	74
45–59	212 (70)	90 (30)	302
60–74	218 (53)	190 (47)	408
75+	95 (40)	141 (60)	236
Total	600	470	1070

Source: Ref. 82.

Cases of pulmonary disease may be due to *M. avium* or *M. intracellulare* (1,2,89); both are common. One report has suggested clinical differences between pulmonary disease caused by the two species (90), but most authors feel this is not clinically important.

B. Trends Over Time

MAC pulmonary disease is increasing in many countries, although increased awareness of the disease may account for some of the increases. Reports from the United States, Canada, Switzerland, and Sweden have documented increases in MAC pulmonary disease over the past decade (84,88,91–93); causes for these increases remain to be elucidated.

V. Disseminated MAC Disease

A. Demographics

Over 98% of cases of disseminated MAC (DMAC) in patients with AIDS are caused by *M. avium* rather than *M. intracellulare* (3,89). This may be due to differential exposure of patients with AIDS to *M. avium* or differential susceptibility of patients with AIDS to *M. avium*. Patients may also harbor several distinct MAC isolates (68). Analyses have suggested that MAC isolates from patients with AIDS are more likely to have plasmids (94–95), but a causal relation between such plasmids and virulence factors leading to disease has not been established. MAC isolates from patients with AIDS with disseminated disease also differ from MAC isolates from patients with cervical lymphadenitis or localized pulmonary disease by antibiotic susceptibility, serotype, and presence of DNA insertion sequences (3,89,96–98).

Surveys of the incidence and prevalence of DMAC have found that 15–24% of patients with AIDS have the disease (99), and 20% of patients with AIDS can be expected to acquire the disease over the course of a year (100–102). Thus, in the United States in 1992, when there were 100,000 AIDS cases, the incidence of DMAC can be estimated at 20,000 cases, making it easily the most common manifestation of human MAC disease.

AIDS is a reportable disease in the United States, and the frequency of DMAC among patients with AIDS can be ascertained by analyzing these reports, although the absolute number of DMAC cases is necessarily underestimated, because diagnoses of DMAC made after AIDS is first diagnosed are incompletely reported. Nonetheless, it can be seen that among patients with AIDS reported to the CDC by 1987, there were no significant gender differences in frequency of DMAC (103). With increasing age, DMAC became somewhat less common, declining from 7.8% in children aged 0–9 years to 3.1% in persons 60 years of age or greater. Hispanics were somewhat less likely to have DMAC (3.8%) than African-Americans (6.2%) or whites (5.6%), but, again, the differences were not marked. There were no significant differences in frequency of MAC among the various HIV transmission categories. In the United States, geographical variability of DMAC was also minimal, with no increase in frequency in the southeast (Fig. 3). Worldwide, DMAC has been reported in 10–25% of patients with AIDS in developed countries (104,105–110) (Table 2). DMAC has been reported from developing countries, but its occurrence is less frequent (111–115). The reasons for decreased frequency of DMAC in developing countries may include decreased exposure, shorter survival of patients with AIDS, or protection by BCG or prior exposure to other mycobacteria. MAC isolates from patients with AIDS also show geographical variability, and this may play a role in differences in disease frequency (3,97).

The most important risk factor for DMAC is the level of CD4$^+$ lymphocytes. DMAC does not occur until the CD4$^+$ cell count declines below 100 cells/mm^3 (100,102,116), and the risk increases as counts decrease (100). A multivariate analysis of risk factors for DMAC in patients with AIDS, including CD4$^+$ count, age, sex, race, and HIV transmission category has shown that the CD4$^+$ cell count was the only significant risk factor for development of DMAC (117).

B. Trends Over Time

In absolute numbers, DMAC has increased annually as the number of AIDS cases has increased. In addition, DMAC has increased as a percentage of

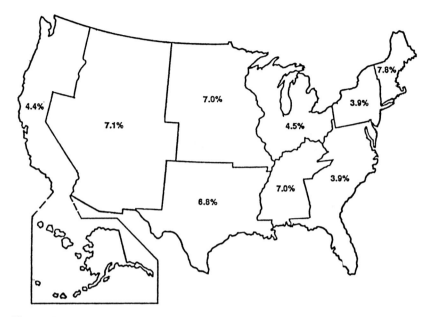

Figure 3   Cases of disseminated nontuberculous mycobacterial disease as a percentage of persons with AIDS by region, as reported to the US Centers for Disease Control, 1987. Greater than 96% of cases were caused by MAC. (From Ref. 120.)

Table 2   Frequency of Disseminated MAC Disease in AIDS by Geographical Area

City/country	Percentage disseminated MAC[a]
Atlanta, Georgia	16.0 (111)
Denver, Colorado	18.0 (121)
New York City	16.0 (122)
Sydney, Australia	24.0 (123)
Berlin, Germany	24.0 (124)
France	12.5 (125)
London	11.0 (126)
Mexico City	9.6 (127)
Uganda	0.0 (128)

[a]Numbers in parentheses refer to reference numbers.

AIDS cases; that is, DMAC is increasing faster than AIDS (99) (Fig. 4). This phenomenon is explained by the increasing percentage of patients with AIDS with low CD4$^+$ cell counts over time. With the increased use of antiretroviral agents and prophylaxis and early therapy of opportunistic infections, more patients with AIDS are surviving to the low CD4$^+$ cell levels where they are susceptible to DMAC.

This phenomenon is particularly notable among homosexual men. In the United States, this population acquired HIV infection before injection drug users and blood product recipients; thus, it has also been the first to have large numbers of persons with low CD4$^+$ cell counts. By 1991, DMAC had become more frequent in men compared to women, whites compared to nonwhites, and homosexuals compared to IV drug users (118). Similarly, among children, cases of HIV acquired through exposure to blood or blood products preceded those acquired through perinatal transmission, and a higher frequency of DMAC has also recently been noted in the former group (135–138).

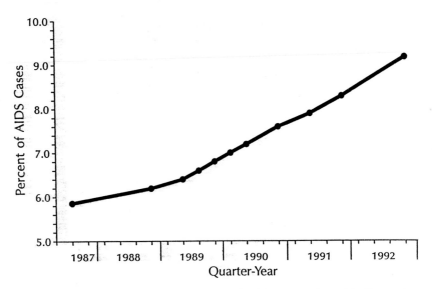

Figure 4 Frequency of disseminated nontuberculous mycobacterial disease in persons with AIDS reported to the US Centers for Disease Control, 1987–1992. Cumulative cases of MAC are shown as a percentage of cumulative AIDS cases reported by that date. Greater than 96% of cases were caused by MAC.

C. Natural History and Survival

Untreated DMAC adversely affects survival of persons with AIDS. In a retrospective analysis, patients with untreated DMAC had a median survival of 4 months after the diagnosis of DMAC (123). Patients with AIDS with DMAC and similar CD4$^+$ counts and histories of antiretroviral therapy and *Pneumocystis* prophylaxis had a significantly shorter median survival, 11 months, than in those without DMAC. This shortened survival in patients with DMAC has been confirmed in several studies (101,124–127). Patients with DMAC who receive antimycobacterial chemotherapy may not have this shortened survival (123), but prospective studies of the effect of therapy on survival are needed.

VI. Conclusions

MAC is a ubiquitous environmental organism that causes three disease syndromes in humans. Each of these disease syndromes—cervical lymphadenitis, pulmonary disease, and disseminated disease in AIDS—is increasing in frequency. The causes of increases of DMAC are clear, but increases in MAC lymphadenitis and MAC pulmonary disease remain unexplained. The environmental reservoirs and routes of acquisition of the organism are unknown for any of the three clinical manifestations. Better understanding of these factors is needed and could contribute to prevention of MAC disease.

References

1. Schaefer WB. Incidence of the serotypes of *Mycobacterium avium* and atypical mycobacteria in human and animal diseases. Am Rev Respir Dis 1968; 97: 18–23.
2. Wolinsky E. Nontuberculous mycobacteria and associated diseases. Am Rev Respir Dis 1979; 119:107–159.
3. Yakrus MA, Good RC. Geographic distribution, frequency, and specimen source of *M. avium* complex serotypes isolated from patients with acquired immunodeficiency syndrome. J Clin Microbiol 1990; 28:926–929.
4. Meissner G, Anz W. Sources of *Mycobacterium avium* complex infection resulting in human diseases. Am Rev Respir Dis 1977; 116:1057–1064.
5. Goslee S, Wolinsky E. Water as a source of potentially pathogenic mycobacteria. Am Rev Respir Dis 1976; 113:287–292.
6. du Moulin GC, Stottmeier KD, Pelletier PA, Tsang AY, Hedley-Whyte J. Concentration of *Mycobacterium avium* by hospital hot water systems. JAMA 1988; 260:1599–1601.

7. Gruft H, Falkinham JO, Parker BC. Recent experience in the epidemiology of disease caused by atypical mycobacteria. Rev Infect Dis 1981; 3:990–996.

8. Falkinham JO, Parker BC, Gruft H. Epidemiology of infection by nontuberculous mycobacteria. I. Geographic distribution in the eastern United States. Am Rev Respir Dis 1980; 121:931–937.

9. Meissner PS, Falkinham JO. Plasmid DNA profiles as epidemiological markers for clinical and environmental isolates of *M. avium*, *M. intracellulare*, and *M. scrofulaceum*. J Infect Dis 1986; 153:325–331.

10. Fry KL, Meissner PS, Falkinham JO. Epidemiology of infection by nontuberculous mycobacteria. VI. Identification and use of epidemiologic markers for studies of *Mycobacterium avium*, *M. intracellulare*, and *M. scrofulaceum*. Am Rev Respir Dis 1986; 134:39–43.

11. Kirschner Jr RA, Parker BC, Falkinham III JO. Epidemiology of infection by nontuberculous mycobacteria. *Mycobacterium avium*, *Mycobacterium intracellulare*, and *Mycobacterium scrofulaceum* in acid, brown-water swamps of the southeastern United States and their association with environmental variables. Am Rev Respir Dis 1992; 145:271–275.

12. Meissner PS, Falkinham III JO. Plasmid DNA profiles as epidemiological markers for clinical and environmental isolates of *Mycobacterium avium*, *Mycobacterium intracellulare*, and *Mycobacterium scrofulaceum*. J Infect Dis 1986; 153:325–331.

13. Byrne SK, Geddes GL, Isaac-Renton JL, Black WA. Comparison of in vitro antimicrobial susceptibilities of *M. avium-M. intracellulare* strains from patients with acquired immunodeficiency syndrome (AIDS), patients without AIDS, and animal sources. Antimicrobial Agents Chemother 1990; 34:1390–1392.

14. Martin EC, Parker BC, Falkinham JO. Epidemiology of infection by nontuberculous mycobacteria. VII. Absence of mycobacteria in southeastern groundwaters. Am Rev Respir Dis 1987; 136:344–348.

15. George KL, Parker BC, Gruft H, Falkinham JO. Epidemiology of infection by nontuberculous mycobacterai. II. Growth and survival in natural waters. Am Rev Respir Dis 1980; 122:89–94.

16. Jucker MT, Falkinham JO. Epidemiology of infection by nontuberculous mycobacteria. IX. Evidence for two DNA homology groups among small plasmids in *Mycobacterium avium*, *Mycobacterium intracellulare*, and *Mycobacterium scrofulaceum*. Am Rev Respir Dis 1990; 142:858–862.

17. Parker BC, Ford MA, Gruft H, Falkinham JO. Epidemiology of infection by nontuberculous mycobacteria. IV. Preferential aerosolization of *Mycobacterium intracellulare* from natural waters. Am Rev Respir Dis 1983; 128:652–656.

18. Kazda J, Hoyte R. Concerning the ecology of *Mycobacterium intracellulare* serotype Davis. Zbl Bakt Hyg 1972; 222(I.Abt Orig A):506–509.

19. Kazda J. The importance of water for the distribution of potentially pathogenic mycobacteria. I. Possibilities for the multiplication of mycobacteria. Zbl Bakt Hyg 1973; 158(I.Abt Orig B):161–169.

20. Portaels F. Contribution a l'etude des mycobacteries de l'environment au Bas-Zaire. The genus Mycobacterium, Proceeds of the Third International Colloquium on Mycobacteria, Prince Leopold Institute of Tropical Medicine, Antwerp, Belgium, 1973:169–183.

21. von Reyn CF, Waddell RD, Eaton T, et al. Isolation of M. avium complex from water in the United States, Finland, Zaire, and Kenya. J Clin Microbiol 1993; 31:3227–3230.

22. Murphey SA, Jungkind DL, Schwartz HG, Adams K. *Mycobacterium avium-intracellulare* in a hospital hot water system: Epidemiological investigation (abstr). In: Abstracts of the 23rd Interscience Conference on Antimicrobial Agents and chemotherapy. Washington, DC: American Society for Microbiology, 1983:1047.

23. Aronson T, Holtzman A, Glover N, et al. Potable water—A source of *Mycobacterium avium* complex infection (abstract U-80). Abstracts of the 93rd Annual Meeting of the American Society for Microbiology. Washington, DC: American Society for Microbiology, 1993:183.

24. von Reyn CF, Maslow JN, Barber TW, et al. Persistent colonization of potable water as a source of *Mycobacterium avium* infection in AIDS. Lancet 1994; 343:1137–1141.

25. Gruft H, Katz J, Blanchard DC. Postulated source of *Mycobacterium intracellulare* infection. Am J Epidemiol 1975; 102:311–318.

26. Gruft H, Falkinham JO, Parker BC. Recent experience in the epidemiology of disease caused by atypical mycobacteria. Rev Infect Dis 1981; 3:990–996.

27. Prichard WD, Thoen CO, Himes EM, Muscoplat CC, Johnson DW. Epidemiology of mycobacterial lymphadenitis in an Idaho swine herd. Am J Epidemiol 1977; 106:222–227.

28. Reznikov M, Dawson DJ. Mycobacteria of the *intracellulare-scrofulaceum* group in soils from the Adelaide area. Pathology 1980; 12:525–528.

29. Reznikov M, Leggo JH. Examination of soil in the Brisbane area for organisms of the *M. avium–intracellulare–scrofulaceum* complex. Pathology 1974; 6: 269–273.

30. Reznikov M, Leggo JH, Dawson DJ. Investigations by seroagglutination of strains of the *M. intracellulare–M. scrofulaceum* group from house-dusts and sputum in southeastern Queensland. Am Rev Respir Dis 1971; 104:951–953.

31. Reznikov M, Leggo JH, Tuffley RE. Further investigations of an outbreak of mycobacterial lymphadenitis at a deep-litter piggery. Aust Vet J 1971; 47: 622–623.

32. Saitanu K. Studies on mycobacteria isolated from animals, with special reference to the agglutination test. Acta Pathol Microbiol Scand 1977; 85(sect B): 303–307.

33. Engbaek HC, Vergmann B, Baess I, Benton MW. *M. avium.* A bacteriological and epidemiological study of *M. avium* isolated from animals and man in Denmark. Part 1: Strains isolated from animals. Acta Pathol Microbiol Scand 1968; 72:277–294.

34. Engbaek HC, Vergmann B, Baess I, Benton MW. *M. avium.* A bacteriological and epidemiological study of *M. avium* isolated from animals and man in Denmark. Part 2: Strains isolated from man. Acta Pathol Microbiol Scand 1968; 72:295–312.

35. Holmberg CA, Henrickson RV, Malaga C, et al. Nontuberculous mycobacterial disease in Rhesus monkeys. Vet Pathol 1982; 19S:9–16.

36. Wolinsky E, Rynearson TK. Mycobacteria in soil and their relation to disease-associated strains. Am Rev Respir Dis 1968; 97:1032–1037.

37. Kubica GP, Bean RE, Palmer JW, Rigdon AL. The isolation of unclassified (atypical) acid-fast bacilli from soil and water samples collected in the state of Georgia (abstr). Am Rev Respir Dis 1961; 84:135–136.

38. Nassos PS, Yajko DM, Gonzalez PC, et al. Soil as a possible reservoir for *M. avium* complex (MAC) infection in patients with AIDS. Abstracts of the 32nd ICAAC, Washington, DC: American Society for Microbiology, 1992:260.

39. Chapman JS, Bernard JS, Speight M. Isolation of mycobacteria from raw milk. Am Rev Respir Dis 1965; 91:351–355.

40. Chapman JS, Speight M. Isolation of atypical mycobacteria from pasteurized milk. Am Rev Respir Dis 1968; 98:1052–1053.

41. Hosty TS, McDurmont CI. Isolation of acid-fast organisms from milk and oysters. Health Lab Sci 1975; 12:16–19.

42. Chapman JS. The atypical mycobacteria. Hosp Pract 1970; 5:69–80.

43. Nel EE. *Mycobacterium avium–intracellulare* complex serovars isolated in South Africa from humans, swine, and the environment. Rev Infect Dis 1981; 3:1013–1020.

44. Edwards LB, Palmer CE. Isolation of "atypical" mycobacteria from healthy persons. Am Rev Respir Dis 1959; 80:747–748.

45. Mills CC. Occurrence of *mycobacterium* other than *Mycobacterium tuberculosis* in the oral cavity and in sputum. Appl Microbiol 1972; 24:307–310.

46. Iseman MD, Corpe RF, O'Brien RJ, et al. Disease due to *Mycobacterium avium–intracellulare.* Chest 1985; 87:139S–149s.

47. Graham DY, Markesich DC, Yoshimura HH. Mycobacteria and inflammatory bowel disease. Results of culture. Gastroenterology 1987; 92:436–442.

48. Portaels F, Larsson L, Smeets P. Isolation of mycobacteria from healthy persons' stools. Int J Lepr 1988; 56:468–471.

49. Edwards LB, Palmer CE. Epidemiologic studies of tuberculin sensitivity. I. Preliminary results with purified protein derivatives prepared from atypical acid-fast organisms. Am J Hyg 1958; 68:213–231.

50. Smith DT. Diagnostic and prognostic significance of the quantitative tuberculin tests. Ann Intern Med 1967; 67:919–946.

51. Edwards LB, Smith DT. Community-wide tuberculin testing study in Pamlico county, North Carolina. Am Rev Respir Dis 1965; 92:43–54.

52. Heubner RE, Schein MF, Cauthen GM, et al. Usefulness of skin testing with mycobacterial antigens in children with cervical lymphadenopathy. Pediatr Infect Dis J 1992; 11:450–456.

53. Magnusson M. Mycobacterial sensitins: where are we now? Rev Infect Dis 1981; 3:944–948.
54. Lind A, Larsson LO, Bentzon MW, et al. Sensitivity to sensitins and tuberculin in Swedish children. I. A study of schoolchildren in an urban area. Tubercle 1991; 72:29–36.
55. Larsson LO, Skoogh B-E, Bentzon, et al. Sensitivity to sensitins and tuberculin in Swedish children. II. A study of preschool children. Tubercle 1991; 72: 37–42.
56. Larsson LO, Bentzon MW, Lind A, et al. Sensitivity to sensitins and tuberculin in Swedish children. Part 5: A study of school children in an inland rural area. Tubercle 1993; 74:371–376.
57. Osman AA, Hakim JG, Luneborg-Nielsen M, et al. Comparative skin testing with PPD tuberculin, *M. avium* and *M. scrofulaceum* in schoolchildren in Saudi Arabia. Tubercle 1994; 75:38–43.
58. von Reyn CF, Barber TW, Arbeit RD, et al. Evidence of previous infection with *M. avium–M. intracellulare* complex among healthy subjects: An international study of dominant mycobacterial skin test reactions. J Infect Dis 1993; 168:1553–1558.
59. von Reyn CF, Green PA, McCormick D, et al. Dual mycobacterial skin testing in patients infected with *Mycobacterium avium* complex or *Mycobacterium tuberculosis*. Clin Infect Dis 1994; 19:15–20.
60. D'Arcy Hart P, Miller CL, Sutherland I, Leslie IW. Sensitivity to avian and human old tuberculin in man in Great Britain. Tubercle 1962; 43:268–286.
61. Bermudez LEM, Wu M, Enkel H, Young LS. Naturally occurring antibodies against *M. avium* complex. Ann Clin Lab Sci 1989; 19:435–443.
62. Morris SL, Bermudez L, Chaparas SD. *M. avium* complex disease in patients with AIDS: Seroreactivity to native and recombinant mycobacterial antigens. J Clin Microbiol 1991; 29:2715–2719.
63. Winter DS, Bernard EM, Gold JWM, Armstrong D. Humoral response to disseminated infection by *M. avium–M. intracellulare* in acquired immunodeficiency syndrome and hairy cell leukemia. J Infect Dis 1985; 151:523–527.
64. Wayne WG, Young LS, Bertram M. Absence of mycobacterial antibody in patients with acquired immune deficiency syndrome. Eur J Clin Microbiol 1986; 5:363–365.
65. Miller RA, Collier AC, Horsburgh Jr CR. Characterization of the humoral immune response to *Mycobacterium avium intracellulare* in patients with and without the acquired immune deficiency syndrome. Abstracts of the 85th Annual meeting of the American Society for Microbiology, Washington, DC, 1985, No. U40.
66. Lee B-Y, Chatterjee D, Bozic C, et al. Prevalence of serum antibody to the type-specific glycopeptidolipid antigens of *M. avium* in human immunodeficiency virus-positive and -negative individuals. J Clin Microbiol 1991; 29: 1026–1029.

67. Horsburgh CR, Chin DP, Yajko DM, et al. Environmental risk factors for acquisition of *Mycobacterium avium* complex in persons with human immunodeficiency virus infection. J Infect Dis 1994; 170:362–367.

68. Arbeit RD, Slutsky A, Barber TW, et al. Genetic diversity among strains of *M. avium* causing monocloncal and polyclonal bacteremia in patients with AIDS. J Infect Dis 1993; 167:1384–1390.

69. Hampson SJ, Portaels F, Thompson J, et al. DNA probes demonstrate a single highly conserved strain of *M. avium* infecting AIDS patients. Lancet 1989; 1: 65–68.

70. von Reyn CF, Arbeit RD, Gilks CF, et al. Risk factors for mycobacteremia among patients with AIDS in developed and developing countries [abstract PO-B07-1186]. In: Abstracts of the Ninth International Conference on AIDS (Berlin). Geneva: International AIDS Society and World Health Organization, 1993; 1:333.

71. O'Brien RJ, Geiter LJ, Snider DE. The epidemiology of nontuberculous mycobacterial diseases in the United States. Results from a national survey. Am Rev Respir Dis 1987; 135:1007–1014.

72. Schaad UB, Votteler TP, McCracken GH, Nelson JD. Management of atypical mycobacterial lymphadenitis in childhood: a review based on 380 cases. J Pediatr 1979; 95:356–360.

73. Altman RP, Margileth AM. Cervical lymphadenopathy from atypical mycobacteria: Diagnosis and surgical treatment. J Pediatr Surg 1975; 10:419–422.

74. Saitz EW. Cervical lymphadenitis caused by atypical mycobacteria. Pediatr Clin North Am 1981; 28:823–839.

75. Lincoln EM, Gilbert LA. Disease in children due to mycobacteria other than *Mycobacterium tuberculosis*. Am Rev Respir Dis 1972; 105:683–714.

76. Taha AM, Davidson PT, Bailey WC. Surgical treatment of atypical mycobacterial lymphadenitis in children. Pediatr Infect Dis 1985; 4:664–667.

77. Spark RP, Fried ML, Bean CK, et al. Nontuberculous mycobacterial adenitis of childhood. The ten-year experience at a community hospital. Am J Dis Children 1988; 142:106–8.

78. Lai KK, Stottmeier KD, Sherman IH, McCabe WR. Mycobacterial cervical lymphadenopathy. Relation of etiologic agents to age. JAMA 1984; 251: 1286–1288.

79. Pransky SM, Reisman BK, Kearns DB, et al. Cervicofacial mycobacterial adenitis in children: endemic to San Diego? Laryngoscope 1990; 100:920–925.

80. Alessi DP, Dudley JP. Atypical mycobacteria-induced cervical adenitis. Arch Otolaryngol Head Neck Surg 1988; 114:664–666.

81. Grange J, Collins C, Yates M. Bacteriological survey of tuberculous lymphadenitis in south-east England: 1973–80. J Epidemiol Commun Health 1982; 36: 157–161.

82. Martin T, Hoeppner VH, Ring ED. Superficial mycobacterial lymphadenitis in Saskatchewan. CMAJ 1988; 138:431–434.

83. Llewelyn DM, Dorman D. Mycobacterial lymphadenitis. Aust Pediatr J 1971; 7:97–102.

84. Wickman K. Clinical significance of nontuberculous mycobacteria. A bacteriological survey of Swedish strains isolated between 1973 and 1981. Scand J Infect Dis 1986; 18:337–344.

85. Romanus V. First experience with BCG discontinuation in Europe. Experience in Sweden 15 years after stopping general BCG vaccination at birth. Bull Int Union Tuberc Lung Dis 1990; 65:32–35.

86. Good RC, Snider DE. Isolation of nontuberculous mycobacteria in the United States. J Infect Dis 1982; 146:829–833.

87. Tsukamura M, Kita N, Shimoide H, et al. Studies on the epidemiology of nontuberculous mycobacteriosis in Japan. Am Rev Respir Dis 1988; 137: 1280–1284.

88. Debrunner M, Salfinger M, Brandli O, von Graevenitz A. Epidemiology and clinical significance of nontuberculous mycobacteria in patients negative for human immunodeficiency virus in Switzerland. Clin Infect Dis 1992; 15: 330–345.

89. Guthertz LS, Damsker B, Bottone EJ, et al., Janda JM. *Mycobacterium avium* and *Mycobacterium intracellulare* infections in patients with and without AIDS. J Infect Dis 1989; 160:1037–1041.

90. Yamori S, Tsukamura M. Comparison of prognosis of pulmonary diseases caused by *M. avium* and by *M. intracellulare*. Chest 1992; 102:89–90.

91. Prince DS, Peterson DD, Steiner RM, et al. Infection with *Mycobacterium avium* complex in patients without predisposing conditions. N Engl J Med 1989; 321:863–868.

92. Contreras MA, Cheung OT, Sanders DE, Goldstein RS. Pulmonary infection with nontuberculous mycobacteria. Am Rev Respir Dis 1988; 137:149–152.

93. du Moulin G, Sherman IH, Hoaglin DC, Stottmeier KD. *Mycobacterium avium* complex, an emerging pathogen in Massachusetts. J Clin Microbiol 1985; 22: 9–12.

94. Jensen AG, Bennedsen J, Rosdahl VT. Plasmid profiles of *M. avium/ intracellular* isolated from patients with AIDS or cervical lymphadenitis and from environmental samples. Scand J Infect Dis 1989; 21:645–649.

95. Crawford JT, Bates JH. Analysis of plasmids in *M. avium–intracellulare* isolates from persons with acquired immunodeficiency syndrome. Am Rev Respir Dis 1986; 134:659–661.

96. Horsburgh CR, Cohn DL, Roberts RB, et al. *Mycobacterium avium–M. intracellulare* isolates from patients with or without acquired immunodeficiency syndrome. Antimicrobial Agents Chemother 1986; 30:955–957.

97. Hoffner SE, Kallenius G, Petrini B, et al. Serovars of *M. avium* complex isolated from patients in Sweden. J Clin Microbiol 1990; 28:1105–1107.

98. Kunze ZM, Portaels F, McFadden JJ. Biologically distinct subtypes of *M. avium* differ in possession of insertion sequence IS901. J Clin Microbiol 1992; 30:2366–2372.

99. Horsburgh CR. *Mycobacterium avium* complex infection in the acquired immunodeficiency syndrome. N Engl J Med 1991; 324:1332–1338.

100. Nightingale SD, Byrd LT, Southern PM, et al. Incidence of *Mycobacterium avium–intracellulare* complex bacteremia in human immunodeficiency virus-positive patients. J Infect Dis 1992; 165:1082–1085.

101. Chaisson RE, Moore RD, Richman DD, et al. Incidence and natural history of *Mycobacterium avium* complex infections in patients with advanced human immunodeficiency virus disease treated with zidovudine. Am Rev Respir Dis 1992; 146:285–289.

102. Nightingale SD, Cameron DW, Gordin FM, et al. Two controlled trials of rifabutin prophylaxis against *Mycobacterium avium* complex infection in AIDS. N Engl J Med 1993; 329:828–833.

103. Horsburgh CR, Selik RM. The epidemiology of disseminated nontuberculous mycobacterial infection in the acquired immunodeficiency syndrome (AIDS). Am Rev Respir Dis 1989; 139:4–7.

104. Havlik JA, Horsburgh CR, Metchock B, et al. Disseminated *Mycobacterium avium* complex infection: clinical identification and epidemiologic trends. J Infect Dis 1992; 165:557–580.

105. Bessesen MT, Berry CD, Johnson MA, et al. Site of origin of disseminated *M. avium* complex infection in AIDS (abstr). In: Program and Abstracts of the 30th Interscience Conference on Antimicrobial Agents and Chemotherapy. Washington DC: American Society for Microbiology, 1990:297.

106. Hawkins CC, Gold JWM, Whimbey E, et al. *Mycobacterium avium* complex infections in patients with the acquired immunodeficiency syndrome. Ann Intern Med 1986; 105:184–188.

107. Hoy J, Mijch A, Sandland M, et al. Quadruple-drug therapy for *Mycobacterium avium–intracellulare* bacteremia in AIDS patients. J Infect Dis 1990; 161:801–805.

108. Peters M, Schurmann D, Rusch-Gerdes S, et al. Serotype pattern of *Mycobacterium avium–intracellulare* isolates from German AIDS patients [abstract]. Am Rev Respir Dis 1991; 143:A281.

109. Dautzenberg B, Chauvin JP, Koulaksezian A, et al. French report on nontuberculosis resistant mycobacteria receiving non-registered drugs (abstr). Am Rev Respir Dis 1993; 147:A116.

110. Gardener TD, Flanagan P, Dryden MS, et al. Disseminated *Mycobacterium avium–intracellulare* infection and red cell hypoplasia in patients with the acquired immune deficiency syndrome. J Infect 1988; 16:135–401.

111. Mohar A, Romo J, Salido F, et al. The spectrum of clinical and pathological manifestations of AIDS in a consecutive series of autopsied patients in Mexico. AIDS 1992; 6:467–473.

112. Okello DO, Sewankambo N, Goodgame, R, et al. Absence of bacteremia with *Mycobacterium avium–intracellulare* in Ugandan patients with AIDS. J Infect Dis 1990; 162:208–210.

113. Levy-Frebault V, Pangon B, Bure A, et al. *Mycobacterium simiae* and *Mycobacterium avium–M.intracellulare* mixed infection in acquired immune deficiency syndrome. J Clin Microbiol 1987; 25:154–157.

114. Barreto JA, Palaci M, Ferrazoli L, et al. Isolation of *Mycobacterium avium* complex from bone marrow aspirates of AIDS patients in Brazil. J Infect Dis 1993; 168:777–779.

115. Yeung KT, Li PCK, Lee SS, Sitt WH. Mycobacterial infection in HIV positive individuals in Hong Kong. Abstracts of the Eighth International Conference on AIDS. Amsterdam: International AIDS Society, 1992; 2:B134.

116. Cameron DW, Schoenfeld D, Schoenfelder J, et al. Short term *Mycobacterium avium* complex bacteremia risk related to CD4 T cell counts in AIDS (Abstract No. PO-B07-1248). Abstracts of the Ninth International Conference on AIDS. Berlin: International Aids Society 1993; 1:343.

117. Horsburgh CR, Wynne B, Bianchine J, et al. Epidemiology of *M. avium* complex bacteremia in patients enrolled in a placebo-controlled study. Abstracts of the Eighth International Conference on AIDS. Amsterdam: International AIDS Society 1992; 2:B118.

118. Horsburgh CR. Recent trends in the epidemiology of disseminated *M. avium* complex infection in patients with AIDS. Frontiers in mycobacteriology: *M. avium*, the modern epidemic. Denver: National Jewish Center for Immunology and Respiratory Medicine, 1992:6.

119. Horsburgh CR, Caldwell MB, Simonds RJ. Epidemiology of disseminated nontuberculous mycobacterial infection in children with AIDS. Pediatr Infect Dis J 1993; 12:219–222.

120. Rutstein RM, Cobb P, McGowan KL, et al. *M. avium–intracellulare complex* infection in HIV-infected children. AIDS 1993; 7:507–512.

121. Hoyt L, Oleske J, Holland B, Connor E. Nontuberculous mycobacteria in children with acquired immunodeficiency syndrome. Pediatr Infect Dis J 1992; 11:354–360.

122. Lewis LL, Butler KM, Husson RN, et al. Defining the population of human immunodeficiency virus-infected children at risk for *M. avium–intracellulare* infection. J Pediatr 1992; 121:677–683.

123. Horsburgh CR, Havlik JA, Ellis DA, et al. Survival of AIDS patients with disseminated *Mycobacterium avium* complex infection with and without antimycobacterial chemotherapy. Am Rev Respir Dis 1991; 144:557–559.

124. Horsburgh CR, Metchock B, Gordon S, et al. Predictors of survival of patients with AIDS and disseminated *Mycobacterium avium* complex disease. J Infect Dis 1994; 170:573–577.

125. Jacobson MA, Hopewell PC, Yajko DM, et al. Natural history of disseminated *Mycobacterium avium* complex infection in AIDS. J Infect Dis 1991; 164:994–998.

126. Kerlikowske KM, Katz MH, Chan AK, Perez-Stable EJ. Antimycobacterial therapy for disseminated *Mycobacterium avium* complex infection in patients with acquired immunodeficiency syndrome. Arch Intern Med 1992; 152:813–817.

127. Church T, Horsburgh R, Brelje T, et al. Effects of disseminated *Mycobacterium avium* complex and its treatment on survival of AIDS patients: An observational study [abstract WS-B10-6]. In: Abstracts of the Ninth International Conference on AIDS (Berlin). Geneva: International AIDS Society and World Health Organization, 1993; 1:53.

128. Okello DO, Sewankambo N, Goodgame R, et al. Absence of bacteremia with *Mycobacterium avium-intracellulare* in Ugandan patients with AIDS. J Infect Dis 1990; 162:208–10.

129. Levy-Frebault V, Pangon B, Bure A, Katlama C, Marche C, David HL. *Mycobacterium simiae* and *Mycobacterium avium-M. intracellulare* mixed infection in acquired immune deficiency syndrome. J Clin Microbiol 1987; 25: 154–7.

130. Barreto JA, Palaci M, Ferrazoli L, et al. Isolation of *Mycobacterium avium* complex from bone marrow aspirates of AIDS patients in Brazil. J Infect Dis 1993; 168:777–9.

131. Yeung KT, Li PCK, Lee SS, Sitt WH. Mycobacterial infection in HIV positive individuals in Hong Kong. Abstracts of the Eighth International Conference on AIDS. Amsterdam; International AIDS Society 1992; 2:B134.

132. Cameron DW, Schoenfeld D, Schoenfelder J, Gordin F, Wynne B, Nightingale S. Short term *Mycobacterium avium* complex bacteremia risk related to CD⁴ T cell counts in AIDS (Abstract No. PO-B07-1248). Abstracts of the Ninth International Conference on AIDS. Berlin; International AIDS Society 1993; 1:343.

133. Horsburgh CR, Wynne B, Bianchine J, et al. Epidemiology of *M. avium* complex bacteremia in patients enrolled in a placebo-controlled study. Abstracts of the Eighth International Conference on AIDS. Amsterdam; International AIDS Society 1992; 2:B118.

134. Horsburgh CR. Recent trends in the epidemiology of disseminated *M. avium* complex infection in patients with AIDS. Frontiers in mycobacteriology: *M. avium*, the modern epidemic. Denver, CO; National Jewish Center for Immunology and Respiratory Medicine 1992: 6.

135. Horsburgh CR, Caldwell MB, Simonds RJ. Epidemiology of disseminated nontuberculous mycobacterial infection in children with AIDS. Pediatr Infect Dis J 1993; 12:219–22.

136. Rutstein RM, Cobb P, McGowan KL, Pinto-Martin J, Starr SE. *M. avium-intracellulare complex* infection in HIV-infected children. AIDS 1993; 7:507–12.

137. Hoyt L, Oleske J, Holland B, Connor E. Nontuberculous mycobacteria in children with acquired immunodeficiency syndrome. Pediatr Infect Dis J 1992; 11: 354–60.

138. Lewis LL, Butler KM, Husson RN, et al. Defining the population of human immunodeficiency virus-infected children at risk for *M. avium-intracellulare* infection. J Pediatr 1992; 121:677–83.

2

Molecular Epidemiology Techniques for the Study of *Mycobacterium avium*–Complex Infection

JOSEPH O. FALKINHAM, III

Virginia Polytechnic Institute and State University
Blacksburg, Virginia

I. Introduction

A. Background

Members of the *Mycobacterium avium* complex are opportunistic human pathogens whose source of infection is most likely the environment (1–3). Based on the fact that isolates of the *M. avium* complex have been recovered from hospital water supply systems (4,5), public bath waters (6) and natural waters (5,7), soils (8), and aerosols (9), it is possible that patients not infected with the human immunodeficiency virus (HIV) and those with acquired immunodeficiency syndrome (AIDS) are being infected from their immediate (i.e., hospital) environment. Proof of this hypothesis requires development of a method which accurately "fingerprints" each *M. avium*–complex strain. It is the objective of this chapter to describe the newer "molecular" tools for fingerprinting *M. avium* complex isolates, their application for epidemiological studies, and the advantages and disadvantages of each type.

The power of molecular typing is illustrated by the first report demonstrating the identity of *M. avium*–complex isolates recovered from patients with AIDS and their environment (3). In that report, large restriction fragments (LRF) of DNA recovered from *M. avium* strains were compared and identical patterns of fragments were found in patient and environmental isolates. The identification of matching isolates was significant because LRF patterns of *M. avium* isolates in nature are quite diverse (3).

A second important outcome of epidemiological studies of *M. avium* by molecular typing methods is the demonstration of the enormous diversity of *M. avium* types. This diversity has been seen in both environmental and patient isolates. Thus, it is likely that there will be little predictive value to studies of individual isolates. Particularly, the progression and characteristics of disease and response to chemotherapy may be unique to each patient and *M. avium* strain.

B. Molecular Epidemiology

Recently, new molecular methods for fingerprinting *M. avium* complex isolates have been described. The molecular markers used for the fingerprint are DNA, RNA, or protein molecules in *M. avium*. These molecular markers include (1) multilocus enzyme electrophoresis (MLEE) (10,11); (2) plasmid DNA typing (12); (3) restriction fragment length polymorphism (RFLP) typing of chromosomal DNA (13,14), 5S ribosomal DNA (rDNA) (15) or 16S rDNA (16); (4) ribosomal DNA spacer sequence analysis (17,18); (5) large restriction fragment (LRF) typing of genomic DNA (19,20); and (6) random amplified polymorphic DNA (RAPD) analysis (21,22).

There is no single characteristic that distinguishes one molecular epidemiological marker from others. Their targets are DNA, RNA, or protein. Rather than focusing on detection of a specific microbiological (e.g., growth or antimicrobial susceptibility) or biochemical (e.g., enzyme activity) characteristic, molecular epidemiological techniques focus on the molecules, and thereby are not limited by differential expression under different growth conditions. For example, all *M. avium*–complex isolates have DNA and rDNA whether they are grown in rich or poor medium. That is not the case for expression of characteristics, such as enzyme activity, used as markers to fingerprint bacterial strains. Thus, every strain can be typed.

C. Applications of Molecular Epidemiology

In addition to the use of molecular epidemiological markers for the identification of the source of *M. avium* complex in infected patients, these techniques can be employed to answer a variety of other questions. Evidence of polyclonal *M. avium*–complex infection was derived by LRF (20) and RFLP (23) analysis of isolates recovered from individual patients with AIDS. RFLP analysis led to discovery of a unique African *M. avium* type distinct from types found in Europe and North America (13,23,24).

It is anticipated that molecular epidemiological markers will be able to determine the route of acquisition of *M. avium* infection in patients with AIDS. It is not sufficient to prove that sputum or fecal *M. avium* isolation precedes disseminated infection; the fingerprint(s) of the blood *M. avium* isolate should be the same as that from either the sputum or fecal samples.

Molecular epidemiological analysis will be quite valuable in identifying the origin and relatedness of drug-resistant *M. avium* isolates. In particular, molecular fingerprinting can be used to determine whether the emergence of drug-resistant *M. avium* during or after antibiotic therapy is a result of mutation, selection of a minor, drug-resistant component of the infecting population, or secondary infection by a drug-resistant isolate from the patient's environment.

II. The Problem of Numbers

The diversity of *M. avium*–complex types recovered from patients and the environment (3,19,20) requires that for adequate epidemiological links to be established many isolates must be recovered from both the patients and environmental samples. For example, detection of polyclonal *M. avium* infection in 3 of 13 patients with AIDS was possible because at least three separate patient isolates were recovered and characterized (20). Using isolates from different specimens, blood, sputum, and feces from individual patients with AIDS, Dawson (25) showed that 38% of Australian patients with AIDS were infected with more than one *M. avium* strain based on serotype. Because of the limited number of isolates tested, those frequencies are likely underestimates of the true frequency of polyclonal *M. avium*–complex infection in AIDS patients.

The number of isolates recovered from patients and from their environment directly influences the probability of identifying environmental *M. avium* strains which match patient isolates. Even if all the colonies on the primary isolation medium have the same morphology, different colonies must be recovered and the isolates typed. It has been our experience that *M. avium* isolates from the same sample having the same colonial morphology can have different plasmid (T. Eaton and J. O. Falkinham, unpublished results) or large restriction fragment profiles (R. D. Arbeit, personal communication, October, 1992).

III. Molecular Epidemiological Markers

A. Multilocus Enzyme Electrophoresis

Background

Enzymes present in lysates of *M. avium*–complex strains can be separated by gel electrophoresis and detected by activity stains in gels. Mutation results in the appearance of electrophoretic variants of individual enzymes, which if they retain enzymatic activity, can be detected on the basis of their different electrophoretic mobility. If the frequency of such electrophoretic variant alleles for individual enzymes is high and if enough different enzymes can be characterized in this fashion, a highly distinctive fingerprint of individual strains can be generated.

Results

A large number of electrophoretic types (ETs) have been identified among strains of the *M. avium* complex indicating the utility of MLEE for epidemiological studies. For example, 31 ETs were found among 58 *M. avium*–complex isolates of serotype 4 (10). This is due to the fact that the average number of alleles per locus in a collection of *M. avium* complex strains was 2.8 (11). Because MLEE is capable of subdividing *M. avium* serotypes (10,11), it may be used to identify the environmental source of *M. avium* infection and determine whether patients are infected with more than a single isolate. To date, however, there have been no epidemiological studies in which this technique has been used.

Applicability, Advantages, and Disadvantages

In both reports of MLEE typing of *M. avium* isolates, the typability of isolates was 100% (10,11). Interpretation of results was problematic in only one case involving detection of esterase activity (10).

At the present time, the stability of the genetic determinants and their alleles are unknown. More than likely the determinants are chromosomal and are expected to be stable. In addition, it is not known whether selection influences the frequencies of alleles in *M. avium* populations. If strong selection occurred in laboratory culture media, a single MLEE type could predominate. That phenomenon could lead to mistaken evidence of identity of

M. avium isolates. That in turn would lead to underestimates of the frequency of polyclonal infection and mistaken evidence that an environmental *M. avium* sample was the source of infection in patients.

Evidence has also not been presented describing the influence of physiological conditions on the presence of the different enzyme activities and their alleles. Such problems are typically shared by epidemiological markers whose manifestation is based on phenotypic expression and not on direct analysis of genotype (i.e., DNA). Possibly some MLEE alleles require different conditions for expression of enzyme activity or lack activity toward the chosen substrate. To a large extent, those uncertainties have been overcome by the use of a large number of enzymes (17 or 20 in the cited studies) and ensuring that strains were grown under identical conditions before isolation of active fractions.

B. Plasmid Typing

Background

Plasmids are distinct extrachromosomal DNA elements inherited in a relatively stable manner from generation to generation. Consequently, they can serve as unique markers for individual strains of mycobacteria. Because plasmids of the same incompatibility group cannot stably coexist in an individual cell, plasmids can be detected by hybridization even if chromosomal DNA is present. Depending on the number of different plasmid homology groups, a highly discriminatory system of strain typing can be developed. In addition to whole plasmids, restriction endonuclease-generated plasmid fragments can be detected using a DNA probe. In this case, each fragment can be used as a character or fingerprint for epidemiological typing.

Results

M. avium complex strains recovered from non–HIV-infected patients are more likely to have plasmids than environmental isolates (2,26). Because *M. avium* plasmids are quite stable (27), they meet one of the important criteria for utility as epidemiological markers. Further, almost all *M. avium*–complex isolates recovered from patients with AIDS carry small (i.e., <25 kb) plasmids (12,28), which by contrast differ from the plasmids isolated and characterized from non–HIV-infected patients and environmental samples which are of wide variation in size (26). The *M. avium*–complex plasmids of less than 25 kb size fall into at least four different groups (I, II, III, and IV) based on DNA-DNA hybridization data (12,29). Plasmid DNA profiles of a number of clinical and environmental *M. avium*–complex strains are shown in Fig. 1.

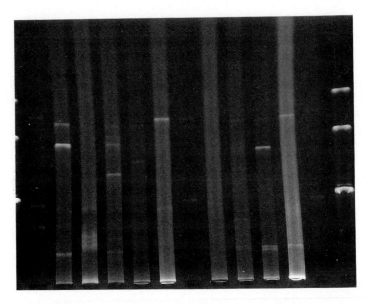

Figure 1   Plasmids of *M. avium*–complex strains separated in 0.7% agarose gel. Lane 1, lambda HindIII restriction fragments; lane 2, pVT2 (12); lane 3, CL25 (chicken litter); lane 4, DE20 (non-HIV patient); lane 5, GA1 (non-HIV⁺ patient); lane 6, GA9 (non-HIV⁺ patient); lane 7, pVT2 (12); lane 8, MD1 (non-HIV⁺ patient); lane 9, MD3 (non-HIV⁺ patient); lane 10, MD22 (non-HIV⁺ patient); lane 11, SC7 (non-HIV⁺ patient); lane 12, VA3 (non-HIV⁺ patient), lane 13, pVT2; lane 14, lambda HindIII restriction fragments.

Plasmid typing has been used to confirm polyclonal *M. avium* infection of patients with AIDS. A study of *M. avium*–complex isolates recovered from patients with AIDS using the plasmids representative of two of the small plasmid homology groups, groups I and II, led to the detection of simultaneous infection with more than a single strain. In 23 patients with AIDS from whom blood cultures were obtained, 9 (39%) had *M. avium*–complex blood isolates with different plasmid DNA compositions (T. Eaton, J. O. Falkinham, and C. F. von Reyn, in preparation). Because only two plasmid DNA probes were used and only 3 *M. avium* isolates were recovered from each patient sample, the frequency of multiple *M. avium*–complex infection judged using the two plasmid probes is likely an underestimation. Further, strains with related plasmids of different size will be scored as having identical plasmid types. Thus, plasmid typing data using a substantial number of patients, samples, and isolates suggest that the true frequency of polyclonal *M. avium* infection in patients with AIDS is very likely higher.

Applicability, Advantages, and Disadvantages

Because plasmid typing can be performed by Dot-Blot hybridization of labeled plasmid probes with total DNA preparations from individual isolates, it is amenable for screening many isolates and is relatively easy, rapid, and inexpensive. However, the utility of plasmid typing is limited by the fact that a significant proportion of environmental and clinical *M. avium* isolates lack plasmids (26).

C. Restriction Fragment Length Polymorphism

Background

Total *M. avium* DNA can be isolated, purified, subjected to restriction endonuclease digestion, and the fragments separated by gel electrophoresis. Fragments containing specific insertion sequences or genes can be identified by hybridization using probes for those sequences. Mutation at sites recognized by restriction endonucleases can be detected by loss, gain or change in size of DNA fragments, hence, restriction fragment length polymorphism.

M. avium–complex sequence employed as targets in RFLP studies include insertion sequences IS900 (13) and IS901 (30) and 5S (15) and 16S (16) ribosomal DNA (rDNA).

Results

RFLP analysis of the *M. avium* complex using IS900 as probe in the *M. paratuberculosis* cloned genomic fragment pMB22 demonstrated the existence of at least four distinct types (13). A majority (70%) of patients with AIDS from the United States and Europe were found to be infected with *M. avium*–complex isolates which belonged to a single RFLP type, *M. avium* RFLP type A. By contrast, *M. avium*–complex isolates recovered from African patients with AIDS were members of a different RFLP type, *M. avium* complex type H (24). Using the same pMB22 probe, Visuvanathan et al. (23) confirmed that the single *M. avium*–complex RFLP type A predominated in isolates recovered from European patients with AIDS. Further, those investigators were able to demonstrate *M. avium*–complex isolates belonging to three different RFLP types from a single patient with AIDS (23).

RFLP analysis of *M. avium*–complex isolates using DNA probes for IS900 and the related insertion sequence IS901 (30) revealed that there exist distinct subtypes of *M. avium.* The majority of *M. avium* isolates from patients with AIDS (81/81) and non–HIV-infected patients (40/44) lacked either IS900 or IS901 and thus belonged to *M. avium*–complex type A. Those were European patients. The eight environmental isolates examined also belonged to *M. avium* RFLP type A (30). Because the probes contained chromosomal DNA sequences which flank the integrated insertion sequence, the probes were capable of hybridizing to genomic DNA (30). Another group of *M. avium*–complex isolates contained the element IS901 (30). Those strains were mostly of animal origin (20 of 27 isolates) and shared a similar RFLP pattern (30). In addition, 4 of 44 non-AIDS *M. avium* isolates had IS901 and shared that same RFLP pattern (i.e., *M. avium* RFLP type A/I). The investigators did not employ the probes to determine whether patient and environmental isolates shared the same RFLP patterns.

RFLP analysis employing the *Escherichia coli* 5S rRNA gene as probe demonstrated that members of the *M. avium* complex had only a single copy of the 5S rRNA gene (15). The diversity of the *M. avium* complex was demonstrated by the fact that of six *M. avium*–complex strains examined, each had a different RFLP pattern (15). This approach has not been employed to study the epidemiology of *M. avium*–complex infection.

RFLP analysis of the sequence of 16S rDNA has been used to infer phylogenetic relationships between members of the *M. avium* complex (16). Though ribosomal RNA sequences are subject to strong selection and are thus less variable than other sequences in bacteria, 16S rRNA amplification by the polymerase chain reaction (PCR) followed by sequencing identified different *M. avium*–complex groups (16). Although only two *M. avium* strains were examined (one 16S sequence pattern), four distinct sequence patterns were found among 17 *M. intracellulare* isolates (16). To date, an RFLP analysis method based on those sequence data has not been published.

Applicability, Advantages, and Disadvantages

RFLP analysis using either insertion plus surrounding sequences as probes or 5S or 16S rDNA genes appears to offer promise for epidemiological studies. However, the utility of this technique may be restricted by the limited number of character states. There are only single copies of IS901 (30), the IS900 flanking regions (13), and the 5S rDNA gene (15) in *M. avium*–complex strains. Consequently, the methods may lack discriminatory power. In addition to that constraint, the stability of the alternative RFLP types is unknown, as is the influence of selection.

D. Ribosomal DNA Spacer Sequence Analysis

Background

Spacer regions in the 16S–23S ribosomal RNA gene cluster (rDNA) have been amplified by the polymerase chain reaction (PCR) and sequenced (17,18). The spacer sequences mutate but are not subject to the same level of stringent selection as are the 16S, 23S, and 5S rRNA sequences. Thus, spacer regions are anticipated to accumulate more mutations and may distinguish closely related strains of *M. avium*.

Results

There are only two reports describing the variation of sequences of the 16S–23S rDNA spacer region. Four sequevars were found in 16 different *M. avium* strains, 1 sequevar shared by 12 *M. intracellulare* strains, and 7 additional sequevars represented by 7 *M. avium*–complex strains (17). These data confirm the diversity of members of the *M. avium* complex demonstrated by other molecular epidemiological markers. In a second report, the same investigators showed that 6 different patterns were found among 21 different *M. avium* complex isolates recovered from patients with AIDS and non–HIV-infected patients (18). Interestingly, four of the patterns were quite different and were found in seven of the isolates, all of pulmonary origin (18). The remaining two sequevars were very similar and found in 13 isolates (18).

Applicability, Advantages, and Disadvantages

Because of the large population size of *M. avium* isolates recovered from patients with AIDS and the environment, strains with spacer sequence differences due to mutation may be quite common. Already analysis of the 16S-23S rDNA spacer region suggests that it will be useful for epidemiological typing. Because the extent of discrimination of strains by this technique has not yet been established, conclusions concerning the significance of shared sequences between patients (18) cannot be made. The major drawback for employing this method of analysis is the time and expense required of DNA sequencing. However, based on the available data, it may be possible to perform RFLP analysis of the 16S–23S rDNA spacer region using restriction endonucleases chosen on the basis of differences in spacer sequence making this a less costly method of analysis.

E. Large Restriction Fragment Typing

Background

Changes in chromosomal DNA sequence due to mutation in sites recognized by restriction endonucleases should be reflected by changes in the sizes of restriction fragments. Rather than cleaving DNA with endonucleases that generate a large number of fragments, cleavage of genomic DNA with restriction endonucleases which seldom cut will yield a limited number of large restriction fragments (LRF). Large genomic fragments can be separated using pulsed field gel electrophoresis (PFGE). The large fragments are protected from breakage by shear forces by carrying out cell lysis and restriction endonuclease digestion in agar plugs (19,20). Because of the reduced number and size of the fragments, coupled with the ability to embed many cells in the agar plugs, the LRF can be seen on gels by ethidium bromide staining without the need for detection by hybridization.

Results

Comparison of LRF of genomic DNA separated by PFGE has proven useful in discriminating *M. avium*–complex strains (3,19,20). Restriction endonucleases are chosen by selection of those expected to infrequently cleave guanine and cytosine (GC)-rich *M. avium*–complex DNA. The "right" enzymes can be selected empirically on the basis of their ability to reproducibly produce between 8 and 20 distinct fragments. Enzymes chosen include ApaII (19) and AapI (20). Studies to date have established the diversity of LRF types among members of the *M. avium* complex recovered from patients (19,20). Further, the LRF patterns appear to be quite stable (19). In addition, LRF pattern analysis has demonstrated the existence of polyclonal *M. avium*–complex infection in patients with AIDS (20). When applied to an epidemiological study, LRF pattern comparison identified *M. avium* isolates recovered from the environment (e.g., water) and from individual patients with AIDS whose LRF fingerprints were identical (3).

Applicability, Advantages, and Disadvantages

LRF analysis may become the "gold standard" of epidemiological markers for members of the *M. avium* complex. Unfortunately it is laborious and time consuming and requires some expensive equipment. Thus, its use may be limited to those instances where preliminary evidence, such as plasmid typing by Dot-Blot, suggests identity of strains from a single source or lack of identity for establishing polyclonal infection. One factor remains to be investigated. It is not yet established whether cut or uncut *M. avium*–complex plasmid DNA (covalently closed circular DNA) molecules enter the gels and contribute to the patterns.

F. Random Amplified Polymorphic DNA Analysis

Background

Single 10-mer primers can be employed to amplify DNA sequences using the polymerase chain reaction (21,22). The resulting PCR products can be separated by agarose gel electrophoresis and appear as distinct bands. Changes in nucleotide sequence should either create or abolish sequences for primer binding through hybridization and hence change the number and size of amplified fragments (21,22).

Results

Rapid amplified polymorphic DNA (RAPD) analysis has been employed to determine if *M. avium* isolates from soil collected in a prison were identical to those recovered from prisoners who had AIDS (L. E. Via and J.O. Falkinham, submitted). First, RAPD patterns for the individual *M. avium* isolates were quite diverse, confirming the genetic diversity of *M. avium*. Second, although no identical isolates were identified, one *M. avium* soil isolate shared 12 of 14 bands with an *M. avium* patient isolate (L. E. Via and J. O. Falkinham, submitted).

Recently, using this technique we have demonstrated that a clarithromycin-resistant *M. avium* isolate which emerged following the institution of clarithromyin therapy in a single patient with AIDS was almost identical to the original, clarithromyin-sensitive *M. avium* isolate (D. M. Jensen and J.O. Falkinham, unpublished results). By contrast in a second patient, the clarithromycin-resistant isolate had a unique RAPD fingerprint (D. M. Jensen and J.O. Falkinham, unpublished results). That strain either represented a clarithromycin-resistant component of the original *M. avium* population which was selected during chemotherapy or represented secondary superinfection with a clarithromycin-resistant *M. avium* strain.

In both these applications of the RAPD typing, the wide diversity of patterns further emphasizes the conclusion that identity of pairs of strains reflects true relationship if not clonal origin.

Applicability, Advantages, and Disadvantages

Although conceptually simple, RAPD analysis has proven to be difficult to perform. Primarily the RAPD technique requires a great deal of skill and care to ensure reproducible results. Further, the enormous amplification potential of PCR leads to appearance of minor products which appear as weak bands. Those minor, weak bands cause difficulty in interpreting the patterns. In some instances the minor, weak bands are not reproducible and thus one criterion for the analysis requires that bands meet some standard for intensity and reproducibility. RAPD bands amplified from DNA isolated from antibiotic-sensitive and antibiotic-resistant *M. avium*–complex isolates are shown in Fig. 2. Note the presence of faint bands and of an amplified band in the DNA-free control lane (Fig. 2).

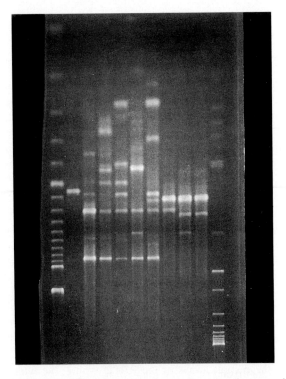

Figure 2   RAPD bands of *M. avium*–complex strains using the same single primer. lane 1, 1 kb ladder; lane 2, *M. avium*, clarithromycin-sensitive (Cla^S, patient with AIDS 1); lane 3, *M. avium* Cla^R (patient with AIDS 1); lane 4, *M. avium* Cla^S; lane 5, *M. avium* Cla^R (patient with AIDS 2); lane 6, *M. avium*, azithromycin-sensitive (Azi^S, patient with AIDS 3); lane 7, *M. avium* Azi^R (patient with AIDS 3); lane 8, *M. avium* Azi^R (patient with AIDS 3); lane 9, *M. avium* Azi^R (patient with AIDS 3); lane 10, no DNA control; lane 11, 100 bp ladder.

It is likely that plasmids do not contribute to band formation, because plasmid DNA is diluted out by the vast excess of chromosomal DNA fragments recovered during DNA isolation (31).

IV. Factors Influencing Results and Interpretation of Molecular Typing

One of the advantages of molecular epidemiology is that the target molecules for characterization are, for the most part, DNA and RNA. Unlike proteins, enzymes, glycopeptidolipids, or the targets of MLEE analysis, the presence of DNA and RNA is not necessarily influenced by growth conditions or medium composition. However, their isolation yields, purity, and susceptibility to experimental manipulation (e.g., nuclease digestion) are influenced by growth conditions.

Although there are advantages to direct examination of DNA or RNA sequences in molecular typing, they too are subject to variation brought about by biological phenomena. Changes in plasmid DNA profiles occur as a result of insertion sequence IS1110 transposition (32) or can occur in colonial variants (33). Further, the stability of different epidemiological markers such as insertion sequences or specific DNA sequences has not yet been established by direct measurement. If markers were unstable, analysis of strains following prolonged laboratory culture could lead to false differences or similarities between strains. Finally, markers may be subject to selection, either during laboratory cultures of in different geographical areas or patient types. The influence of selection on markers used for molecular epidemiology of *M. avium* is unknown.

Internal positive and negative standards and a quality assurance program are necessary whenever performing any of the molecular epidemiological typing techniques. Each technique is subject to unique variations and controls must be included at every step.

If a molecular typing method employs a probe (e.g., RFLP) or primer (e.g., RAPD), the characteristics of that nucleic acid sequence (e.g., G+C composition, length) and the conditions for the reaction between that element and the target DNA or RNA (e.g., hybridization stringency) will directly influence the results. Preliminary experiments to identify the required nucleic acid sequence and the reaction conditions should not be modified when many individual samples are analyzed.

The interpretation of results of a number of molecular epidemiological methods involves analysis of band patterns on gels. Caution should be taken in analysis because of the possibility that a single DNA band can consist of fragments of the same size but different sequence. Usually this can be detected by increased intensity of bands (e.g., twice the amount of DNA) compared with a band of equal size in a molecular weight standard. However, band intensity is not necessarily proportional to size of DNA fragments. That problem can be partially overcome by including ethidium bromide in the gel buffer rather than staining separated DNA fragments after electrophoresis (34).

V. Methods of Analysis of Molecular Epidemiological Data

A. Methods of Analysis

A number of different techniques have been employed to present and analyze data generated by the use of molecular epidemiological markers. The simplest has been comparison by eye as exemplified by RFLP (13,23) and LRF (19,20) typing of *M. avium* strains. If all the bands are the same, the strains are identical and from the same clone. However, identity has not been attained in all instances and investigators have suggested different criteria for attribution of strains to a single type. A study applying plasmid restriction fragment and LRF analyses to characterize methicillin-resistant strains of *Staphylococcus aureus* responsible for nosocomial outbreaks in hospitals considered that isolates were members of the same subtype if 90% or more of the bands matched (35).

There are a number of computational methods which provide a numerical value for the relationship between strains. One is the coefficient of similarity (CS) (36), where, CS = 2 $\times$ (number of matching bands/total number of bands in both strains). Similarity indexes between strains can be calculated using a computer program described by Scott et al. (37). A method for estimating the nucleotide sequence divergency from RAPD data, as well as the limitations and criteria that must be met when employing RAPD data has been published (38). A number of different methods have been used for expressing the relationships between *M. avium*–complex strains illustrated by RFLP analysis of 5S rRNA (15). Genetic diversity of enzyme loci used in MLEE analysis of *M. avium*–complex strains can also be calculated (10).

Often, the analysis of relationships between strains is presented graphically in the form of a dendrogram. Phylogenetic trees can be constructed (39) and confidence limits for such trees calculated (40). The relationship between individual *M. avium* strains illuminated by MLEE was shown in a dendrograms (10,11). Phylogenetic trees were constructed to show the relationships between members of the *M. avium* complex based on 16S rRNA (16) and 16S-23S rDNA spacer sequences (17).

B. Discrimination Index

Recently, a method for assessing the discriminatory power of different typing schemes was presented (41,42). The value for a calculated discrimination index is directly proportional to the number of different types and is based on the probability that two unrelated strains sampled from a test population will be placed into different typing groups (41,42). The greater the number of types, the greater the discrimination index (41,42). However, if many strains fall into a single type, the value for the index falls (41,42).

VI. Comparison of Conventional and Molecular Epidemiological Markers

A. Conventional Epidemiological Markers

A variety of typing methods and systems have been developed for typing members of the *M. avium* complex. They include (1) biotyping (43,44), (2) serotyping (45–47), and (3) phage typing (48).

Biotyping using pigmentation and urease and catalase activity measurements can discriminate between *M. avium*–complex strains (43,44). Unfortunately, biotyping is the method most likely to be influenced by growth conditions.

Though there are a large number of *M. avium* serotypes, the narrow range of *M. avium* serotypes identified from patients with AIDS (45–47) limits the utility of serotyping in this patient population. Further, not all *M. avium* isolates can be serotyped (i.e., typeability is between 77 and 87%). Despite those limitations, Dawson (25) demonstrated polyclonal *M. avium*–complex infection in Australian patients with AIDS and Hoffner et al. (47) demonstrated that Swedish patients with AIDS were infected with a different spectrum of *M. avium* serotypes compared with Swedish children with lymphadenitis.

Because of the variety of *M. avium* phages, phage typing offers good discrimination (48). Unfortunately, only 78 of 235 clinical isolates (33%) could be typed (48). Most *M. avium*–complex strains were phage resistant, particularly environmental isolates (48). Of the 26 AIDS and 40 environmental isolates included in one study, only 27% and 3%, respectively, could be typed with this method (48).

B. Comparison of Conventional and Molecular Epidemiological Typing

Molecular typing methods for *M. avium* have become necessary because of the weak or absent ability of conventional typing methods to discriminate strains. It is not yet clear whether the molecular typing methods involving analysis of DNA will meet the criteria necessary for practical clinical application (49). Much of the work describing molecular epidemiological markers is developmental and has consisted of feasibility studies which necessarily used small numbers of strains. Consequently, the small numbers prevent calculation of discrimination indices (41,42). For RFLP typing using either chromosomal (13) or 5S rRNA (15) probes, weak discrimination between strains was due to the predominance of a single class. Analysis of LRF patterns may, as suggested above, become the "gold standard" for *M. avium* typing. Unfortunately, the labor intensity and cost of LRF typing requires that it be used in conjunction with some other technique (e.g., plasmid typing).

Interpretation of typing results from existing studies is limited because of a number of confounding factors. These include (1) small population sizes, (2) strains comprising each study population were isolated from different geographical regions which has been shown to influence serotype (47) and RFLP type (13), and (3) study populations were made up of different proportions of *M. avium*–complex species or included *M. paratuberculosis* (15).

In spite of those limitations, new insights into *M. avium* epidemiology and genetics can be generated from a comparison of results of epidemiological typing. In Table 1 are data on RFLP typing (using IS901), plasmid typing, and serotyping of a large collection of human, animal, and environmental

Table 1   RFLP, Plasmid, and Serological Types of the *Mycobacterium avium* Complex

Type	IS901	pLR7 (%)	Serotype	Source[a]
A	–	59	4, 6, 8	AIDS (81/81) Non-AIDS (40/44) Environment (8/8) Animals (4/66)
A/I	+	0	1, 2, 3	AIDS (0/81) Non-AIDS (4/44) Environment (0/8) Animals (62/66)

[a]Number of strains with the characteristic/total strains tested.
Source: Data from Ref. 30.

isolates of the *M. avium* complex (30). The data demonstrate that there are two populations of *M. avium*: one group infecting man and a second group infecting animals. Further, the data suggest that the source of human *M. avium* infection is in the environment. Finally, plasmid pLR7 (representative of one plasmid homology group common in patients with AIDS [12,28]) is absent in members of the A/I RFLP type (30), which belong to serotypes 1, 2, and 3. This suggests that IS901 and pLR7 cannot coexist in the same cytoplasm and that pLR7 may be involved in virulence in humans (28).

VII. Application of Molecular Epidemiology to *M. avium* Complex

There are a number of immediate and important problems for which molecular epidemiological approaches can provide the information needed to guide the choice of a solution(s). These include (1) the failure of chemotherapy to clear patients of *M avium* complex, even when the isolate appears susceptible to drug concentrations achieved in blood or tissue; (2) identification of the source of *M. avium*–complex strains infecting patients with AIDS; (3) establishment of the number of *M. avium* complex in a particular source (i.e., colony-forming units per milliliter of water) which poses a direct risk to AIDS patients; and (4) identification of virulence genes and antibiotic-resistance genes.

One potential explanation for the failure of in vitro antibiotic susceptibility to correlate with chemotherapeutic success in the treatment of *M. avium* complex may be the high frequency of polyclonal infection. It is common to recover and perform susceptibility studies on a single isolate from a sample. Further, it has been established that a substantial proportion of patients with AIDS are infected with more than one *M. avium*–complex strain (20,23,25). Finally, it is likely that two isolates in the same patient differ in antibiotic susceptibility (2). If those three conditions were met, employing an antibiotic based on susceptibility testing of only one isolate, and the antibiotic was chosen based on susceptibility of a single strain, treatment failure and continued infection could be due to resistance of the other untested strain. Studies must be performed to determine the true frequency of polyclonal *M. avium*–complex infection in patients with AIDS. Such studies require that at least 5, and even better 10, individual *M. avium*–complex isolates from each sample be isolated and characterized by some molecular technique.

Because of the relative antibiotic resistance of *M. avium*–complex isolates, prevention of *M. avium*–complex infection in patients with AIDS may reduce the morbidity and mortality of infection. Toward that end, molecular epidemiological approaches can serve to assist identification of the sources of *M. avium*–complex isolates which have infected patients with AIDS (3).

Following the identification of possible sources of *M. avium*–complex organisms, a study relating the number of *M. avium* types in a single source with the probability of infection in patients with AIDS can be initiated. That study is of importance because a survey of the literature demonstrates that *M. avium*–complex organisms have been isolated from almost every possible environmental source. Such a study would relate infection with exposure to possible sources, where the number of each *M. avium* type in each source could be determined.

Molecular epidemiological approaches will serve to identify the route of infection in disseminated *M. avium* disease. One major question is whether disseminated disease due to *M. avium* complex results from primary infection in the gastrointestinal tract or lungs? Evidence to date suggests that primary *M. avium* infection in either the lungs or gastrointestinal tract is equally likely to result in disseminated infection (50). Proof that one, or both, are sources for disseminated infection will require molecular typing methods.

Molecular epidemiological approaches will be of value in determining whether *M. avium* disease is due to reactivation following remote infection or a new exposure and infection. Evidence that patient isolates did not share related fingerprints with environmental *M. avium* strains would be evidence supporting the hypothesis that infection occurred previously. However, these data could also be explained by a failure to identify and sample the true source of *M. avium*.

Finally, the molecular markers may serve as tools to identify virulence or antibiotic-resistance genes in members of the *M. avium* complex. Molecular characterization of a large collection of individual *M. avium*–complex isolates which differ in virulence could lead to identification of DNA sequences which are significantly associated with virulence (or nonvirulence). Identification of antibiotic-resistance genes would employ antibiotic-sensitive strains recovered from patients and the antibiotic-resistant strains that emerge during therapy, because those strains are possibly related (D. M. Jensen and J. O. Falkinham, unpublished results). For identifying virulence determinants, individuals of the same species (i.e., *M. avium* defined by DNA probe) yet differing in virulence in any of the available animal models (e.g., beige mouse) would be compared. Both studies would require a large enough population of strains (i.e., virulent and nonvirulent or antibiotic-resistant and sensitive) to ensure that differences not associated with either virulence or resistance would not obscure differences in molecular markers (e.g., RFLP or RAPD patterns) associated with virulence.

References

1. Wolinsky E. Nontuberculous mycobacteria and associated diseases. Am Rev Respir Dis 1979; 119:107–159.

2. Fry KL, Meissner PS, Falkinham JO III. Epidemiology of infection by nontuberculous mycobacteria. VI. Identification and use of epidemiologic markers for studies of *Mycobacterium avium, M. intracellulare* and *M. scrofulaceum.* Am Rev Respir Dis 1986; 134:39–43.

3. von Reyn CF, Maslow JN, Barber TW, et al. Persistent colonisation of potable water as a source of *Mycobacterium avium* infection in AIDS. Lancet 1994; 343:1137–1141.

4. duMoulin GC, Stottmeier KD, Pelletier PA, et al. Concentration of *Mycobacterium avium* by hospital hot water systems. JAMA 1988; 260:1599–1601.

5. von Reyn CF, Waddell RD, Eaton T, et al. Isolation of *Mycobacterium avium* complex from water in the United States, Finland, Zaire, and Kenya. J Clin Microbiol 1993; 31:3227–3230.

6. Saito H, Tsukamura M. *Mycobacterium intracellulare* from public bath water. Jpn J Microbiol 1976; 20:561–563.

7. Falkinham JO III, Parker BC, Gruft H. Epidemiology of infection by nontuberculous mycobacteria. I. Geographic distribution in the eastern United States. Am Rev Respir Dis 1980; 121:931–937.

8. Brooks RW, Parker BC, Gruft H, Falkinham JO, III. Epidemiology of infection by nontuberculosis mycobacteria. V. Numbers in eastern United States soils and correlations with soil characteristics. Am Rev Respir Dis 1984; 130:630–633.

9. Wendt SL, George KL, Parker BC, et al. Epidemiology of infection by nontuberculous mycobacteria. III. Isolation of potentially pathogenic mycobacteria from aerosols. Am Rev Respir Dis 1980; 122:259–263.

10. Yakrus MA, Reeves MW, Hunter SB. Characterization of isolates of *Mycobacterium avium* serotypes 4 and 8 from patients with AIDS by multilocus enzyme electrophoresis. J Clin Microbiol 1992; 30:1474–1478.

11. Wasem CF, McCarthy CM, Murray LW. Multilocus enzyme electrophoresis analysis of the *Mycobacterium avium* complex and other mycobacteria. J Clin Microbiol 1991; 29:264–271.

12. Jucker MT, Falkinham JO III. Epidemiology of nontuberculous mycobacteria. IX. Evidence for two DNA homology groups among small plasmids in *Mycobacterium avium, M. intracellulare* and *M. scrofulaceum.* Am Rev Respir Dis 1990; 142:858–862.

13. Hampson SJ, Thompson J, Moss MT, et al. DNA probes demonstrate a single highly conserved strain of *Mycobacterium avium* infecting AIDS patients. Lancet 1989; i:65–69.

14. Lévy-Frébault VV, Thorel M.-F., Varnerot A, Gicquel B. DNA polymorphism in *Mycobacterium paratuberculosis*, ''wood pigeon mycobacteria,'' and related

mycobacteria analyzed by field inversion gel electrophoresis. J Clin Microbiol 1989; 27:2823–2826.

15. Chiodini RJ. Characterization of *Mycobacterium paratuberculosis* and organisms of the *Mycobacterium avium* complex by restriction polymorphism of the rRNA gene region. J Clin Microbiol 1990; 28:489–494.

16. Böddinghaus B, Wolters J, Heikens W, Böttger EC. Phylogenetic analysis and identification of different serovars of *Mycobacterium intracellulare* at the molecular level. FEMS Microbiol Lett 1990; 70:197–204.

17. Frothingham R, Wilson KH. Sequence-based differentiation of strains in the *Mycobacterium avium* complex. J Bacteriol 1993; 175:2818–2825.

18. Forthingham R, Wilson KH. Molecular phylogeny of the *Mycobacterium avium* complex demonstrates clinically meaningful divisions. J Infect Dis 1994; 169: 305–312.

19. Mazurek GH, Hartman S, Zhang Y, et al. Large DNA restriction fragment polymorphism in the *Mycobacterium avium–Mycobacterium intracellulare* complex: A potential epidemiologic tool. J Clin Microbiol 1993; 31:390–394.

20. Arbeit RD, Slutsky A, Barber TW, et al. Genetic diversity among strains of *Mycobacterium avium* causing monoclonal and polyclonal bacteremia in patients with AIDS. J Infect Dis 1993; 167:1384–1390.

21. Welsh J, McClelland M. Fingerprinting genomes using PCR with arbitrary primers. Nucl Acids Res 1990; 18:7213–7218.

22. Palittapongarnpim P, Chomcy S, Fanning S, Kunimoto D. DNA fragment length polymorphism analysis of *Mycobacterium tuberculosis* isolates by arbitrary primed polymerase chain reaction. J Infect Dis 1992; 167:975–978.

23. Visuvanathan S, Holton J, Nye P, et al. Typing by DNA probe of mycobacterial species isolated from patients with AIDS. J Inf 1992; 25:259–265.

24. Kunze ZM, Portaels F, McFadden JJ. DNA probes to investigate epidemiology of mycobacterial infections in AIDS. 2nd International Meeting on Bacterial Epidemiological Markers, Rhodes, Greece, Apr 8–11, 1990.

25. Dawson DJ. Infection with *Mycobacterium avium* complex in Australian patients with AIDS. Med J Aust 1990; 153:466–468.

26. Meissner PS, Falkinham JO III. Plasmid DNA profiles as epidemiologic markers for clinical and environmental isolates of *Mycobacterium avium, M. intracellulare* and *M. scrofulaceum.* J Infect Dis 1986; 153:325–331.

27. Crawford JT, Falkinham JO, III. Plasmids of the *Mycobacterium avium* complex. In: McFadden JJ, ed. Molecular biology of the Mycobacteria. Surrey, England: Surrey University Press, 1990:97–119.

28. Crawford JT, Bates JH. Analysis of plasmids in *Mycobacterium avium–intracellulare* isolates from persons with acquired immunodeficiency syndrome. Am Rev Respir Dis 1986; 134:659–661.

29. Jucker MT. Relationship of Plasmids in *Mycobacterium avium, Mycobacterium intracellulare,* and *Mycobacterium scrofulaceum.* PhD. dissertation, Virginia Polytechnic Institute and State University, Blacksburg, VA, 1991.

30. Kunze ZM, Portaels F, McFadden JJ. Biologically distinct subtypes of *Mycobacterium avium* differ in possession of insertion sequence IS901. J Clin Microbiol 1992; 30:2366–2372.

31. Elaichouni A, Vanemmelo J, Claeys G, et al. Study of the influence of plasmids on the arbitrary primer polymerase chain reaction fingerprint of *Escherichia coli* strains. FEMS Microbiol Lett 1994; 115:335–359.

32. Hernandez M, Hellyer T, Dale JW. Characterisation of IS1110, a highly mobile element from a clinical isolate *Mycobacterium avium*. 126th Annual Meeting of the Society for General Microbiology, Exeter, England, Sept 7–9, 1993.

33. Erardi FX, Meissner PS, Falkinham JO, III. Simple method for obtaining mycobacterial clones with altered plasmid profiles. Plasmid 1985; 13:220.

34. Hartley JL, Xu L. DNA mass ladder: estimation of PCR products in gels. Focus 1994; 16:52–53.

35. Branchini ML, Morthland VH, Tresoldi AT, et al. Application of genomic DNA subtyping by pulsed field gel electrophoresis and restriction enzyme analysis of plasmid DNA to characterize methicillin-resistant *Staphylococcus aureus* from two nosocomial outbreaks. Diagn Microbiol Infect Dis 1993; 17:275–281.

36. Dice KR. Measures of the amount of ecological association between species. Ecology 1945; 26:297–302.

37. Scott DA, Welt M, Leung FC. A computer program to aid in calculating similarity indexes from DNA fingerprints. BioTechniques 1993; 14:980–983.

38. Clark AG, Lanigan CMS. Prospects for estimating nucleotide divergence with RAPDs. Mol Biol Evol 1993; 10:1096–1111.

39. Fitch WM, Margoliash E. Construction of phylogenetic trees. Science 1967; 155: 279–284.

40. Felsenstein J. Confidence limits on phylogenies: an approach using the bootstrap. Evolution 1985; 39:783–791.

41. Hunter PR, Gaston MA. Numerical index of the discriminatory ability of typing systems: an application of Simpson's index of diversity. J Clin Microbiol 1988; 26:2465–2466.

42. Hunter PR. Reproducibility and indices of discriminatory power of microbial typing methods. J Clin Microbiol 1990; 28:1903–1905.

43. Hawkins JE. Scotochromogenic mycobacteria which appear intermediate between *Mycobacterium avium–intracellulare* and *Mycobacterium scrofulaceum*. Am Rev Respir Dis 1977; 166:963–964.

44. Portaels F. Difficulties encountered in identification of *M. avium–M. intracellulare, M. scrofulaceum* and related strains. Am Rev Respir Dis 1978; 188:969.

45. Horsburgh CR Jr, Cohn DL, Roberts RB, et al. *Mycobacterium avium–M. intracellulare* isolates from patients with or without acquired immunodeficiency syndrome. Antimicrob Agents Chemother 1986; 30:955–957.

46. Yakrus MA, Good RC. Geographic distribution, frequency, and specimen source of *Mycobacterium avium* complex serotypes isolated from patients with acquired immunodeficiency syndrome. J Clin Microbiol 1990; 28:926–929.

47. Hoffner SE, Källenius G, Petrini B, et al. Serovars of Mycobacterium avium complex isolated from patients in Sweden. J Clin Microbiol 1990; 28:1105–1107.
48. Crawford JT, Bates JH. Phage typing of the Mycobacterium avium–intracellulare–scrofulaceum complex. Am Rev Respir Dis 1985; 132:386–389.
49. Maslow JN, Mulligan ME, Arbeit RD. Molecular epidemiology: Application of contemporary techniques to the typing of microorganisms. Clin Infect Dis 1993; 17:153–164.
50. Jacobson MA, Hopewell PC, Yajko DM, et al. Natural history of disseminated Mycobacterium avium complex infection in AIDS. J Infect Dis 1991; 164:994–998.

3

Pulmonary Disease Due to *Mycobacterium avium* Complex

MICHAEL D. ISEMAN

University of Colorado School of Medicine
Denver, Colorado

I. Introduction

Pulmonary disease due to organisms of the *M. avium* complex (pulmonary MAC or P-MAC), notably *M. avium M. intracellulare*, has been recognized with increasing frequency throughout the latter half of the twentieth century. To some extent this may reflect improved laboratory capacity to distinguish MAC from *M. tuberculosis* or increased awareness on the part of clinicians of the pathogenic potential of these microbes; that is, isolates are not routinely dismissed as commensal. However, it is my belief that this is a significant trend associated with several changes in the ecosystems associated with life in modern industrialized societies: widespread use of tobacco, diminishing rates of true tuberculosis, altered systems of potable water, and the supplanting of tub bathing by showering.

II. Epidemiology

Since isolation of MAC from clinical specimens does not require public health notification (unlike tuberculosis [TB]) systematic data on the frequency

45

of recovery, rates of disease, or deaths due to MAC are not available. The most quantitative data on MAC in the United States were derived in a Centers for Disease Control (CDC) survey from 1981–1983 in which the prevalence of disease was estimated to be 1.28 cases per 100,000 population (1) and a review of patients from an Health Maintenance Organization in Oregon from 1975 to 1986 in which the annual incidence was 0.98 cases per 100,000 (2). A retrospective analysis of patients with disease due to MAC or TB in two Philadelphia hospitals from 1975 to 1987 demonstrated that as TB receded in these institutions, P-MAC cases rose steadily over this period (3).

Anecdotal reports in scientific communications have obvious limitations. Nonetheless, the observations of clinicians* from across the United States who comment on substantial and steady increases in the numbers of cases of P-MAC encountered in their communities or practices are impressive. Analogously, a recent report by Kennedy and Weber described 21 patients in Virginia with pulmonary mycobacterial diseases seen in a private practice from 1990 to 1992 (4). Of these cases, 16 involved MAC and only one was associated with *M. tuberculosis*. The investigators also documented a rising number of respiratory isolates from a regional hospital that were positive for nontuberculous mycobacteria from 1980 to 1991, with 32 of 47 cases involving MAC. Although such reports are not ideal methodologically, they suggest that more patients with P-MAC are being seen in diverse communities and regions.

Early series of P-MAC disease indicated the preponderance of the cases occurring among males, most of whom had preexisting lung disorders (5,6). However, more recent reports have noted a preponderance of females, including many without apparent underlying disorders (2–4). In the 1981–1983 CDC survey, 43.9% of MAC pulmonary cases were in females (1). In the series from Philadelphia, 64 cases with associated lung diseases were described, with 50% of these patients being female. By contrast, among their 21 cases without recognized predisposing conditions, 81% were females (3). Similarly, among the Oregon cases, there were 29 patients with P-MAC, 18 of whom (62%) were females. Predisposing diseases were noted overall in 12 (41%) of these patients; among males 8 of 11 (73%) had underlying disorders, whereas among females only 4 of 18 (22%) were so affected.

---

*The National Jewish Center provides free telephone consultation service regarding patients with complicated mycobacterial disease; annually we receive over 700 calls. Thus, we have corresponded with physicians from the contiguous 48 states, Alaska, and Hawaii regarding patients with pulmonary MAC.

Among the series from Virginia, 12 of 16 patients (75%) were females; 10 of these 12 were nonsmokers. By contrast, all four of the males were smokers or ex-smokers.

Notable also among the various reports of P-MAC were the relative paucity of P-MAC among nonwhites. In the CDC survey, 85% of MAC cases were reported in whites; in the 29 cases from Oregon, 28 were in whites (97%); race was not reported in the Philadelphia or Virginia series. Again, owing to the absence of ideal data, it is not possible to conclude that there are racial differences in susceptibility to P-MAC. An alternative explanation could include higher rates of disease due to *M. tuberculosis* involving those nonwhite Americans who are particularly susceptible to mycobacterial lung disease. Certainly for tertiary institutions, skewed patterns of referral could also explain disproportionate racial representation.

III. Transmission

The routes of transmission of MAC in pulmonary disease have not been determined. The leading possibilities are fine particle aerosol or aspiration, and it is possible that both contribute. Falkinham and coworkers demonstrated that environmental strains of MAC which more closely resembled human disease–derived strains were more likely to come out of suspension when the liquid was agitated (7); from this observation, the investigators speculated that wave action in brackish coastal waters generated MAC in an aerosol likely to be inhaled by those living near the ocean. This would be consistent with the intense level of skin test reactivity—over 75% of recruits reacting to PPD-B—among US Navy recruits residing in selected coastal counties of North and South Carolina, Georgia, Florida, Alabama, Mississippi, Louisiana, and Texas. This would also be consistent with the geographical preponderance of P-MAC in the southeastern United States during the period 1950–1970.

As noted above, cases of P-MAC have been widely reported across the United States in recent years. A plausible hypothesis to explain this redistribution of infection/disease would be MAC contamination of potable water systems. MAC has been recovered on various occasions from institutional hot water systems (8–10). Recently, in a survey of home potable water in Westchester, New York (11), MAC organisms were recovered in 32% of the 77 homes studied, sometimes including more than one serotype. MAC organisms can transiently tolerate temperatures as high as 70°C (9). Formerly, hot water systems employed temperatures as high as 71°C; however, to both conserve energy and prevent scalding accidents, modern systems raise water temperatures to only 49–60°C (12). Thus, it is possible that MAC bacilli survive in substantial numbers in these systems, are aerosolized during showering, and are inhaled during such exposures.

Over the past three decades, there has been a substantial change in the hygienic practices of Americans. During this period, there has been a shift from tub bathing toward showering: the American Society of Heating, Refrigerating, and Air-Conditioning Engineers, Inc. (ASHRAE) estimates that virtually all US males and 90% of females employ showering as their primary means of hygiene (13). An over recent decades, there has been a steady increase in the use of closed or partially enclosed stalls for showering. Thus, it is my conjecture that aerosolized MAC derived from potable water systems may be the route of infection for an unknown portion of persons with P-MAC. In particular, the pattern of diffuse, subpleural nodular disease reported in several recent series would be most compatible with delivery of MAC by aerosols. The best analogy for this scenario occurred in the West Haven, Connecticut, Veterans Administration Hospital (VAH) where a number of patients who were admitted on repeated occasions for exacerbation of chronic obstructive pulmonary disease developed nodular granulomatous lung disease due to *M. xenopi* (14). Investigators found the hot water system of the VAH was contaminated with *M. xenopi* and inferred that the infections has been acquired through exposure to the showers. VonReyn and colleagues recently described seven patients with acquired immunodeficiency syndrome (AIDS) who had disseminated MAC and appeared to have been infected from institutional water systems, a scenario which is consistent with this hypothesis, although the portal of entry in these cases was postulated to be the alimentary canal (10).

IV. Other Conditions Associated with P-MAC

A substantial portion, if not a clear majority, of P-MAC cases occurs in persons with predisposing lung conditions. Historically, the initial reports from the United States emphasized the roles of cigarette-related chronic bronchitis and emphysema, previous tuberculosis, or other infections that resulted in bronchiectasis, pneumoconioses, or fibrotic lung disorders associated with rheumatoid arthritis or ankylosing spondylitis (5,6,15).

Pectus excavatum, or abnormal narrowing of the chest in the anteroposterior axis, thoracic scoliosis, and mitral valve prolapse (MVP) were found in variable frequencies in a prior series of patients with P-MAC from our institution (16); our subsequent experience confirms these apparent relationships (Fig. 1A and B). These cardiothoracic anomalies were most commonly seen in female patients and typically found with nodular-bronchiectatic disease, often with prominent right middle lobe and lingular involvement (Fig. 1C and D). I believe that these patients probably will be found to have genetically determined abnormalities of connective tissue, possibly subsets of the fibrillin disorders currently seen to be associated with Marfan's syndrome (17,18). Historically, the vulnerability of persons with these features to mycobacterial disease has been long recognized: both Hippocrates and Galen commented on "phthisical" chest types with similar findings. Indeed, at the turn of the twentieth century, Tyson (19) described two variations. One of these sounded Marfan-like: "alar" . . . "Narrow, shallow, and long, the angles of the scapulae projecting like wings behind, the proper ratio between the antero-posterior and transverse diameters being preserved . . . ribs droop or are unduly oblique . . . the throat is prominent, the neck long, and the head bent forward." The other variation was mindful of pectus excavatum: "flat" . . . "the antero-posterior diameter is disproportionately short, owing to the absence of convexity in the cartilages, which are sometimes even depressed, carrying with them the sternum and producing a form of chest which, on section, is kidney-shaped."

In addition to these associated conditions, patients with cystic fibrosis (CF) have been noted with increasing frequency to be colonized with MAC and, in some cases, develop disease caused by MAC (20,21). Obviously as improved care of patients with CF results in extended survival, we may anticipate rising numbers of cases in which MAC (or other environmental mycobacteria) are recovered from respiratory secretions and produce invasive disease.

Other underlying lung disorders that we at The National Jewish Center for Immunology and Respiratory Medicine (NJC) have noted to be in apparent association with P-MAC include alpha$_1$-antitrypsin deficiency, tracheobronchomegaly, pulmonary thromboembolism, prior histoplasmosis, and previous radiation therapy for breast cancer. Heterozygous, phenotype MZ, alpha$_1$-antitrypsin deficiency with mild airflow limitation, subtle hyperinflation, and insignificant prior history of cigarette use has been seen in three middle-aged women with P-MAC in the last decade at NJC; they manifested the nodular, bronchiectatic variety of disease (see below). In addition, several patients with tracheobronchomegaly (Mounier-Kuhn syndrome) with bronchiectasis were noted to have invasive P-MAC. Also, we have seen a small group of patients with chronic, unresolved thrombosis following pulmonary embolism who subsequently developed P-MAC. In these cases, P-MAC pre-

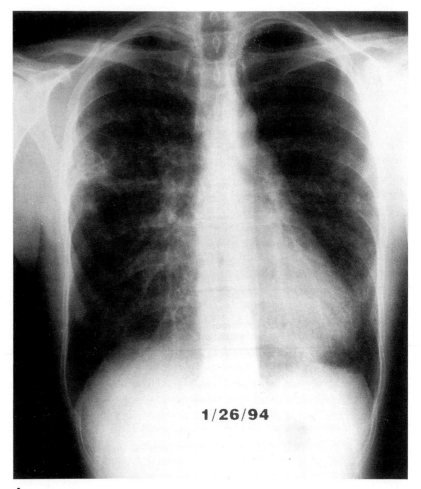

1/26/94

A

Figure 1 A, B: PA and lateral chest x-ray views of a 48-year-old woman with P-MAC. A thin-walled cavity is seen near the chest wall in the anterior segment of the right upper lobe. On the frontal view the cardiac silhouette is prominent; however, as seen in (C), this is due to displacement of the heart into the left hemithorax by a severe pectus excavatum deformity. On the lateral view, the depth of the excavatum depression can be seen; the distance from the posterior aspect of the xiphisternum to the anterior surface of the vertebrae, 4.7 cm, falls well below the lower limits of normal for women, 9.2 cm (26). In addition to a slender habitus, "straight back," and subtle rotatory scoliosis, the patient has documented mitral valve prolapse.

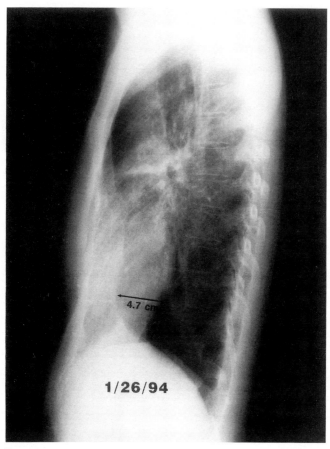

B

sented with extensive destruction of lung parenchyma. Eight cases were seen of invasive, destructive P-MAC in the hemithorax of women who had undergone radiation therapy for breast cancer; we suspect the ionizing irradiation had resulted in lung damage that increased vulnerability to MAC. And we have recently noted a potential association between prior infection with *Histoplasma capsulatum* and vulnerability to MAC lung disease (22). Among certain patients we have observed large, calcified peribronchial lymph nodes

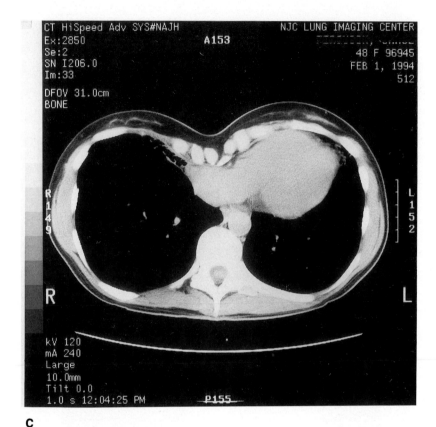

C

Figure 1 Continued. C,D: Computed tomographic images of this 48-year-old woman demonstrate the extreme pectus excavatum deformity which has displaced the heart into the left hemithorax. As seen on the lung window, (D), there is dense saccular bronchiectasis involving the anterior portions of the medial segment of the right middle lobe and the inferior segment of the lingula.

surrounding and/or impinging on airways that subserve lung regions involved with MAC (Fig. 2). We suspect prior histoplasmosis facilitates MAC by causing parenchymal scarring with bronchiectasis and/or impaired drainage due to bronchial compromise. Although we do not have direct evidence that these calcified nodes are due to histoplasmosis, we infer this is so because P-MAC

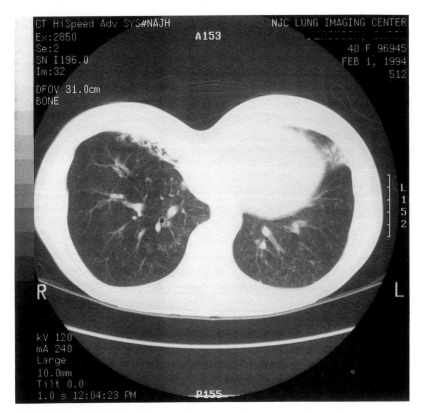

D

is not seen in association with such calcifications except for patients who
have resided for considerable periods in regions indigenous for *H. capsulatum*
infection; also splenic calcifications typical of histoplasmosis were seen
among several patients in this group.

V. Clinicoradiographic Presentations of P-MAC

Although there may be considerable overlap or transition between these forms
of P-MAC, there are several distinctive patterns of P-MAC which can provide
useful diagnostic, therapeutic, or prognostic information.

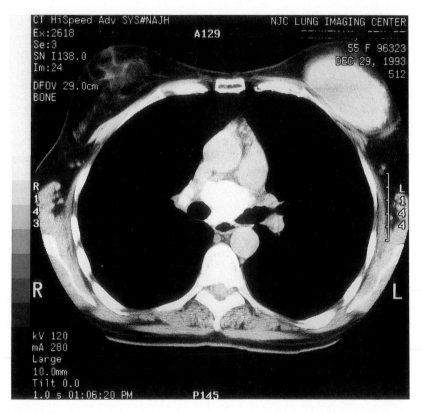

Figure 2 Computed tomographic lung scan of 45-year-old woman from Arkansas with P-MAC, primarily involving the right middle lobe and superior segment of the right lower lobe. We believe the massive, dense, subcarinal calcification represents prior infection with *Histoplasma capsulatum* the sequelae of which predispose to P-MAC (23). Incidentally, the patient also experienced modest dysphagia, presumably associated with impingement of calcified lymph node mass on the esophagus.

A. Cavitary/Destructive Form

Particularly among persons with underlying lung diseases, P-MAC may present with extensive lobar or multilobar dense, necrotizing inflammation (Fig. 3A and B). The radiographic appearance of these processes may demonstrate coarse, fibronodular infiltration or homogeneous pneumonic shadowing with a prominent air bronchogram effect. Cavitation, single or multiple, is common. Early there may be unilateral involvement, but with the passage of time, bilateral disease is more common. In such cases, all lobes may be involved, although upper zone disease is more prominent. Broad, scalloped thickening of the apical pleura is characteristic but not pathognomic of this type of P-MAC; effusions are not demonstrable (Fig. 3A).

Clinically, patients with the cavitary/destructive form of P-MAC tend to have rather prominent respiratory and constitutional symptoms, including productive cough, hemoptysis, dyspnea, fever, sweats, malaise, anorexia, and weight loss. Vague, deep, nonpleuritic chest pain is reported by a minority of patients. Very rarely, classic pleuritic chest pain is reported; among these patients coarse, snowshoe-type pleural friction rubs may be heard in the absence of demonstrable effusions.

Sputum microscopy from patients with untreated cavitary disease typically shows numerous acid-fast bacilli (AFB); indeed, for patients with obvious cavitary lesions who have not received chemotherapy, negative sputum smears for AFB should raise serious doubts about a mycobacterial etiology (23,24). This is an important distinction from those with nodular bronchiectatic disease whose respiratory secretions are uncommonly smear positive and typically yield sparsely and irregularly positive culture results (23). Pulmonary function testing varies according to underlying lung disorders. Leukocytosis or a left shift of the neutrophil series is uncommon. Nonspecific markers of inflammation and inanition include moderate elevation of the erythrocyte sedimentation rate (ESR) and lowered albumin and cholesterol levels. The tuberculin skin test employing purified protein derivative T (PPD-T) (the only mycobacterial antigen currently approved for intradermal testing by the Food and Drug Administration) is nonreactive or yields small reactions, 4 mm or less, in the majority of cases (25); however, 4 of 22 patients with culture-proven MAC disease in a recent series gave a greater than 10 mm indurated reaction to PPD-T, reaffirming the marginal specificity of skin testing for mycobacterial infections (26).

B. Multinodular Bronchiectatic Form

Recently there has been increasing recognition of a distinct form of P-MAC largely involving women without underlying lung diseases and negative or minimal cigarette smoking histories. In the report from two Philadelphia hospitals, which embraced a 10-year period from 1978 to 1987, 85 patients were diagnosed with P-MAC (3). Twenty-one of these cases did not have apparent underlying lung disease identified; 17 of them (81%) were in females. The most common radiographic pattern seen among these patients was multiple, discrete pulmonary nodules (71%); the infiltrates were either diffuse or localized, prominently involving the anterior segment of the right upper lobe.

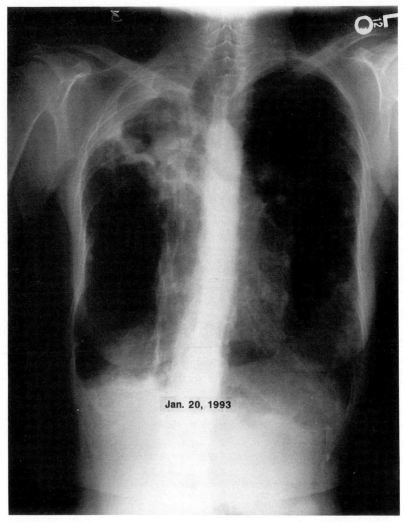

A

Figure 3 A, B: Posteroanterior and lateral chest radiographic views of cavitary-destructive P-MAC. The right upper lobe has been totally destroyed and sloughed out, resulting in a "lobar cavitation." Note thick, scalloped pleural capping along the apical-lateral surfaces and severe volume loss.

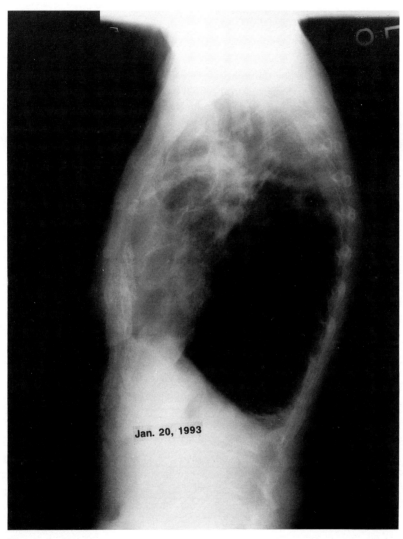

Jan. 20, 1993

B

Similarly, in the series from Oregon, 29 cases of P-MAC were identified from 1975 to 1986 (2). Of this group, 18 (62%) were female, and—among the female patients—there were significant trends toward less underlying lung disease (22 vs 73% in males) and toward less extensive, noncavitary lung disease. One-third of these females presented with disease, nodular and bronchiectatic, localized to the right middle lobe (RML) and/or lingula. This is analogous to our experience with RML-lingular disease among female patients (16,23). Also, 11 of 12 (92%) female patients with MAC from Virginia had prominent or isolated RML involvement; the other had disease in the lingula and elsewhere (4).

A group from the Mayo Clinic reported that among patients with sputum culture-positive P-MAC, 40 of 62 cases were associated with bronchiectasis and that 39 of these 40 patients had nodular infiltrates (27). Notably, 35 of the patients had a pattern of multiple small nodules; none of these patients had preexisting risk factors and 29 (83%) of them were women. The close association between MAC and nodular and bronchiectatic lung disease was affirmed by a second study from the Mayo Clinic in which there was an association between certain findings on computed tomographic scans (CTS) of patients with bronchiectesis and P-MAC (28). In a retrospective analysis of 100 cases in which the CTS showed bronchiectasis, 24 patients had multiple pulmonary nodules and 19 of these had nodules in the same lobe with bronchiectasis. Cultures for pathogens were not performed consistently in all cases, but among the 15 (of 24) patients who were cultured for mycobacteria, 8 were positive for MAC. The investigators concluded that, in their series, CTS findings of bronchiectasis with multiple small nodules predicted positive MAC cultures with a sensitivity of 80%, a specificity of 87%, and an accuracy of 86%.

The clinical presentations of patients with the nodular bronchiectatic variety of P-MAC is generally more insidious and subtle than for those with the destructive cavitary variety. As noted in the previous series, cough and expectoration are the usual complaints; fever, sweats, chills, and weight loss are uncommon and typically mild when reported. However, we have noted a characteristic malaise marked by a prominent sense of lethargy and diminished energy; this varies from day-to-day but may exert a profound effect on quality of life. Not uncommonly, such patients have been evaluated for chronic fatigue syndrome because of the prolonged disabling effects of this response. Over time, patients may complain of diminished exercise tolerance, dyspnea, and curtailment of activity, ascribable more to respiratory impairment than the malaise noted above. Sputum characteristically is thick, tenacious, discolored but not foul; intermittent blood streaking is common but gross hemoptysis rare. Microbiologically, such patients may at various times shed rapid-growing mycobacteria or *Pseudomonas* species in their sputum, as well as MAC. In some cases, these organisms appear to function as co-pathogens and may require specific therapy for optimum outcome.

C. Transition/Combination Forms

Although patients with the nodular bronchiectatic form of P-MAC noted above tend to stay within that pattern for extended periods, we and others have seen patients who begin with radiographically localized disease marked by a segmental nodular appearance with cylindrical or saccular bronchiectesis and progress to lobar, destructive cavitary disease (29). I have been impressed, in particular, by a small but memorable group of patients who begin with the "right-middle lobe syndrome" variant of P-MAC and, untreated, go on over months to years to develop extensive disease throughout the lungs, resulting in respiratory insufficiency (Fig. 4A and B).

D. Bullitis

An unusual variant of P-MAC is disease within large cystic or bullous spaces within the lung parenchyma. Most of such patients have either underlying cigarette-induced emphysema or pneumoconiotic fibrosis.

E. Solitary Pulmonary Nodule

Rarely, P-MAC may present as an asymptomatic solitary pulmonary nodule. In these cases, the differential diagnosis usually is focused on lung cancer and biopsy or resection is performed, yielding the diagnosis. When there is truly only a solitary nodule and it has been resected, it has been suggested that drug therapy is not indicated (30). However, the number of cases and the duration for which these patients were followed up are not adequate to assure that these patients are not at increased risk for subsequent invasion by MAC, and I recommend that such patients undergo postoperative radiographic and symptomatic surveillance for several years.

VI. Criteria and Procedures Used for Diagnosis of P-MAC

In 1990, the American Thoracic Society (ATS) published a statement on the diagnosis and treatment of disease due to mycobacteria other than tuberculosis (31). I have substantial disagreements with this document which, I be-

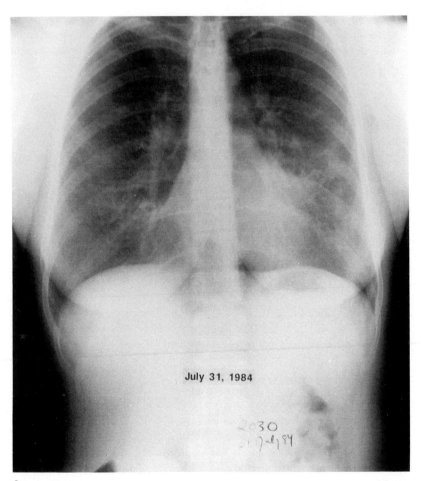

July 31, 1984

A

Figure 4   Posteroanterior chest radiographic view of 65-year-old woman who had P-MAC disease localized to the lingula and right middle lobe in 1984 (A). Therapy was initiated in 1984 but abandoned after a few weeks due to drug intolerance. When the patient next was evaluated in 1992 for P-MAC (B), both upper lobes were extensively damaged and the patient, a nonsmoker, had developed oxygen-dependent respiratory insufficiency. The lingular and right middle lobe infiltrates seen in 1984 were no longer apparent due to cephalad retraction as the upper lobes were destroyed.

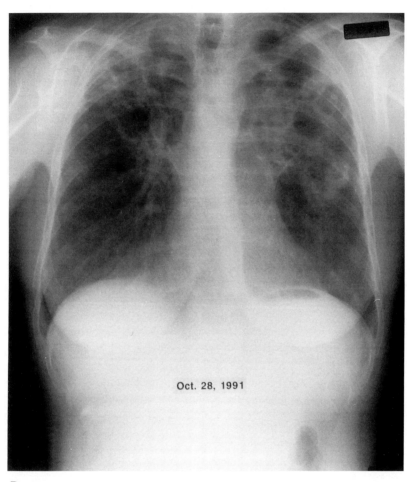

Oct. 28, 1991

B

lieve, sets overly stringent criteria for diagnosis which can result in delayed diagnosis, belated treatment, and heightened morbidity.

In this document, which dealt with various mycobacteria, including MAC, it was stated that:

> A single positive sputum culture does not suffice to diagnosis *disease.* Furthermore, some patients with multiple positive sputum cultures may not need drug therapy ... "colonization" has been seen most often with *M. avium*

complex. It is characterized by the presence of noncavitary, stable, and usually minimal radiographic disease associated with sporadic excretion of organisms from the respiratory tract. Recognition of this syndrome is important because drug therapy may not be required (31).

The document goes on to state that in the presence of a cavitary infiltrate on chest radiograph,

> definite NTM [nontuberculous mycobacteria] disease is considered to be present when: (1) two or more sputum samples (or sputum and bronchial washing) are acid-fast bacilli smear-positive and/or result in moderate to heavy growth of NTM on culture; (2) other reasonable causes for the disease process have been excluded, e.g., fungal disease, malignancy, tuberculosis, etc.

This is a reasonable construct and generally will result in suitable sensitivity and specificity for the diagnosis of *cavitary* P-MAC.

However, the document then sets criteria for the diagnosis of noncavitary disease which in my opinion are too rigid:

> (1) two or more sputums (or sputum and a bronchial washing) are AFB smear-positive and/or result in moderate to heavy growth on culture; (2) failure of the sputum cultures to convert to negative with either bronchial hygiene of 2 weeks of specific mycobacterial drug therapy; (3) other reasonable causes for the disease have been excluded (Ref. 31, p. 941).

In my experience, a substantial portion of patients who have the multinodular bronchiectatic variety of P-MAC would fail to meet these criteria, specifically the requirement for AFB smear positivity or moderate to heavy growth on cultures. Also, the stipulation that cultures remain positive after 2 weeks of drug therapy is too restrictive. Certainly, if these conditions are met, they confirm the diagnosis. But dismissing those who fail the criteria as merely colonized will result in failure to recognize numerous patients who have early-stage but nonetheless clinically important pulmonary disease due to MAC.

The ATS statement claims that 75% of patients with P-MAC have cavitary infiltrates. But this is circular reasoning that flows from their diagnostic criteria. As noted in the above discussion, a majority of recent case series (2,4,28) had features of multinodular bronchiectatic P-MAC as the dominant pattern. Certainly, in one recent experience at NJC, we have seen a preponderance of such cases (32). By employing the overly restrictive ATS criteria, it has been made to appear as though most P-MAC is of the destructive cavitary variety. But based on the more recent literature as well as my experience, I believe the nodular bronchiectatic variety is substantially more prevalent in this era.

VII. Medical Management of P-MAC Disease

A. Background

Historically, chemotherapy of P-MAC has been fraught with controversy. There have been no well-controlled studies even to document that treatment is better than no treatment, although virtually all authorities would concur that therapy is definitely indicated in the destructive cavitary type disease described above. Furthermore, there have been no careful trials that compared "regimen A with regimen B," nor are there clear-cut data to indicate whether in vitro susceptibility testing is useful in choosing drugs or regimens. Hence, any recommendations for therapy will inherently represent an amalgam of "clinical experience," published but uncontrolled observations, extrapolations from in vitro investigations, and analogies to the experiences with *M. tuberculosis* in which controlled studies have been performed.

B. Outcome Measures

In large measure, drug therapy of P-MAC has been associated with disappointing outcome. There has been an inevitable tendency to contrast the results of MAC treatment with modern therapy of pulmonary tuberculosis. Short-course chemotherapy of drug-susceptible tuberculosis yields 100% response rates, minimal drug intolerance, less than 5% lifetime relapse rates, and— unassailably—prolongation of life. Hence, when the experience with MAC treatment is viewed from this perspective, the results look rather dismal. Owing to the intrinsically greater resistance of MAC to antimicrobial agents as well as its propensity to afflict persons with preexisting lung disorders, the utility of P-MAC treatment should—I submit—be viewed through a wider prism.

Functionally, treatment efficacy can be seen in terms of these variables: symptomatic relief, initial bacteriological response (conversion of sputum cultures to negative or failure to do so), radiographic course (improving, unchanged, worsening), drug consequences (toxicity, side effects, and financial burdens), respiratory physiology (improving, stable, or worsening), recurrence (relapse rates after treatment is discontinued), and mortality (does treatment prevent or delay premature death due to P-MAC).

When considered in these terms, I believe chemotherapy does offer considerable benefits for a wide array of patients.

C. Current American Thoracic Society Guidelines

In the 1990 American Thoracic Society Statement on Nontuberculous Mycobacteria, a standard three- or four-drug regimen was advocated for initial therapy of P-MAC (31) which consisted of isoniazid (INH), rifampin (RIF), and ethambutol (EMB) with streptomycin (SM) to be given for 3–6 months for patients with more extensive disease. This was based in some measure on the success of this regimen among a group of 46 patients in Texas, 91% of whom converted their sputum cultures to negative (33).

Our group took exception to several aspects of these recommendations, however (34). We had previously shown that INH was not active in vitro singly or in combination against clinical isolates of MAC (35); and because of the modest but clinically significant risk of INH toxicity—particularly in older persons—we discouraged its use. Subsequently, another group reported INH to have in vitro synergy with streptomycin and found favorable effects when INH-SM were used in an in vivo murine model (36); however, owing to the limited number of strains in which this relationship has been demonstrated and the absence of human clinical data to support these findings, the importance of in vitro synergy between these two agents is unclear.

The ATS statement also indicated that in vitro susceptibility testing of clinical isolates was not relevant to the selection of drugs. Although we conceded that standard solid-agar methods employed for *M. tuberculosis* did have shortcomings, we argued that more quantitative liquid medium methods did reveal patterns of in vitro susceptibility that correlated broadly with clinical experience (34). Furthermore, we argued that our prior series of P-MAC cases demonstrated a statistically significant relationship between in vitro susceptibility and response to therapy (37). Similarly, Tsukamura and colleagues in Japan had shown that response to treatment related to pretreatment in vitro susceptibility and that during treatment minimal inhibitory concentrations to the drugs employed drifted upward, indicating killing of vulnerable populations (38).

D. Principles in Chemotherapy

The utility of in vitro susceptibility testing in selecting drugs for the treatment of MAC disease remains a confusing morass of uncontrolled reports. Unfortunately, given the extraordinary array of variables involved with P-MAC, including extent of MAC disease, in vitro resistance patterns, extent and nature of underlying lung disorders, patients' tolerance of or adherence to medications, absorption or other pharmacokinetic parameters, and potential for exogenous reinfection, it will be extremely difficult to conduct a prospective trial. Perhaps the only mechanism by which such a study could be conducted would be a multicenter collaborative project on the model of the AIDS Clinical Trials Group studies of treatment of disseminated MAC disease; unfortunately, no such mechanism currently exists for evaluation of treatments for P-MAC, and there appears to be little interest on the part of national organizations or the pharmaceutical industry to sponsor such endeavors.

Thus, we are left with a largely descriptive literature of "clinical experience" to guide in the choice of therapy. Table 1 includes the results of selected reports of the outcome of treatment of P-MAC. As seen, initial response rates range widely, 55–100%, and relapse rates between 10 and 38% were noted. In general, better outcomes were seen when more agents were employed, but no clear pattern of efficacy can be discerned.

E. Current Medications

The most promising recent development in the therapy of MAC disease has been the discovery of the macrolide clarithromycin. A related compound, azithromycin, is also active against these mycobacteria, but its clinical utility has been less well studied. Clarithromycin is quite active in vitro; among 49 *M. avium* strains from bacteremic patients with AIDS, broth-determined MICs ranged from 0.12 to 1.0, with 43 of the isolates in the 0.25–0.50 range (39). In addition, ex vivo human macrophage studies demonstrated that a single 2-hr pulsed exposure of clarithromycin at 3.0 mg/ml resulted in total inhibition of intracellular MAC for 4 days and very slow resumption of growth between days 4 and 7 (40). The clinical utility of clarithromycin in pulmonary MAC in persons negative for human immunodeficiency virus (HIV) has been suggested by reports from France in which it was used in combination with other drugs (41) and from Texas in which it was employed as monotherapy (42). The study from Texas was highly instructive. Of 30 enrolled patients, 20 completed treatment with clarithromycin administered at 500 mg orally twice daily for 4 months. Among the 19 patients with pretreatment MICs ≤8 mg/ml, 58% became culture negative and another 21% showed substantial reductions in the numbers of cultivable mycobacteria. Despite monotherapy, only 3 of the 19 (16%) patients developed resistance to clarithromycin.

We have also had a favorable experience with clarithromycin in the management of P-MAC at the National Jewish Center. Although we have not studied it in a prospective manner, we have been impressed that a great majority of the clinical isolates—a mixture of *M. avium* and *M. intracellulare*—from patients with P-MAC have MICs ≤0.5 mg/ml, that true toxic reactions are very rare, and that with patience in adjusting the dosage and timing nearly all patients can tolerate the drug. However, it has not

Table 1 Results of Medical Treatment of Pulmonary MAC Disease

Report	Initial response (%)	Relapse (%)	Overall response (%)	Comments
Arkansas, 1979 (63)	68/85 (80)	16/68 (24)	39/85 (46)	4–5 drugs; no RIF
Milwaukee, 1979 (64)	46/82 (56)	9/46 (20)	37/82 (45)	2–5 drugs; rare RIF
Wales, 1981 (65)	22/40 (55)	3/22 (14)	19/40 (48)	Better response with more drugs
NJC, 1981 (5)	63/81 (78)	10/63 (16)	53/81 (65)	5–6 drugs; high rates of death from MAC ±/or underlying disease
Alabama, 1984 (65)	52/86 (60)	10/52 (20)	42/86 (49)	Better response with more drugs.
Texas, 1986 (40)	42/46 (91)	4/22 (18)	Unclear	All cavitary. Only 22 available for follow. Failure and relapse seen with gastrectomy.
Texas, 1986 (66)	32/54 (59)	11/32 (34)	Unclear	Better response with more drugs and less extensive disease.
NJC, 1987 (45)	52/76 (68)	6/52 (12)	46/76 (61)	5–6 drugs; correlation with in vitro susceptibility.
Philadelphia, 1989 (3)	21/21 (100)	8/21 (38)	13/21 (62)	Mostly nodular bronchiectatic disease.
Oregon, 1991 (2)	11/12 (92)	1/10 (10)	10/12 (83)	3–5 drugs; better outcome in females w/o cavitary disease.

resulted in predictable, dramatic clinical responses such as those observed with drug-susceptible tuberculosis even when combined with aggressive, multidrug regimens.

Rifampin and ethambutol have been the most frequently administered drugs in our recent P-MAC cases. This reflects both the probability of in vitro susceptibility and low levels of toxicity. According to Heifets' tentative criteria, 19% of the National Jewish Center clinical isolates were susceptible to rifampin and 67% to ethambutol (34). Furthermore, additive or synergistic action of these drugs in combination against the great majority of MAC isolates has been shown (43).

However, recent observations about potentially significant reductions in clarithromycin serum levels when administered with rifampin have raised questions about the advisability of the routine use of rifamycins (59). Furthermore, rifampin's capacity to induce the cytochrome P-450 enzymatic pathways results in accelerated clearance of numerous other medications, as well as endogenous hormones, including cortisol and estrogens (44–46). Hence, in patients receiving polypharmacy for other conditions or individuals with marginal ovarian or adrenal function, rifampin may prove problematic.

Other rifamycins, including rifabutin and rifapentine, are active in vitro versus MAC. Rifabutin has not been compared with rifampin in a controlled trial in P-MAC. The CDC reported on the results of rifabutin used largely for patients with P-MAC who had failed other therapy (47). Rifabutin was used in 150-g, 300-g, and 450-mg dosage. There was a trend toward improved response with the higher dose, 44 versus 30% with low dose. However, the drug did not have an overall significant effect on outcome. Uveitis has been reported in association with rifabutin when given with clarithromycin and ethambutol (48,49) and with fluconazole (50,51). Both clarithromycin and fluconazole impair hepatic catabolism of rifabutin, and probably result in toxic elevations of rifabutin levels. Regarding combined effect with ethambutol, additive and synergistic effects are comparable to those seen with rifampin (43). Enzyme induction and drug interaction effects of rifabutin appear similar to but less intense than those seen with rifampin.

Ethambutol probably plays a substantial role in P-MAC therapy. In addition to its intrinsic activity, the drug has a well-documented effect enhancing rifamycin activity (43) and possibly augmenting the effects of clarithromycin. In the laboratory at NJC, clarithromycin and ethambutol have a predictable additive effect; for example, if the clarithromycin and ethambutol MICs for a given strain are 0.5 and 4.0 mg/ml, respectively, the resultant MICs when the drugs are combined are 0.25 and 2.0 mg, respectively (L. Heifets, unpublished data, 1993–1994). As suggested by a Swedish group, ethambutol may mediate the effect by interference with cell wall permeability (52). Generally well tolerated orally, ethambutol's major potential toxicity is retrobulbar neuritis. This complication is dose and duration dependent and has been reported infrequently in patients treated for tuberculosis. However, there have been anecdotal reports of impaired vision in elderly patients P-MAC receiving ethambutol for relatively short periods, emphasizing the need for careful patient education and careful monitoring in such patients. However, we have used extended courses of this drug in older persons and —with monthly tests of color vision (Ishihara plates) and acuity (Snellen tests)—have not observed major deterioration.

The decision to employ injectable agents is complex and involves such issues as extent and course of disease, strain susceptibility, prior therapy, age of patient, renal status, auditory or vestibular function, and patient attitudes. We use streptomycin or amikacin for patients with cavitary, destructive, rapidly progressive, highly symptomatic disease. This is based on the empirical observations that regimens containing such agents have been associated with more favorable response rates (53). Also, in a semiquantitative manner, there is a broad correlation between therapeutic efficacy and the number of agents employed in a regimen (see references in Table 1). We have also used these agents for patients with the nodular bronchiectatic variety of disease when the principal symptom is relentless coughing; in such instances, we have added the injectable agents when patients failed to respond to the initial oral regimen. Analogous to infectious bronchiectasis in patients with cystic fibrosis, we also have employed nebulized administration of amikacin or kanamycin in selected patients with nodular bronchiectatic MAC disease to diminish toxicity and avoid parenteral administration. However, our experience to date is too limited to comment on its utility.

Renal and auditory or vestibular toxicity due to aminoglycoside antibiotics are largely dependent on dosage and age. Recent experience indicates that short dosing intervals to a greater extent than high peak levels may accelerate the appearance of these toxicities (54). Indeed, Sbarbaro et al. gave streptomycin twice weekly at doses of 27 mg/kg for up to 18 months with less than 10% serious toxicity among patients receiving directly observed tuberculosis therapy (55). Because mycobacteria multiply very slowly in comparison with the gram-negative bacteria for which these drugs are typically given, dosing intervals may be extended considerably without evident loss of efficacy, allowing longer use of these agents (see Table 2 for details of dose and rhythm of administration). Thus, we have used these drugs even in patients in their eighth and ninth decades. In such cases, we are very

Table 2 Suggested Regimen for Pulmonary MAC

Initial Phase (2–4 months)	Continuation (20–22 months)	Comments
Clarithromycin 500 mg po bid	Clarithromycin 750 mg po qd	Dysgeusia; GI symptoms
Ethambutol 20–25 mg/kg po qd	Ethambutol 15 mg/kg po qd	Monitor vision
Clofazimine 200 mg po qd	Clofazimine 100 mg po qd	Reduce dose for GI symptoms or excess pigment
Amikacin or Streptomycin 15 mg/kg IV or IM thrice weekly		Monitor levels and toxicity, particularly in elderly

careful to establish baseline pharmacokinetic parameters and to monitor frequently and carefully for organ damage.

Clofazimine has been employed in the treatment of P-MAC because of a reasonable probability of in vitro activity and a favorable toxicity profile (56). Predictably, all patients receiving this drug for a month or more develop obvious skin pigmentation, which is initially bronze in hue and shifts toward sienna or slate color with extended use. However, with cessation of therapy, the compound is gradually leached from the skin (the half-life in tissue is approximately 70 days) and normal skin tones are restored. The other major side effect of clofazimine is gastrointestinal distress. Usually this appears several months into therapy and is believed to be due to progressive deposition of the drug in the bowel epithelium; rarely it occurs early, with the drug behaving as a direct irritant. Clofazimine may be deposited in ocular structures but has not been associated with visual impairment in our experience.

Ciprofloxacin is the most active in vitro of the currently available fluoroquinolone antibiotics, with 28% of the NJC clinical isolates deemed susceptible by the criteria of Heifets. Our experience with long-term, high-dose administration of ciprofloxacin has indicated a low frequency of toxicity, with only 7% of persons requiring cessation of the drug (57). However, the side effects are not inconsequential, with common reports of agitation, tremulousness, nausea, insomnia, and disturbing dreams. Therefore, we limit ciprofloxacin use to cases with documented in vitro susceptibility, extensive or progressive disease, and resistance to or intolerance of the major drugs noted above.

Formerly, we employed ethionamide and cycloserine routinely in the treatment of P-MAC disease (5). However, we have now restricted their use to cases in which there is proven in vitro susceptibility to them and resistance to or intolerance of the other agents noted above. Ethionamide has an extremely high likelihood of gastrointestinal side effects, including nausea, anorexia, griping discomfort, diarrhea, and profound dysgeusia; depression, hypothyroidism, and arthralgias are also seen. Cycloserine has no gastrointestinal effects but poses risks for potentially severe central nervous system effects, including clouded sensorium, depression, suicidal ideation, thought disorders, and both focal and generalized seizures. In large measure, these manifestations are dependent on serum concentrations. Careful monitoring of serum levels to keep peak concentrations between 25 and 30 mg/ml may diminish these complications in most patients. We administer pyridoxine (vitamin B_6), 30–50 mg, with each 250-mg dose of cycloserine in an effort to reduce cycloserine toxicity; however, the utility of this practice is unproven. Obviously, cycloserine should be used with considerable caution in persons with preexisting mental conditions or seizure disorders. The drug is cleared by the kidneys, so doses must be reduced and levels followed closely in the presence of renal impairment.

F. Selecting Treatment Regimens

In most cases, clinicians must begin treatment of patients with MAC disease without the benefit of drug susceptibility testing. In such cases, treatment will be based on an analysis of the prior probability of drug activity, the nature of the disease, and patient variables that determine the likelihood of acceptance and tolerance of the medication/regimen. In other instances, drug susceptibility results are available. Although some contend that such information is not useful, we feel that there is sufficient clinical experience to endorse in vitro susceptibility testing when radiometric broth-dilution techniques are utilized (34).

Until recently our choice for empirical therapy has been a four-drug regimen comprising clarithromycin, rifampin, ethambutol, and an aminoglycoside or clofazimine. Dosage of medications (other than clarithromycin for which we had no assay) was adjusted after pharmacokinetic assays (58). Clarithromycin dosage was determined by gastrointestinal tolerance. During the initial phase of treatment, the usual dose has been 500 mg twice daily. In the continuation phase of treatment, we attempt to reduce medication to once daily for purposes of adherence and to diminish side effects.

However, recent data have raised questions about the suitability of this regimen. Using assays provided by Abbott Laboratories (Abbott Park, IL),

Wallace and colleagues have shown the simultaneous administration of rifampin or rifabutin resulted in substantial reductions of clarithromycin serum levels (59). In this study, patients were given clarithromycin alone, 500 mg, twice daily for 4 months; subsequently, other drugs were added, including rifampin or rifabutin, 600 mg daily. Mean serum levels of clarithromycin alone were 5.4 ± 2.1 mg/ml; following addition of rifampin, the levels fell to 0.7 ± 0.6 mg/ml and of rifabutin to 2.2 ± 1.5 mg/ml. The apparent mechanism of this drug interaction relates to activity of one of the cytochrome P-450 enzyme pathways. Macrolides, which are metabolized predominately through this system, progressively inhibit the P-450 pathway when given at higher doses, resulting in nonlinear build-up of the drug levels. The rifamycins overcome this inhibition, actually accelerating the catabolism of macrolides, including clarithromycin. As the investigators indicate, the levels of a metabolite which has some activity against MAC, 14-OH clarithromycin, remains in the same range with or without the rifamycins. This may in some measure compensate for the dramatic reduction in the primary compound. However, these findings cast doubt on the advisability of this combination of agents.

Further troubling is the observation that clarithromycin, by slowing enzymatic degradation, results in increased tissue levels of rifabutin which may be responsible for some complications, including uveitis, when these drugs are used together (see above). Until further study clarifies the clinical importance of these drug interactions, my judgment is that simultaneous use of clarithromycin and rifampin or rifabutin is not generally advisable.

Based on the various considerations delineated, my current recommendations for initial treatment of patients with P-MAC are represented in Tables 2 and 3. As noted in the text, the employment of injectable agents poses significant organizational issues for drug delivery. However, these agents do appear to augment response rates modestly and should be considered for patients with extensive or highly symptomatic disease. By using peripherally inserted central catheters, in-home intravenous therapy can be accomplished in most instances. Alternative agents are employed when there is major intolerance to the primary agents, treatment failure, and/or acquired resistance.

G. Duration of Treatment

In the absence of controlled studies, it is difficult to identify an ideal length of therapy. Data indicate that 12 months is too short for patients with asymptomatic cavitary disease (60). Our practice at NJC has been to target 24 months but adjust according to extent of disease, response to treatment, tolerance of medication, and overall medical status. Our concern has been that

Table 3 Alternative Medications for Pulmonary MAC

Drug	Dose	Comments
Rifampin	450–600 mg po qd	Multiple drug interactions, including clarithromycin
Rifabutin	300–450 mg po qd	Drug interactions; uveitis with clarithromycin and fluconazole
Ciprofloxacin	500–750 mg po qd	GI and CNS effects; give in morning to avoid insomnia
Ethionamide	250 mg po bid to qid	Potentially severe GI distress
Cycloserine	250 mg po bid	Monitor levels; CNS effects; supplement with pyridoxine

premature discontinuation of therapy will result in reactivation and further lung damage. Thus, for patients with marginal respiratory reserve, there is reluctance to jeopardize their ventilatory status by permitting recrudescence. Among those patients to whom therapy is a continuously unpleasant, disruptive experience, we attempt to persevere through a minimum of 18 months. For some patients who have been slow to respond, who have marginal respiratory reserve, and/or who feel much better on therapy than they did before, therapy may be extended beyond 24 months.

When termination of therapy is anticipated, it is appropriate to emphasize to patients that there is a modest risk for reactivation (see Table 1). I usually explain to the patient that there is the potential for recurrence and indicate signs and symptoms which might mark this event (most patients are all too familiar with these manifestations). Periodic surveillance of objective markers is encouraged, including sputa for smear and culture and chest radiographs or CT scans for patients with the nodular bronchectatic variety of disease. In an effort to reassure, we stress that patients who experience relapses usually respond well to retreatment (especially if they did well on initial therapy). Over the course of many months or years of therapy, however, progressive resistance to the drugs employed may evolve.

VIII. Resectional Surgery

Because of the inherent drug resistance of MAC and the often frustrating results of chemotherapy, resectional surgery to control the infection has been employed frequently, albeit in an uncontrolled manner. There have been two recent series of reporting lung resection as an adjunct to treatment of P-MAC, one from Duke University in 1983 (61) and one from NJC in 1991 (62). The selection criteria and types of surgery in the Duke series were not well described; from among 175 patients with P-MAC, 37 were selected for surgery. Long-term follow-up was available for 33 of these patients, 31 of whom had a favorable response. Among the patients at NJC, we have observed highly divergent results. From 1983 to 1990, 33 patients with P-MAC underwent resectional procedures in efforts to control the infection. Complication rates in this group were substantially higher than a simultaneous series of patients undergoing surgery for multidrug-resistant tuberculosis; among these 33 patients there were 7 bronchopleural fistulae, 4 prolonged air leaks, and 2 chronic respiratory failures. The bronchopleural fistulae occurred following right pneumonectomy and were associated with these risk factors: prior therapeutic irradiation to that hemithorax, peristently positive preoperative sputum mycobacterial cultures, and polymicrobial superinfection of the damaged lung.

The best results occurred with resection of localized bronchiectasis of the right middle lobe and/or lingula (see Fig. 1). However, even in these cases, there was a pattern of persistent or recurrent postoperative bronchiectasis that required aggressive ongoing medical attention. In several cases, *Pseudomonas aeruginosa* appeared to be the dominant pathogen associated with continued inflammation. In others, no pathogens were recovered, including MAC as multiple AFB cultures of sputum and bronchial washes remained negative; however, several patients responded to reinstitution or modification of antimycobacterial therapy.

The decision to perform resectional surgery in P-MAC cases remains problematic. On the favorable side of the balance, surgery can help control debilitating constitutional symptoms associated with uncontrolled infection, eliminate potentially hazardous hemoptysis, and—possibly—halt the ongoing risk of contamination of undiseased lung from infected foci. However, there is a significant risk of serious operative morbidity, including lethal respiratory insufficiency associated with bronchopleural fistulae. All patients undergoing surgery (except for emergent resection to control life-threatening hemoptysis) should receive 3–4 months of intensive preoperative chemotherapy and must be treated for an extended postoperative period. Some patients will accede to surgery in the hope that they can escape medical treatment which they find very difficult to tolerate; but this is not an acceptable situation, for failure to take medication after surgery will almost certainly result in recurrence of the infection, obviating the benefits of the resection.

References

1. O'Brien R, Geiter L, Snider D Jr. The epidemiology of nontuberculous myco-bacterial diseases in the United States. Results from a national survey. Am Rev Respir Dis 1987; 135:1007–1014.
2. Reich J, Johnson R. *Mycobacterium avium* complex pulmonary disease. Inci-dence, presentation, and response to therapy in a community setting. Am Rev Respir Dis 1991; 143:1381–1385.
3. Prince D, Peterson D, Steiner R, et al. Infection with *Mycobacterium avium* complex in patients without predisposing conditions. N Engl J Med 1989; 321(13):863–868.
4. Kennedy T, Weber D. Nontuberculous mycobacteria: An underappreciated cause of geriatric lung disease. Am J Respir Crit Care Med 1994; 149:1654–1658.
5. Davidson P, Khanijo V, Goble M, Moulding T. Treatment of disease due to *Mycobacterium intracellulare*. Rev Infect Dis 1981; 3(5):1052–1059.
6. Rosenzweig D, Schlueter D. Spectrum of clinical disease in pulmonary infection with *Mycobacterium avium–intracellulare*. Rev Infect Dis 1981; 3(5):1046–1051.
7. Parker B, Ford M, Gruft H, Falkinham J III. Epidemiology of infection by nontuberculous mycobacteria. IV. Preferential aerosolization of *Mycobacterium intracellulare* from natural waters. Am Rev Respir Dis 1983; 128:652–656.
8. duMoulin G, Stottmeier K. Waterborne mycobacteria: An increasing threat to health. Demographic patterns, larger immunodeficient populations, and the prev-alence of mycobacteria in water systems contribute to a rising problem. ASM News 1986; 52(10):525–529.
9. duMoulin G, Stottmeier K, Pelletier P, et al. Concentration of *Mycobacterium avium* by hospital hot water systems. JAMA 1988; 260(11):1599–1601.
10. vonReyn C, Maslow J, Barber T, et al. Persistent colonisation of potable water as a source of *Mycobacterium avium* infection in AIDS. Lancet 1994; 343: 1137–1141.
11. Montecalvo M, Forester G, Tsang A, et al. Colonisation of potable water with *Mycobacterium avium* complex in homes of HIV-Infected persons. Lancet 1994; 343:1639.
12. Sullivan, Sullivan. as cited in Ref. 10.
13. Rozier D. Member ASHRAE, consultant to the National Jewish Center for Im-munology and Respiratory Medicine (personal communication), 1994.
14. Costrini A, Mahler D, Gross W, et al. Clinical and roentgenographic features of nosocomial pulmonary disease due to *Mycobacterium xenopi*. Am Rev Respir Dis 1981; 123:104–109.
15. Contreras M, Cheung O, Sanders D, Goldstein R. Pulmonary infection with nontuberculous mycobacteria. Am Rev Respir Dis 1988; 137:149–152.
16. Iseman M, Buschman D, Ackerson L. Pectus excavatum and scoliosis: Thoracic anomalies associated with pulmonary disease due to *M. avium* complex. Am Rev Respir Dis 1991; 144:914–916.

17. Francke U, Furthmayr H. Marfan's Syndrome and other disorders of fibrillin. N Engl J Med 1994; 330(19):1384–1385.

18. Pereira L, Levran O, Ramirez F, et al. A molecular approach to the stratification of cardiovascular risk in families with Marfan's syndrome. N Engl J Med 1994; 331(3):148–153.

19. Tyson J. The Practice of Medicine. Philadelphia: Blakiston's, 1906:241.

20. Kilby J, Gilligan P, Yankaskas J, et al. Nontuberculous mycobacteria in adult patients with cystic fibrosis. Chest 1992; 102:70–75.

21. Aitken M, Burke W, McDonald G, et al. Nontuberculous mycobacterial disease in adult cystic fibrosis patients. Chest 1993; 103:1096–1099.

22. Chan, E, Iseman M. Does prior infection with Histoplasma capsulatum predispose to pulmonary *Mycobacterium avium* complex infection? Am J Respir Crit Care Med 1994;

23. Lynch D, Simone P, Fox M, et al. CT features of pulmonary *Mycobacterium avium* complex infection: Comparison with Mycobacterium tuberculosis, and correlation with sputum positivity. J Computer Assist Tomogr 1994;

24. Tsukamura M. Diagnosis of disease caused by *Mycobacterium avium* complex. Chest 1991; 99(3):667–669.

25. vonReyn C, Barber T, Arbeit R, et al. Evidence of previous infection with *Mycobacterium avium–Mycobacterium intracellulare* complex among healthy subjects: An international study of dominant mycobacterial skin test reactions. J Infect Dis 1993; 168:1553–1558.

26. vonReyn C, Green P, McCormick D, et al. Dual skin testing with *Mycobacterium avium* sensitin and purified protein derivative: An open study of patients with M. avium complex infection or tuberculosis. Clin Infect Dis 1994; 19:15–20.

27. Hartman T, Swensen S, Williams D. *Mycobacterium avium–intracellulare* complex: Evaluation with CT. Radiology 1993; 187:1–4.

28. Swenson S, Hartman T, Williams D. Computed tomographic diagnosis of *Mycobacterium avium–intracellulare* complex in patients with bronchiectasis. Chest 1994; 105:49–52.

29. Tanaka E, Lee W, Yuba Y, et al. Computed tomography findings of pulmonary infections caused by *Mycobacterium avium* complex in patients without predisposing conditions (abstr). Am J Respir Crit Care Med 1994; 149:A109.

30. Gribetz A, Damsker B, Bottone E, et al. Solitary pulmonary nodules due to nontuberculous mycobacterial infection. Am J Med 1981; 70:39–43.

31. American Thoracic Society. Diagnosis and treatment of disease caused by nontuberculous mycobacteria. Am Rev Respir Dis 1990; 142:940–953.

32. Iseman M. *Mycobacterium avium* complex and the normal host. The other side of the coin (editorial). N Engl J Med 1989; 321(13):896–898.

33. Ahn C, Ahn S, Anderson R, et al. A four-drug regimen for initial treatment of cavitary disease caused by *Mycobacterium avium* complex. Am Rev Respir Dis 1986; 134:438–441.

34. Heifets L, Iseman M. Individualized therapy versus standard regimens in the treatment of *Mycobacterium avium* infections. Am Rev Respir Dis 1991; 144:1–2.

35. Heifets L, Iseman M. Choice of antimicrobial agents for *M. avium* disease based on quantitative tests of drug susceptibility. N Engl J Med 1990; 323(6):419–420.

36. Reddy M, Gangadharam P, Srinivasan S. In vitro and in vivo synergistic effect of isoniazid with streptomycin and clofazimine against *Mycobacterium avium* complex (MAC). Tubercle Lung Disease 1994; 75:208–212.

37. Horsburgh C, Mason U, Heifets L, et al. Response to therapy of pulmonary *Mycobacterium avium intracellulare* infection correlates with results of in vitro susceptibility testing. Am Rev Respir Dis 1987; 135:418–421.

38. Tsukamura M. Evidence that antituberculosis drugs are really effective in the treatment of pulmonary infection caused by *Mycobacterium avium* complex. Am Rev Respir Dis 1988; 137:144–148.

39. Heifets L, Lindholm-Levy P, Comstock R. Clarithromycin minimal inhibitory and bactericidal concentrations against *Mycobacterium avium*. Am Rev Respir Dis 1992; 145:856–858.

40. Mor N, Heifets L. Inhibition of intracellular growth of *Mycobacterium avium* by one pulsed exposure of infected macrophages to clarithromycin. Antimicrob Agents Chemother 1993; 37:1380–1382.

41. Dautzenberg B, Breux J, Febvre M, et al. Clarithromycin containing regimens for mycobacterial infections in 55 non-AIDS patients (abstr). Am Rev Respir Dis 1992: 145:A809.

42. Wallace R Jr., Brown B, Griffith D, et al. Initial clarithromycin monotherapy for *Mycobacterium avium–intracellulare* complex lung disease. Am J Respir Crit Care Med 1994; 149:1335–1341.

43. Heifets L, Iseman M, Lindholm-Levy P. Combinations of rifampin or rifabutin plus ethambutol against *Mycobacterium avium* complex: Bactericidal synergistic, and bacteriostatic additive or synergistic effects. Am Rev Respir Dis 1988; 137:711–715.

44. Baciewicz A, Self T. Rifampin drug interactions. Arch Intern Med 1984; 144: 1667–1671.

45. Borcherding S, Baciewicz A, Self T. Update on rifampin drug interactions II. Arch Intern Med 1992; 152:711–716.

46. Wilkins E, Hnizdo E, Cope A. Addisonian crisis induced by treatment with rifampicin. Tubercle 1989; 70:69–73.

47. O'Brien R, Geiter L, Lyle M. Rifabutin (ansamycin LM427) for the treatment of pulmonary *Mycobacterium avium* complex. Am Rev Respir Dis 1990; 141: 821–826.

48. Shafran S, Deschenes J, Miller M, et al. Uveitis and pseudojaundice during a regimen of clarithromycin, rifabutin, and ethambutol. N Engl J Med 1994; 330: 438–439.

49. Frank M, Graham M, Wispelway B. Rifabutin and uveitis. N Engl J Med 1994; 330:868.

50. Narang P, Trapnell C, Schoenfelder J, et al. Fluconazole and enhanced effect of rifabutin prophylaxis. N Engl J Med 1994; 330:1316–1317.

51. Fuller J, Stanfield L, Craven D. Rifabutin prophylaxis and uveitis. N Engl J Med 1994; 330:1315–1316.
52. Kallenius G, Svenson S, Hoffner S. Ethambutol: A key for *Mycobacterium avium* complex chemotherapy? (letter). Am Rev Respir Dis 1989; 140:264.
53. Tsukamura M, Ichiyama S, Miyachi T. Superiority of enviomycin or streptomycin over ethambutol in initial treatment of lung disease caused by *Mycobacterium avium* complex. Chest 1989; 95:1056–1058.
54. Levison M. New dosing regimes for aminoglycoside antibiotics. Ann Intern Med 1992; 117:693–694.
55. Hudson L, Sbarbaro J. Twice weekly tuberculosis chemotherapy. JAMA 1973; 223:139–143.
56. Lindholm-Levy P, Heifets L. Clofazimine and other rimino-compounds: Minimal inhibitory and minimal bactericidal concentrations at different pHs for *Mycobacterium avium* complex. Tubercle 1988; 69:179–186.
57. Berning S, Madsen L, Iseman M, Peloquin C. Long-term safety of ofloxacin and ciprofloxacin in the treatment of mycobacterial infections. Am J Respir Crit Care Med 1994;
58. Peloquin C. Antituberculosis Drugs: Pharmacokinetics. In: Heifets L, ed. Drug Susceptibility in the Chemotherapy of Mycobacterial Infections. Boca Raton, FL: CRC Press, 1991:59–88.
59. Wallace R Jr., Brown B, Griffith D, et al. Reduced serum levels of clarithromycin in patients on multidrug regimens including rifampin or rifabutin for treatment of *Mycobacterium avium–intracellulare*. J Infect Dis 1994; 171:747–750.
60. Hunter A, Campbell I, Jenkins P, Smith A. Treatment of pulmonary infections caused by mycobacteria of the *Mycobacterium avium–intracellulare* complex. Thorax 1981; 36:326–329.
61. Moran J, Alexander L, Staub E, et al. Long-term results of pulmonary resection for atypical mycobacterial disease. Ann Thorac Surg 1983; 35(6):597–604.
62. Pomerantz M, Madsen L, Goble M, Iseman M. Surgical management of resistant mycobacterial tuberculosis and other mycobacterial pulmonary infections. Ann Thorac Surg 1991; 52:1108–1112.
63. Dutt A, Stead W. Long-term results of medical treatment in *Mycobacterium intracellulare* infection. Am J Med 1979; 67:449–453.
64. Rosenzweig D. Pulmonary mycobacterial infections due to *Mycobacterium intracellulare–avium* complex. Clinical features and course in 100 consecutive cases. Chest 1979; 75:115–119.
65. Barnard M, Hawkins E, Bass J. Pulmonary disease due to *Mycobacterium avium–intracellulare* in Alabama 1970–1980. Am Rev Respir Dis 1984; 129: A187.
66. Etzkorn E, Aldarondo S, McAllister C, et al. Medical therapy of *Mycobacterium avium–intracellulare* pulmonary disease. Am Rev Respir Dis 1986; 134:442–445.

4

Clinical Disease in Human Immunodeficiency Virus–Infected Persons

WILLIAM J. BURMAN

University of Colorado Health Sciences
Center
Denver, Colorado

DAVID L. COHN

Denver Health and Hospitals and
University of Colorado Health Sciences
Center
Denver, Colorado

I. Introduction

Disseminated *Mycobacterium avium*–complex infection (DMAC) was noted as an opportunistic infection in the first series of patients in 1981 with the newly described acquired immunodeficiency syndrome (AIDS); one patient died of a progressive febrile illness, DMAC (1). Since then DMAC has become one of the most common opportunistic infections in AIDS (2,3). The numbers of cases of DMAC have increased dramatically, in part due to the increased numbers of patients with AIDS. In addition, owing to the success of prophylaxis and treatment of other opportunistic illnesses, DMAC has assumed an even greater role as a pathogen in late-stage AIDS (4). The efficacy of treatment was unclear in early studies of DMAC (5), but with more potent, multidrug regimens, there is increasing evidence that therapy improves symptoms (6) and prolongs survival (7,8). The introduction of the macrolide antibiotics may improve the prognosis of patients with DMAC even more (9,10). Therefore, the recognition and diagnosis of DMAC have become very important issues for the clinician caring for individuals with AIDS.

II. Pathogenesis and Pathology of DMAC

Mycobacterium avium complex (MAC) is a common environmental organism (11). The likely portals of entry for these organisms are the gastrointestinal and respiratory tracts. Of the many strains of MAC in the environment, only a limited number have been found in patients with DMAC (12). Strains that cause disseminated disease in AIDS have the capacity to bind and penetrate epithelial cells (13). In animal models, organisms which penetrate the mucosa are quickly phagocytosed by submucosal macrophages (14). In immunocom-

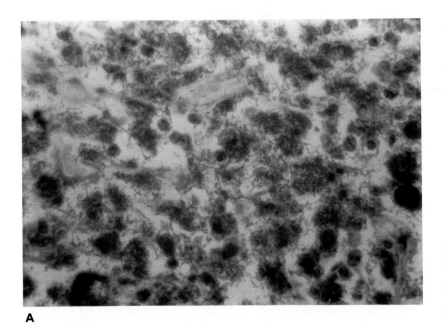

A

Figure 1 A, Abundant intracellular mycobacteria in an intraabdominal lymph node of a patient with disseminated MAC at autopsy. The tissue is stained with Ziehl-Nielsen and mycobacteria appear as dark-staining masses which nearly obliterate details of cellular architecure (400×). B, Gross appearance of the enlarged mesenteric lymph nodes.

petent hosts, the infection is probably contained in the wall of the gut or respiratory tract by a cellular immune response.

In late-stage AIDS, the ability to contain intracellular organisms is severely impaired. This is reflected in the histopathology of DMAC in AIDS. Rather than the well-formed granulomata with scant numbers of visible organisms that characterize the histopathology of mycobacterial infections in immunocompetent individuals, in patients with DMAC granulomata are poorly formed or even absent, and acid-fast bacilli are abundant (15) (Fig. 1A). In some patients, the load of mycobacteria is so great that enlarged nodes are largely composed of the accumulated organisms (Fig. 1B).

The pathology of autopsy cases of DMAC is characterized by prominent involvement of intra-abdominal and, to a lesser extent, intrathoracic lymph nodes (16,17). This suggests that in AIDS, owing to the inability to mount an effective cellular immune response, MAC infection spreads to regional lymph nodes and then to the bloodstream. Localized MAC infection of the gastrointestinal or respiratory tract is seldom recognized in patients with AIDS. For example, some patients with DMAC have an enteritis pre-

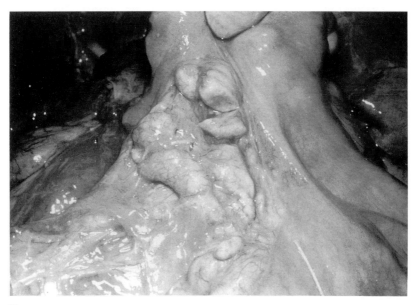

B

sentation with abdominal pain and diarrhea. Endoscopic biopsies in such patients often show prominent infiltration of the duodenal (18–22) or rectal (23) mucosa with MAC, suggesting a primary infection of the gastrointestinal tract. However, almost all patients with this clinical syndrome have positive blood cultures (18–23), demonstrating that dissemination occurs early in the course of infection in patients with AIDS. This is corroborated by two recent autopsy series which showed that MAC bacteremia can occur without identifiable established tissue infection (24,25).

The reticuloendothelial system is one of the major defense mechanisms in bacteremia. Therefore, it is not surprising that the liver and spleen are very commonly involved in DMAC (16,17). There may be marked enlargement of the liver and spleen with macroscopic miliary granulomata (Fig. 2). The bone marrow is almost always culture positive in later stages of DMAC, but prominent histopathological involvement is unusual (17). Acid-fast bacilli are

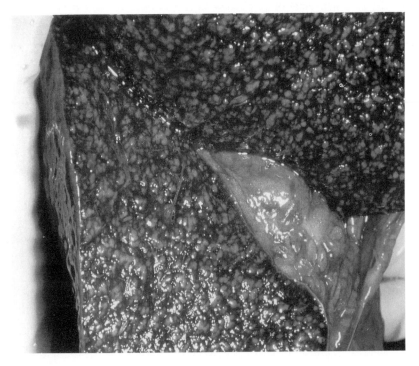

Figure 2   Macroscopic miliary granulomata in the spleen of a patient with disseminated MAC at autopsy.

visible in the lungs in a minority of patients at autopsy, but in contrast to MAC disease in immunocompetent patients, significant pulmonary pathology is almost always due to an alternative coexisting disease (17). Similarly, minor involvement of the central nervous system has been seen at autopsy in a few patients with widely disseminated disease (16), but it is doubtful that DMAC causes clinically significant neurological disease.

Early reports suggested that once established bacteremia with MAC was constant (26,27). However, this suggestion was based on relatively few cases and further studies have shown that MAC bacteremia can be intermittent. Two DMAC treatment trials required two successive positive blood cultures prior to enrollment; 7 of 60 patients had two negative blood cultures following an initial positive culture (28). The natural history of patients with transient MAC bacteremia is still being defined, but one report suggests that such patients have fewer symptoms and laboratory abnormalities referable to DMAC and that they survive longer than patients with sustained MAC bacteremia (28). Most of these patients eventually had a recurrence of MAC bacteremia (28), suggesting that such patients were detected earlier in the course of MAC infection (Fig. 3).

III. Clinical Presentation of DMAC in AIDS

A. Common Presenting Features of DMAC

In an early review article, Young et al. (29) summarized the most common clinical presentation of DMAC, ''. . . high fever, often associated with drenching night sweats, in a setting of progressive inanition, progressive weakness, diarrhea, and overall clinical deterioration.'' Although subsequent studies have not contradicted this classic description of DMAC, they have shown that with increasing awareness of this infection fewer patients have this degree of illness at the time of diagnosis. Formulating an accurate picture of the clinical presentation of this illness has been complicated by the overrepresentation of severe cases in the published literature, the nonspecificity of the symptoms and signs of DMAC, and the significant incidence of concurrent opportunistic infections. The array of symptoms and signs associated with the clinical presentation of DMAC is shown in Table 1.

Two factors have led to the overrepresentation of severe cases of DMAC in the literature. The clinical presentation is described in greatest detail in early reports of this syndrome (30–33). However, owing to the lack of familiarity with the disease and its most valuable diagnostic test, mycobacterial blood culture, these reports were biased toward the severe end of

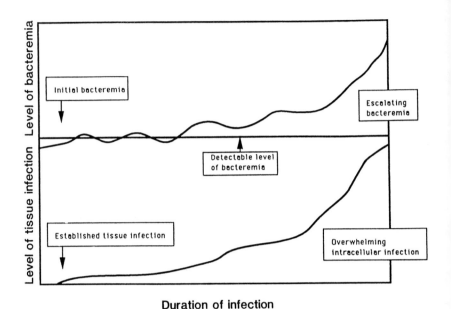

Figure 3 Schematic representation of the proposed pathogenesis of disseminated MAC, with initial transient bacteremia, followed by an increasing tissue burden of infection and continuous bacteremia. (From Ref. 123, with permission.)

the disease spectrum. Supporting evidence is that most patients in early reports had fever, often for weeks to months, before the diagnosis of DMAC (30–33). A much different picture comes from a recently completed rifabutin prophylaxis trial (34). Patients in this study had monthly mycobacterial blood cultures regardless of symptoms. Of the 102 patients in the placebo arm of this trial who developed DMAC, only 51% reported significant fever prior to the diagnosis of DMAC. In addition, the median number of days of fever before the positive blood culture was just 2 days. Another common, but problematic, source of data on the clinical presentation of DMAC has been patients entered into clinical trials of DMAC treatment (35–40). Two studies of DMAC therapy required two consecutive positive blood cultures to be eligible for enrollment (39,40). Then, symptoms recorded at the time of enrollment into the study represent the symptoms of DMAC that have been untreated for a significant period of time (at least long enough for two suc-

Table 1 Clinical Presentation of DMAC in AIDS

Common
fever
anemia
night sweats
weight loss
abdominal pain
diarrhea
elevated alkaline phosphatase
hepatosplenomegaly
Unusual
pulmonary disease
peripheral lymphadenopathy
acalculous cholecystitis
cutaneous lesions
Rare
osteomyelitis/septic arthritis
pyomyositis
sepsis syndrome/metabolic acidosis
pleural/pericardial disease
central nervous system disease

Source: Refs. 43–58.

cessive blood cultures to grow) rather than the symptoms that were present at the time of the original evaluation.

Two additional problems complicate the attempt to formulate an accurate picture of the clinical presentation of DMAC—the nonspecificity of the common symptoms and the frequency of concurrent illnesses. Fever, night sweats, weight loss, and fatigue are common symptoms in a group of patients with late-stage AIDS. Havlik et al. (2) did a cross-sectional study of the association of symptoms and common laboratory tests with the presence of DMAC. Patients with AIDS, excluding those with known DMAC, completed an inventory of symptoms and had a mycobacterial blood culture and routine laboratory tests performed. Factors that were significantly associated with the presence of a positive blood culture for MAC were fever, weight loss, diarrhea, anemia (defined as a hematocrit <26), and an increased alkaline phosphatase (defined as >3 times normal). Interestingly enough, the factor with the best discriminating value was anemia.

Patients with severely depressed CD4 cell counts are predisposed to many infections and malignancies. It is not unusual to diagnose two or more opportunistic illnesses in a short period of time. For example, in our series of 227 patients with DMAC, 18% were diagnosed with another opportunistic infection within 2 weeks of the diagnosis of DMAC, and others had bacterial infections coincident with the diagnosis of DMAC (unpublished data). In such patients, it is difficult to discern the symptoms and laboratory abnormalities due to DMAC from those due to the concurrent infection.

A more complete description of the clinical presentation of DMAC is derived from prospective studies in which blood cultures are drawn regardless of symptoms (41). Also helpful are studies which report the presentation of all patients with DMAC, not a select group who were entered into a clinical trial (42). The data from these types of studies are only available in preliminary form, but the picture that emerges is that the classic symptoms of unrelenting fevers, drenching night sweats, and severe wasting probably represent relatively late manifestations of this infection. Earlier manifestations appear to be fatigue, a decline in functional status, anemia, and an elevation of alkaline phosphatase (34).

It is also important to recognize that patients with DMAC may have only a few of the associated symptoms, signs, and laboratory abnormalities. For example, patients may present with anemia and weight loss, yet have no fever or abdominal symptoms (43). Indeed, in a review of 116 consecutive cases of DMAC, Horsburgh et al. (42) found an inverse correlation between fever and anemia as manifestations of DMAC. In addition to the classic febrile illness, syndromes that may be caused by DMAC include intrahepatic cholestasis (44–46), acalculous cholecystitis (47), unexplained anemia (43), enteritis (23), and diffuse lymphadenopathy (48). It is unclear if these differences in clinical presentation are due to the stage in the illness at the time of diagnosis, differences in the host, or differences in the infecting strain of MAC.

B. Unusual Presenting Features of DMAC

Unusual manifestations of DMAC include endophthalmitis (49), cutaneous lesions (50,51), osteomyelitis and septic arthritis (52), cavitary lung disease (53), and a destructive oral lesion (54). Infrequently, MAC involvement of lymph nodes (38) or the spleen (55) results in the formation of an abscess. Abdominal pain is a common symptom of DMAC; occasionally, the presentation is of sufficient severity to result in laparotomy (56,57). MAC has been isolated from the cerebrospinal fluid of patients with disseminated disease

(58), although it is unclear whether this represents significant infection of the central nervous system. The isolation of MAC from the cerebrospinal fluid of a patient with central nervous system disease is evidence of DMAC, but a concomitant pathogen is a more likely cause of meningitis or brain abscess. This is in contrast to more the virulent mycobacteria, *M. tuberculosis* (59) and *M. kansasii* (60,61), which clearly cause severe infections of the central nervous system in patients with AIDS. Recently, there have been case reports of DMAC presenting as a severe sepsis syndrome with metabolic acidosis (62). Owing to the broad spectrum of antimicrobial agents given to these patients, it is possible though that the sepsis syndrome was due to a bacterial infection which was treated but not detected by blood culture. Further complicating the interpretation of this report is that severe metabolic acidosis has been reported in patients with AIDS without an identifiable infection (63). If DMAC can cause sepsis and metabolic acidosis in AIDS, it is much less common than sepsis due to pyogenic bacteria, fungi (histoplasmosis, blastomycosis), and tuberculosis (64).

C. Localized MAC Infection in AIDS

Though MAC infection in AIDS is usually disseminated at the time of diagnosis, localized forms of the disease have been recognized. Skin and soft tissue involvement can present as localized lymphadenopathy (65), pyomyositis (66), or as subcutaneous abscesses, sometimes with a sporotrichoid distribution (67). However, these cutaneous presentations are more common with other mycobacterial infections such as *M. haemophilum* (68) or *M. marinum* (69). Localized lymphadenopathy is much more common in tuberculosis (70), and empiric treatment of AFB-positive adenopathy should be directed at *M. tuberculosis* rather than MAC. Histologically, the localized lymphadenopathy may mimic a spindle cell tumor (48), causing diagnostic confusion. Endobronchial lesions adjacent to enlarged mediastinal or hilar nodes can occur in the absence of systemic disease (71). The interpretation of pulmonary parenchymal lesions (infiltrates, nodules, or cavities) in the setting of a positive sputum culture for MAC is difficult. Our experience, and the limited information in the literature (17,72), is that parenchymal lesions are much more likely to be due to a concomitant infection or malignancy than MAC. It is not clear whether MAC can cause symptomatic enteritis in the absence of disseminated disease; nearly all of the reported cases had positive blood or bone marrow cultures at the time of diagnosis of MAC enteritis (18–23).

IV. Laboratory Manifestations of DMAC

A. Blood Tests

The population of patients at risk for DMAC is also at risk for many other complications of AIDS. Furthermore, laboratory abnormalities, such as lymphopenia, mild anemia, or moderate elevations of lactate dehydrogenase (LDH), are common in patients with late-stage AIDS even in the absence of an opportunistic infection or malignancy. However, two laboratory abnormalities, moderate to severe anemia and an elevated serum alkaline phosphatase, are associated with DMAC and may be helpful in suggesting this diagnosis. In addition, these two abnormalities offer some insight into the pathogenesis of this infection.

Anemia

Though anemia was seldom mentioned in early reports of DMAC, it is a prominent manifestation of this infection. In 1988, Gardener et al. (43) reported eight cases of DMAC, all of whom had a hemoglobin level of less than 10 g/dl. More recent reports have confirmed the association of anemia and DMAC. In the study by Horsburgh et al. (42) of consecutive DMAC cases, 76% had a hematocrit <26 at the time of diagnosis of DMAC, making anemia second only to fever as a manifestation of this infection. In their cross-sectional study, Havlik et al. (2) demonstrated the specificity of the association of anemia with DMAC; 9 of 15 DMAC patients had a hematocrit <26, although only 4 of 50 controls with CD4 cell counts <100/mm^3 had anemia of this magnitude. The data from the placebo arm of the rifabutin prophylaxis trial offer the clearest evidence of the association of anemia and DMAC (34). Of the 102 patients in the placebo arm who developed DMAC, 67% had a decrease in hemoglobin of 10% or greater. In contrast, a decrease in hemoglobin of this degree was much less common in patients who did not develop DMAC. In addition, anemia may be a valuable early sign of DMAC. Anemia preceded the positive blood culture for MAC in most patients (61 of 69), and the median time from the decrease in hemoglobin to the diagnosis of DMAC was 53 days (34).

A study of red blood cell transfusion in patients with AIDS provides further support for the association of DMAC and anemia (73). DMAC was the most common factor in those requiring transfusion. The relative risk for transfusion associated with a positive blood culture for MAC was 5.2 compared with a control group of patients with AIDS with negative mycobacterial blood cultures. The association of anemia with DMAC is strong enough that it has become our practice to do mycobacterial blood cultures on patients with AIDS who develop unexplained anemia (hematocrit <26) whether or not there are symptoms of DMAC.

The effect of DMAC on the bone marrow appears to be relatively selective for the erythroid line and not simply due to dense infiltration of the marrow by the organism. The bone marrow in patients with DMAC is generally normo- or hypercellular rather than aplastic (43). Although lymphopenia is almost universal and thrombocytopenia is common in patients with DMAC, these changes appear to be due to late-stage AIDS and are not specifically associated with DMAC (74). Studies of bone marrow biopsies of patients with DMAC support the clinical evidence of the selective effect of DMAC on the erythroid line. Gardiner et al. (43) reported marked hypoplasia of the erythroid series in 5 of 5 patients with DMAC as compared with 3 of 19 bone marrow examinations on patients with AIDS without DMAC. Gascon et al. (75) extended these histological observations by demonstrating a marked decrease in erythroid precursor growth in cell culture of the bone marrow in patients with DMAC when compared with samples from normal individuals and patients with AIDS without DMAC. Furthermore, they demonstrated that a soluble factor released from MAC-infected macrophages inhibited in vitro growth of erythroid precursors from the control groups. Therefore, it appears that the anemia of DMAC (and possibly other intracellular pathogens) is due to the elaboration of a specific inhibitor of erythroid precursors (as yet unidentified) from infected macrophages.

The initial studies of the anemia of DMAC did not find an improvement in the severity of anemia with treatment (74). It has been our impression though that the use of a clarithromycin-containing regimen has been associated with a significant decrease in the transfusion requirements of patients with DMAC in our clinic. The response of anemia to treatment in a recent patient is shown in Figure 4.

Elevated Alkaline Phosphatase

Elevation in alkaline phosphatase is the other laboratory manifestation which is associated with DMAC. In Havlik's study (2), 4 of 14 patients with DMAC had an alkaline phosphatase >3 times normal as opposed to 0 of 50 in the control group. Gordin et al. (34) noted a 50% increase in alkaline phosphatase in 53% of patients developing DMAC in the placebo arm of rifabutin prophylaxis study. The elevation in alkaline phosphatase may be a later manifestation of DMAC than anemia; in almost one third of the patients, the increase occurred after the diagnosis of DMAC (34). Although other oppor-

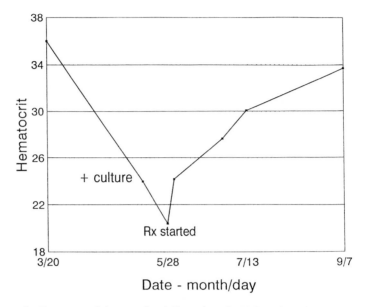

Figure 4   Response of the anemia of disseminated MAC to therapy with clarithromycin, clofazimine, and ethambutol.

tunistic infections and malignancies can cause marked elevations in alkaline
phosphatase, DMAC appears to be one of the most common causes (76).
The alkaline phosphatase appears to be of hepatobiliary origin in that it is
usually associated with an elevated gamma glutamyl transferase (GGT) level.
In addition, one autopsy series noted a close correlation between elevations
of alkaline phosphatase and hepatomegaly (45). The elevated alkaline phosphatase is most likely due to intrahepatic cholestasis from granulomata
containing MAC. DMAC also appears to cause inflammation of the gallbladder in some patients, resulting in the clinical syndrome of acalculous
cholecystitis (47).

B. Radiographic Manifestations

The most common radiographic manifestations of DMAC are the demonstration of hepatomegaly, splenomegaly, and intra-abdominal adenopathy by
computed tomography (CT) (77) or ultrasound (78). Although these tests
have not been performed systematically in a series of patients with DMAC,
abnormalities on abdominal CT appear to be very common. Nyberg et al.

(77) reviewed abdominal CT scans on 17 patients with DMAC (of 31 patients diagnosed with DMAC during the time period of the study). Splenomegaly and an increased number of visible intra-abdominal lymph nodes were seen in all 17 cases; in 82% of the cases, the nodes were enlarged as well. Both retroperitoneal and mesenteric adenopathy occurred; individual patients may have a marked preponderance of involvement in one area. Areas of focal attenuation, suggesting necrosis, can be seen in the liver, spleen, and enlarged lymph nodes of patients with DMAC (79,80), although this occurs much more often in disseminated tuberculosis (79). Hepatomegaly is common; occasionally, the liver is markedly enlarged (77). Thickening of the bowel wall may also be seen on CT of the abdomen (79). None of these findings are specific to DMAC, being seen in patients with other disseminated mycobacterial and fungal infections and in intra-abdominal malignancies. The chest radiograph is often abnormal in patients with DMAC, although in the majority of cases, a concomitant pulmonary infection or malignancy is responsible for the changes (17,72). A finding that can be due to DMAC is intrathoracic adenopathy (72) (Fig. 5). Pulmonary parenchymal lesions (infiltrates,

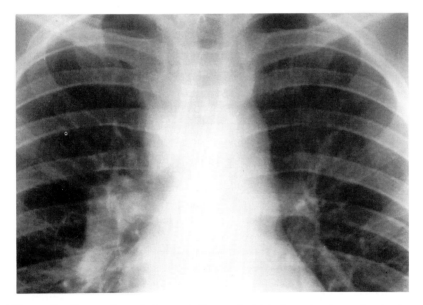

Figure 5 Chest radiograph demonstrating marked intrathoracic adenopathy due to disseminated MAC. Blood cultures were positive for MAC and the enlarged nodes became smaller with therapy.

nodules, or cavities) or are unlikely to be due to DMAC (17,72), and if such lesions are present, our practice is to proceed with an evaluation and not ascribe them to DMAC.

As mentioned previously, there is a subset of patients with DMAC who have prominent gastrointestinal manifestations. Upper gastrointestinal radiography in such patients may show thickening of the mucosal folds of the small bowel (20). Some of these patients have a distinctive endoscopic appearance as well, with small white nodules in the duodenum (21,22).

V. Diagnosis

With improvements in culture techniques, mycobacterial blood culture has become a sensitive diagnostic test for DMAC. There are occasional patients in whom blood cultures are negative, but liver or bone marrow biopsy specimens are positive. Of 12 prospectively studied patients with fevers despite a routine evaluation, 8 had mycobacterial infections diagnosed after a standard evaluation of liver and bone marrow biopsy and mycobacterial blood culture; 6 of the 8 infections were detected by blood culture (81). Autopsy series also indicate the sensitivity of blood culture. In the largest study, of those who had appropriate premortem cultures, the blood culture was positive in 86% of patients diagnosed with DMAC (5).

A number of blood culture systems are sensitive in detecting mycobacteremia (82). Features common to these systems are lysis of blood cells and culturing the lysed material on solid media or in a liquid broth with radiometric detection of growth. The two most commonly used systems have been the Bactec* (Becton-Dickinson Diagnostic Instrument Systems, Sparks, MD) (liquid medium with radiometric detection) and the Wampole Isolator* (Wampole Laboratories, Cranbury, NJ) (lysis/centrifugation). In comparative studies, neither system is ideal; in the largest such study 63 of 72 positive cultures were positive in both systems, 5 were detected in Bactec alone, and 4 by the Isolator system alone (83). We use the Bactec system and also culture a portion of the lysed material on solid media (Middlebrook 711/Mitchison bi-plates and Lowenstein-Jensen slants). In 197 cases of DMAC diagnosed with this system, 24 (12%) were negative in the Bactec, yet positive on solid media, illustrating the advantages of using two culture methods (W.J. Burman and D.L. Cohn, unpublished data). The Bactec system involves less specimen manipulation than the Wampole Isolator and detects growth more quickly

---

*Bactec and Isolator are registered trademarks.

(83). The Wampole Isolator allows quantitation of mycobacteremia, which appears to have prognostic significance (42).

A single blood culture is very sensitive, detecting 88–91% (84) of cases which were detected by paired blood cultures. Discordant results occur in patients with low colony counts; that is, those with early disease (84). Therefore, a single blood culture is adequate; this may be repeated if the initial culture is negative and the patient is still symptomatic. In patients with very high-grade infection, organisms can be seen on an acid-fast stain of a blood smear. However, in a prospective study, only 4% of patients who were culture positive had positive blood smears (84). Therefore, it is difficult to recommend routine acid-fast staining and examination of blood smears in patients suspected of having DMAC.

VI. Significance of MAC Isolation from Nonsterile Sites and the Value of Screening Cultures

The pathogenesis of DMAC is thought to involve local infection in the respiratory tract or gut followed by dissemination. Therefore, isolation of MAC from one of these sites might represent the early stages of this process or be evidence of infection which has already disseminated. As a result, some have argued that the isolation of MAC from a nonsterile site should be treated as evidence of infection regardless of blood culture results. In a small, nonrandomized study, patients with positive sputum or stool cultures for MAC were treated with a multidrug regimen (36). None developed disseminated disease, suggesting that treatment of local infection in the gut or respiratory tract prevents disseminated disease.

Routine cultures of sputum and stool might be used to screen patients for early, localized disease. However, MAC can transiently colonize the respiratory tract or gut. Many positive cultures for MAC in immunocompetent individuals appear to represent colonization rather than infection (86). Even in severely immunocompromised patients, that is, those with AIDS and less CD4 cell counts <50 mm^3, it appears that MAC can transiently colonize the respiratory tract (86). Furthermore, the rates of adverse side effects of multidrug therapy of MAC are significant, leading others to advocate that positive cultures for MAC from nonsterile sites should be ignored (87).

Two recently completed prospective studies address this controversy. Chin et al. (88) studied patients with CD4 cells counts <50 mm^3 who had mycobacterial blood cultures obtained. Blood culture–negative patients were followed prospectively, with repeat sputum, stool, and blood cultures at 3-

month intervals. The incidence of DMAC in this population was high: 44% per year. Patients with a previous sputum or stool MAC isolate had an even higher incidence: 61 and 58%, respectively. In a Cox regression analysis, the relative hazard for developing DMAC associated with a positive sputum culture or stool culture was 2.3 and 6.0, respectively. This is strong evidence that a positive culture for MAC from a nonsterile site is a marker for a higher risk of progression to DMAC in a population of patients with late-stage AIDS. However, most patients who developed DMAC did not have a preceding positive sputum or stool culture; the sensitivity of a positive culture from either site was only 33%. Furthermore, the population studied was at very high risk for DMAC. It is very likely that the positive predictive value of a positive culture from a nonsterile site, 55% in this study, would be significantly lower in patients with higher CD4 cell counts. Havlik et al. (86) did a very similar study in patients at lower risk for DMAC—those with CD4 cell counts <200. They confirmed the poor sensitivity of screening sputum and stool cultures; 79% of patients who developed DMAC had negative screening cultures. In addition, the interval from a positive screening culture to the development of DMAC could be long: up to 8 months (86).

How should the results of these studies affect clinical practice? The clear result of both studies is that screening cultures of sputum and stool are insensitive ways to detect the patient at high risk for developing DMAC. In addition, although neither of these studies included a cost analysis, the cost of routine screening mycobacterial cultures would be significant. The existing data argue strongly that sputum and/or stool cultures not be used to screen for DMAC.

The more common situation is the patient who has positive sputum or stool cultures in tests done as part of the evaluation of an illness for which another cause was eventually found; for example, the patient who has a positive sputum culture for MAC found during bronchoscopy for diagnosis of *Pneumocystis carinii* pneumonia. This finding should prompt a clinical evaluation for the possibility that the patient might have concurrent DMAC. Many patients with a positive blood culture have simultaneous positive sputum or stool cultures (86). In these patients, the positive sputum or stool culture can be viewed as a sign of disseminated infection. Thus, a patient who has a positive stool or sputum culture for MAC should be evaluated for signs or symptoms compatible with DMAC. Those with a low CD4 cell count and any signs of clinical deterioration should have a mycobacterial blood culture. On the other hand, those with a higher CD4 cell count or lack of symptoms probably need no further evaluation.

The management of the late-stage patient who has MAC in sputum or stool culture, but a negative blood culture, remains controversial. The recent demonstration of the efficacy of DMAC prophylaxis (41) further complicates the issue. Should such patients be placed on prophylaxis? If so, will a single medication be sufficient in a patient who already has MAC colonization or local infection? These patients blur the line between prophylaxis and treatment. At present, in the absence of proven benefit of antimycobacterial therapy in this situation, and recognizing that multidrug regimens are associated with a significant incidence of adverse side effects and that colonization may precede DMAC by a considerable length of time (86), we consider such patients candidates for prophylaxis, but we do not start standard multidrug antimycobacterial therapy.

An alternative screening procedure is the use of blood cultures in high-risk individuals. Rather than attempt to detect localized MAC infection, screening blood cultures would allow early diagnosis of disseminated disease. A nonrandomized study reported the yield of monthly blood cultures in all patients with AIDS (3). The risk of DMAC was highly dependent on CD4 cell count, but the overall yield of screening blood cultures for MAC in patients without symptoms associated with DMAC was 1%. Whether patients respond better to therapy when the infection is detected earlier is unknown. Antimycobacterial therapy may be more effective when applied to a lower burden of organisms (42). On the other hand, compliance with a multidrug regimen may be lower in a group of patients who are minimally symptomatic (89). No cost analysis was included in this study, but with the cost of detecting DMAC in the short interval between initial bacteremia and the development of symptoms may be quite high. Furthermore, if MAC prophylaxis comes into widespread use, the yield of screening blood cultures will be even lower, particularly if the macrolides prove to be a more effective form of prophylaxis than rifabutin. At this time, the strategy of screening blood cultures for DMAC does not appear to be warranted in clinical practice (90).

VII. Differential Diagnosis of DMAC and Disseminated Infection with Other Mycobacteria

A. Tuberculosis

Although this review has concentrated on DMAC, in many parts of the world the most common mycobacterial disease in HIV-infected individuals is tuberculosis (91). The clinical distinction of MAC disease and tuberculosis is crucial, since the public health implications and therapeutic approach to the two infections are so different. In the early stages of HIV infection, tuberculosis presents much as it does in immunocompetent hosts, with localized pulmonary, pleural, or nodal involvement (92); DMAC is seldom in the differential diagnosis of such patients.

In late-stage HIV infection, tuberculosis frequently presents as a disseminated disease (64). However, there are clinical features, summarized in Table 2, that can help distinguish disseminated tuberculosis from DMAC. In general, disseminated tuberculosis is a more severe, rapidly progressive disease than DMAC. Even when disseminated, tuberculosis often has pulmonary involvement (64,70). Cavitary lesions are uncommon, but localized pneumonitis or miliary disease should suggest tuberculosis in the patient with a sputum smear positive for acid-fast bacilli. Pleural and/or pericardial involvement appear to be relatively common manifestations of tuberculosis at all stages of HIV infection (64), whereas they are rarely seen in DMAC. Adenopathy is common in both tuberculosis and DMAC, but features that suggest tuberculosis include large, asymmetrical peripheral lymph nodes (70) and necrotic or abscessed nodes (79). Involvement of the central nervous system, with meningitis or brain abscesses, is common in tuberculosis in AIDS (59,64) but is not a feature of DMAC. These clinical features are often sufficient to guide empiric therapy while awaiting the results of definitive laboratory identification of the involved mycobacterial species. Given the increased virulence and infectiousness of tuberculosis, if there is uncertainty based on the clinical presentation, it is best to use antimicrobial agents specifically directed at *M. tuberculosis*.

B. Other Mycobacteria

Approximately 95% of the disease due to nontuberculous mycobacteria in AIDS is caused by MAC (93). Other mycobacteria though can cause severe disease and may be important in different geographical regions. There are

Table 2 Potential Distinguishing Characteristics of Clinical Presentations of DMAC and Tuberculosis in AIDS

	DMAC	Tuberculosis
Radiographic pulmonary involvement	Unusual	Common
Sputum AFB-smear positive	Unusual	Common
Pleural/pericardial involvement	Rare	Common
Central nervous system involvement	Rare, if at all	Common
Localized adenopathy	Unusual	Common
Necrosis in nodes, liver, or spleen	Unusual	Common

Source: Refs. 71 and 80.

many similarities in the clinical presentation of MAC disease and other my-cobacterial infections in AIDS. Most of these species (*M. kansasii, M. gen-avense, M. fortuitum, M. haemophilum, M. xenopi, M. simiae,* and *M. gor-donae*) can cause disseminated disease characterized by hepatosplenomegaly and intra-abdominal adenopathy. However, there can be aspects of the clinical presentation which suggest a particular mycobacterial species. These differences can be very helpful in guiding empiric therapy and suggesting the need for special culture techniques or laboratory procedures (Table 3).

Geographical differences appear to affect the array and relative importance of various nontuberculous, non-MAC mycobacteria in causing disease in individuals with AIDS. In areas of the southern and central United States, *M. kansasii* is relatively common (94), whereas in Colorado, *M. genavense* was more common than *M. kansasii* (95). *M. xenopi* appears to be more common in Europe (96,97) and *M. simiae* has been reported most often from Israel (98) and Africa (99,100). Most cases of *M. haemophilum* have been reported from New York (68). There is little doubt that other species of mycobacteria will be found to cause disease in patients with AIDS as diagnostic tests improve and the HIV epidemic spreads around the world.

M. kansasii appears to be intermediate between *M. tuberculosis* and MAC in its inherent pathogenicity and clinical manifestations. Patients with HIV and *M. kansasii* infection usually have AIDS, although CD4 cell counts are not as uniformly low as in patients with DMAC (101). Pulmonary involvement is common and many patients have radiographic features that suggest mycobacterial infection—upper zone involvement and the presence of

Table 3 Clinical Features of Other Nontuberculous Mycobacterial Infections in AIDS

Organism	Stage of HIV	Common, sites	Special procedures
M. kansasii	CD4 < 200	Lung, pleura, central nervous system, disseminated	None
M. genavense	CD4 < 50	Intraabdominal nodes, liver, disseminated	Slow growth in broth, identification by gene probe
M. haemophilum	CD4 < 200	Skin, joints, bone	Incubate at 32 degrees, iron-supplemented medium

Source: Refs. 61, 62, 69, 95, 96, and 102–113.

cavities (101). In late-stage HIV infection, *M. kansasii* infection is often disseminated, although like tuberculosis, pulmonary involvement remains common, often with diffuse infiltrates (102). Pleural disease (103) and central nervous system involvement (60,61) are other similarities with tuberculosis. Coinfection with *M. kansasii* and MAC has been reported (94); one patient had a positive blood culture for MAC and a brain abscess due to *M. kansasii* (104), illustrating the differences in the pathogenicity of these two organisms.

M. genavense was initially described in a patient with AIDS who had fever and wasting (105). Multiple biopsy specimens showed acid-fast bacilli, but a very slowly growing mycobacterium was only found in liquid culture, and could not be subcultured on solid media. Since then, 33 additional cases have been reported (95,106–109). Nearly all of these cases presented with an illness much like DMAC, with fever, diarrhea, and wasting. Imaging studies have shown prominent enlargement of intra-abdominal lymph nodes, liver, and spleen (95). The organism grows slowly in the Bactec System; the median time to detectable growth in one series was 42 days (95), and the growth index may be lower than usually considered positive (95). The microbiology laboratory should be notified if *M. genavense* is suspected so that cultures can be held longer and bottles with a borderline growth index can be further evaluated. The definitive identification is by polymerase chain reaction of the 16S rRNA gene (106). The incidence of *M. genavense* infection is not clear; given the difficulties in culturing this organism, it is very likely that cases have been missed. In our clinic, this organism caused 4% of disseminated nontuberculous mycobacterial infections, which is second only to MAC (95).

M. haemophilum is associated with a relatively specific clinical syndrome in individuals with late-stage HIV infection. This organism almost always involves the skin, soft tissues, joints, and/or bone (68,110–112). Ulcerating or nodular skin lesions, often with tenosynovitis or arthritis, are the most common presenting features. In addition, there is often radiographic evidence of osteomyelitis in association with arthritis or skin lesions (68,110). Unusual manifestations that have been reported include intra-abdominal adenopathy (110) and progressive pulmonary infiltrates (68) without skin lesions. This organism also can be difficult to culture in that it requires iron-supplemented media and grows best at 32°C (112) (probably explaining its predilection for the skin and soft tissues of the extremities). *M. marinum*, another organism with a low optimal growth temperature, can cause lesions very similar to *M. haemophilum* (69). Finally, *M. ulcerans*, an organism which is common in west Africa and is closely related to *M. marinum*, has recently been reported to cause a nodular cutaneous infection in a patient with HIV infection (113). In all three cases, the laboratory needs to be notified so that specific media and incubation temperatures are used. *M. fortuitum* also appears to have a predilection for involving the skin and soft tissues (114).

Infection with *M. xenopi* (96,97,115,116), *M. gordonae* (117–119), *M. malmoense* (120), and *M. simiae* (98–100) have all been reported in patients with late-stage AIDS. Both disseminated disease, very similar to DMAC, and pulmonary disease have been described. These organisms do not require special conditions for successful culture and the most common clinical question is the significance of their isolation from a nonsterile site. *M. gordonae* is a common laboratory contaminant, but in a patient with AIDS with a compatible clinical syndrome, its isolation may indicate disease.

Mixed infections, in which two mycobacterial species grow from blood culture, also occur in this severely immunocompromised population (94,99,104). In fact, patients with DMAC can be bacteremic with several genetically distinct strains of MAC itself (121). Although the clinical significance of this phenomenon is not yet clear, it is possible that mixed infections may confound the interpretation of antimicrobial susceptibilities if only one of the infecting strains or species is tested.

VIII. Conclusions

DMAC is one of the most common opportunistic infections in patients with AIDS. Its presentation is generally subacute, with fever, abdominal pain, diarrhea, and weight loss. The findings of unexplained anemia and/or an increased alkaline phosphatase can also be helpful in suggesting DMAC. Characteristic radiographic findings are intra-abdominal or intrathoracic adenopathy, splenomegaly, and hepatomegaly. Diagnosis by blood culture is sensitive and relatively rapid. Other mycobacteria, both tuberculous and nontuberculous, can cause similar syndromes. The presence of central nervous system or serosal involvement or necrotic lymphadenopathy suggests tuberculosis or *M. kansasii*. Skin, soft tissue, and/or bone involvement suggest *M. haemophilum* or *M. marinum*. Smear-positive but culture-negative disseminated disease suggests *M. genavense*. Recognition of these clinical manifestations of disseminated mycobacterial infections in HIV-infected persons may lead to prompt diagnosis and potentially effective therapeutic interventions.

References

1. Masur H, Michelis MA, Greene JB, et al. An outbreak of community-acquired Pneumocystis carinii pneumonia: Initial manifestation of cellular immune dysfunction. N Engl J Med 1981; 305:1431–1438.

2. Havlik JA Jr, Horsburgh CR Jr, Metchock B, et al. Disseminated *Mycobacterium avium* complex infection: Clinical identification and epidemiologic trends. J Infect Dis 1992; 165:577–580.
3. Nightingale SD, Byrd LT, Southern PM, et al. Incidence of *Mycobacterium avium–intracellulare* complex bacteremia in human immunodeficiency virus–positive patients. J Infect Dis 1992; 165:1082–1085.
4. Hoover DR, Saah AJ, Bacellar H, et al. Clinical manifestations of AIDS in the era of Pneumocystis prophylaxis. N Engl J Med 1993; 329:1922–1926.
5. Hawkins CC, Gold JWM, Whimbey E, et al. *Mycobacterium avium* complex infections in patients with the acquired immunodeficiency syndrome. Ann Intern Med 1986; 105:184–188.
6. Jacobson MA, Yajko D, Northfelt D, et al. Randomized trial of rifampin, ethambutol, and ciprofloxacin for AIDS patients with disseminated *Mycobacterium avium* complex infection. J Infect Dis 1993; 168:112–119.
7. Horsburgh CR Jr, Havlik JA, Ellis DE, et al. Survival of patients with acquired immunodeficiency syndrome and disseminated *Mycobacterium avium* complex infection with and without antimycobacterial chemotherapy. Am Rev Respir Dis 1991; 144:557–559.
8. Kerlikowske KM, Katz MH, Chan AK, Perez-Stable EJ. Antimycobacterial therapy for disseminated *Mycobacterium avium* complex infection in patients with acquired immunodeficiency syndrome. Arch Intern Med 1992; 152:813–817.
9. Dautzenberg B, Truffot C, Legris S, et al. Activity of clarithromycin against *Mycobacterium avium* infection in patients with the acquired immune deficiency syndrome: A controlled clinical trial. Am Rev Respir Dis 1991; 144:564–569.
10. Young LS, Wiviott L, Wu M, et al. Azithromycin for treatment of *Mycobacterium avium–intracellulare* complex infection in patients with AIDS. Lancet 1991; 338:1107–1109.
11. Von Reyn CF, Waddell RD, Eaton T, et al. Isolation of *Mycobacterium avium* complex from water in the United States, Finland, Zaire, and Kenya. J Clin Microbiol 1993; 31:3227–3230.
12. Yakrus MA, Good RC. Geographic distribution, frequency, and specimen source of *Mycobacterium avium* complex serotypes isolated from patients with acquired immunodeficiency syndrome. J Clin Microbiol 1990; 28:926–929.
13. Bermudez LE, Young LS. *Mycobacterium avium* complex adherence to mucosal cells: a possible role of virulence. 29th Interscience Conference on Antimicrobial Agents and Chemotherapy, Washington, DC, 1989; abstract 247.
14. Bermudez LE, Petrovsky M, Kolonoski P, Young LS. An animal model of *Mycobacterium avium* complex disseminated infection after colonization of the intestinal tract. J Infect Dis 1992; 165:75–79.
15. Solis OG, Belmonte AH, Ramaswamy G, Tchertkoff V. Pseudogaucher cells in *Mycobacterium avium intracellulare* infections in acquired immune deficiency syndrome (AIDS). Am J Clin Pathol 1986; 85:233–235.

16. Klatt EC, Jensen DF, Meyer PR. Pathology of *Mycobacterium avium–intracellulare* infection in acquired immunodeficiency syndrome. Hum Pathol 1987; 18:709–714.

17. Wallace JM, Hannah JB. *Mycobacterium avium* complex infection in patients with the acquired immunodeficiency syndrome: A clinicopathologic study. Chest 1988; 93:926–931.

18. Strom RL, Gruninger RP. AIDS with *Mycobacterium avium–intracellulare* lesions resembling those of Whipple's disease (letter). N Engl J Med 1983; 309: 1323–1324.

19. Roth RI, Owen RL, Keren DF, Volberding PA. Intestinal infection with *Mycobacterium avium* in acquired immune deficiency syndrome (AIDS): Histological and clinical comparison with Whipple's disease. Dig Dis Sci 1985; 30: 497–504.

20. Vincent ME, Robbins AH. *Mycobacterium avium–intracellulare* complex enteritis; Pseudo-Whipple disease in AIDS. AJR 1985; 144:921–922.

21. Gray JR, Rabeneck L. Atypical mycobacterial infection of the gastrointestinal tract in AIDS patients. Am J Gastroenterol 1989; 84:1521–1524.

22. Monsour HP Jr, Quigley EMM, Markin RS, et al. Endoscopy in the diagnosis of gastrointestinal *Mycobacterium avium–intracellulare* infection. J Clin Gastroenterol 1991; 13:20–24.

23. Wolke A, Meyers S, Adelsberg BR, et al. *Mycobacterium avium–intracellulare*–associated colitis in a patient with the acquired immunodeficiency syndrome. J Clin Gastroenterol 1984; 6:225–229.

24. Torriani FJ, McCutchan JA, Bozette SA, et al. Autopsy findings in AIDS patients with *Mycobacterium avium* complex bacteremia. J Infect Dis 1994; 170: 1601–1605.

25. Hoika R, Brodt HR, Keul HG, et al. Clinical and post-mortem findings of MAC infection in 292 autopsied AIDS patients. 9th International Conference on AIDS, Berlin, 1993; abstract PO-B07-1253.

26. Macher AM, Kovacs JA, Gill V, et al. Bacteremia due to *Mycobacterium avium–intracellulare* in the acquired immunodeficiency syndrome. Ann Intern Med 1983; 99:782–785.

27. Wong B, Edwards FF, Keihn TE, et al. Continuous high-grade *Mycobacterium avium–intracellulare* bacteremia in patients with the acquired immunodeficiency syndrome. Am J Med 1985; 78:35–40.

28. Kemper C, Havlir D, Bartok AE, et al. Transient bacteremia due to *Mycobacterium avium* complex in patients with AIDS. Frontiers in Mycobacteriology, Vail, CO, 1992; abstract 17.

29. Young LS, Interlied CB, Berlin OG, Gottlieb MS. Mycobacterial infections in AIDS patients, with an emphasis on the *Mycobacterium avium* complex. Rev Infect Dis 1986; 8:1024–1033.

30. Greene JB, Sidhu GS, Lewin S, et al. *Mycobacterium avium–intracellulare*: A cause of disseminated life-threatening infection in homosexuals and drug abusers. Ann Intern Med 1982; 97:539–546.

31. Sohn CC, Schroff RW, Kliewer KE, et al. Disseminated *Mycobacterium avium–intracellulare* infection in homosexual men with acquired cell-mediated immunodeficiency: A histologic and immunologic study of two cases. Am J Clin Pathol 1983; 79:247–252.

32. Polis MA, Tuazon CU. Clues to the early diagnosis of *Mycobacterium avium–intracellulare* infection in patients with acquired immunodeficiency syndrome. Arch Pathol Lab Med 1985; 109:465–466.

33. Elliot JL, Hoppes WL, Platt MS, et al. The acquired immunodeficiency syndrome and *Mycobacterium avium–intracellulare* bacteremia in a patient with hemophilia. Ann Intern Med 1983; 98:290–293.

34. Gordin F, Cohn D, Sullam P, et al. The occurrence of *Mycobacterium avium* complex (MAC) bacteremia in a standardized cohort of AIDS patients. 33rd Interscience Conference on Antimicrobial Agents and Chemotherapy, New Orleans, LA, 1993; abstract 1405.

35. Masur H, Tuazon C, Gill V, et al. Effect of combined clofazimine and ansamycin therapy on *Mycobacterium avium–Mycobacterium intracellulare* bacteremia in patients with AIDS. J Infect Dis 1987; 155:127–129.

36. Agins BD, Berman DS, Spicehandler, D, et al. Effect of combined therapy with ansamycin, clofazimine, ethambutol, and isoniazid for *Mycobacterium avium* infection in patients with AIDS. J Infect Dis 1989; 159:784–787.

37. Hoy J, Mijch A, Sandland M, et al. Quadruple-drug therapy for *Mycobacterium avium–intracellulare* bacteremia in AIDS patients. J Infect Dis 1990; 161: 801–805.

38. Benson CA, Kessler HA, Pottge JC Jr, Trenholme GM. Successful treatment of acquired immunodeficiency syndrome-related *Mycobacterium avium* complex disease with a multiple drug regimen including amikacin. Arch Intern Med 1991; 151:582–585.

39. Chiu J, Nussbaum J, Bozzette S, et al. Treatment of disseminated *Mycobacterium avium* complex infection in AIDS with amikacin, ethambutol, rifampin, and ciprofloxacin: California Collaborative Treatment Group. Ann Intern Med 1990; 13:358–361.

40. Kemper CA, Meng T, Nussbaum J, et al. Treatment of *Mycobacterium avium* complex bacteremia in AIDS with a four-drug oral regimen: rifampin, ethambutol, clofazimine, and ciprofloxacin. Ann Intern Med 1992; 116:466–472.

41. Nightingale SD, Cameron DW, Gordin FM, et al. Two controlled trials of rifabutin prophylaxis against *Mycobacterium avium* complex infection in AIDS. N Engl J Med 1993; 329:828–833.

42. Horsburgh CR Jr, Metchock B, Gordon SM, et al. Thompson SE III. Predictors of survival in patients with AIDS and disseminated *Mycobacterium avium* complex disease. J Infect Dis 1994; 170:578–584.

43. Gardener TD, Flanagan P, Dryden MS, et al. Disseminated *Mycobacterium avium–intracellulare* infection and red cell hypoplasia in patients with the acquired immune deficiency syndrome. J Infect 1988; 16:135–140.

44. Orenstein MS, Tavitian A, Yonk B, et al. Granulomatous involvement of the liver in patients with AIDS. Gut 1985; 26:1220–1225.
45. Glasgow BJ, Anders K, Layfield LJ, et al. Clinical and pathologic findings of the liver in the acquired immune deficiency syndrome (AIDS). Am J Clin Pathol 1985; 83:582–588.
46. Cappell MS, Schwartz MS, Sempica L. Clinical utility of liver biopsy in patients with serum antibodies to the human immunodeficiency virus. Am J Med 1990; 88:123–130.
47. Salvato P, Thompson C, Stroud S, et al. Acalculous cholecystitis in HIV infection. 9th International Conference on AIDS, Berlin, 1993; abstract PO-B19-1829.
48. Umlas J, Federman M, Crawford C, et al. Spindle cell pseudotumor due to *Mycobacterium avium–intracellulare* in patients with acquired immunodeficiency syndrome (AIDS): Positive staining of mycobacteria for cytoskeleton filaments. Am J Surg Pathol 1991; 15:1181–1187.
49. Cohen KI, Saragas SJ. Endophthalmitis due to *Mycobacterium avium* in a patient with AIDS. Ann Opthalmol 1990; 22:47–51.
50. Lugo-Janer G, Cruz A, Sanchez JL. Disseminated cutaneous infection caused by *Mycobacterium avium* complex. Arch Dermatol 1990; 126:1108–1110.
51. Clark JA, Margolis DM. A cutaneous lesion in a patient with AIDS: An unusual presentation of infection due to *Mycobacterium avium* complex. Clin Infect Dis 1993; 16:555–557.
52. Blumenthal DR, Zucker JR, Hawkins CC. *Mycobacterium avium* complex–induced septic arthritis and osteomyelitis in a patient with the acquired immunodeficiency syndrome (letter). Arthritis Rheum 1990; 33:757–758.
53. Miller RF, Birley HDL, Fogarty P, Semple SJG. Cavitary lung disease caused by *Mycobacterium avium–intracellulare* in AIDS patients. Respir Med 1990; 84:409–411.
54. Volpe F, Schwimmer A, Barr C. Oral manifestation of disseminated *Mycobacterium avium intracellulare* in a patient with AIDS. Oral Surg Oral Med Oral Pathol 1985; 60:567–570.
55. D'Amore TF, Gomez-Hermosillo L, Raviglione MC, et al. Splenic abscess caused by *Mycobacterium avium–intracellulare* in a patient with AIDS. Infect Med 1991; May:47–49.
56. Angelici A, Palumbo P, Piermattei A, et al. Explorative laparotomy for diagnosis of abdominal painful syndromes in HIV positive patients. 9th International Conference on AIDS, Berlin, 1993; abstract PO-B19-1869.
57. Mauss S, Armbrecht CH, Szelenyi H, et al. Abdominal MAC infection as a reason for acute abdomen. 9th International Conference on AIDS, Berlin, 1993; abstract PO-B07-1236.
58. Jacob CN, Henein SS, Heurich AE, Kamholz S. Nontuberculous mycobacterial infection of the central nervous system in patients with AIDS. South Med J 1193; 86:638–640.

59. Berenguer J, Moreno S, Laguna F, et al. Tuberculous meningitis in patients infected with the human immunodeficiency virus. N Engl J Med 1992; 326: 668–672.

60. Gordon SM, Blumberg HM. *Mycobacterium kansasii* brain abscess in a patient with AIDS (letter). Clin Infect Dis 1992; 14:789–790.

61. Bergen GA, Yangco BG, Adelman HM. Central nervous system infection with *Mycobacterium kansasii* (letter). Ann Intern Med 1993; 118:396.

62. Billaud E, Canfere I, Merrien D, Moinard D. Acute severe sepsis syndrome due to *Mycobacterium avium* in two AIDS patients. 9th International Conference on AIDS, Berlin, 1993; abstract PO-B07-1188.

63. Chattha G, Arieff AI, Cummings C, Tierney LM Jr. Lactic acidosis complicating the acquired immunodeficiency syndrome. Ann Intern Med 1993; 118: 37–39.

64. Schafer RW, Kim DS, Weiss JP, Quale JM. Extrapulmonary tuberculosis in patients with human immunodeficiency virus infection. Medicine 1991; 70: 384–397.

65. Barbaro DJ, Orcutt VL, Coldiron BM. *Mycobacterium avium–Mycobacterium intracellulare* infection limited to the skin and lymph nodes in patients with AIDS. Rev Infect Dis 1989; 11:625–628.

66. Miralles CD, Bregman Z. Necrotizing pyomyositis caused by *Mycobacterium avium* complex in a patient with AIDS (letter). Clin Infect Dis 1994; 18:833–834.

67. Piketty C, Danic DL, Weiss L, et al. Sporotrichosis-like infection caused by *Mycobacterium avium* in the acquired immunodeficiency syndrome. Arch Dermatol 1993; 129:1343–1344.

68. Strauss WL, Ostroff SM, Jernigan DB, et al. Clinical and epidemiologic characteristics of *Mycobacterium haemophilum*, an emerging pathogen of immunocompromised patients. Ann Intern Med 1994; 14:1195–1200.

69. Bonnett E, Debat-Zoguereh D, Petit N, et al. Clarithromycin: A potent agent against infections due to *Mycobacterium marinum*. Clin Infect Dis 1994; 18: 664–666.

70. Modilevsky T, Sattler FR, Barnes PF. Mycobacterial disease in patients with human immunodeficiency virus infection. Arch Intern Med 1989; 149:2201–2205.

71. Packer SJ, Cesario T, Williams JH. *Mycobacterium avium* complex infection presenting as endobronchial lesions in immunocompromised patients. Ann Intern Med 1988; 109:389–393.

72. Marinelli DL, Albelda SM, Williams TM, et al. Nontuberculous mycobacterial infection in AIDS: clinical, pathologic, and radiographic features. Radiology 1986; 160:77–82.

73. Jacobson MA, Peiperl L, Volberding PA, et al. Red cell transfusion therapy for anemia in patients with AIDS and ARC: Incidence, associated factors, and outcome. Transfusion 1990; 30:133–137.

74. Sathe SS, Gascone P, Lo W, et al. Severe anemia is an important negative predictor for survival with disseminated *Mycobacterium avium–intracellulare* in acquired immunodeficiency syndrome. Am Rev Respir Dis 1990; 142: 1306–1312.

75. Gascon P, Sathe SS, Rameshwar P. Impaired erythopoiesis in the acquired immunodeficiency syndrome with disseminated *Mycobacterium avium* complex. Am J Med 1993; 94:41–48.

76. Veitch MG, Lucas CR. Association of very high alkaline phosphatase levels with *Mycobacterium avium* complex bacteremia in advanced HIV disease. 8th International Conference on AIDS, Amsterdam, 1992; abstract PuB 7571.

77. Nyberg DA, Federle MP, Jeffrey RB, et al. Abdominal CT findings of disseminated *Mycobacterium avium–intracellulare* in AIDS. AJR 1985; 145:297–299.

78. Watton CW, McCarty M, Tomlinson D, et al. Ultrasound findings in hepatic mycobacterial infections in patients with acquired immune deficiency syndrome (AIDS). Clin Radiol 1993; 47:36–38.

79. Radin DR. Intraabdominal Mycobacterium tuberculosis vs *Mycobacterium avium–intracellulare* infections in patients with AIDS: Distinction based on CT findings. AJR 1991; 156:487–491.

80. Bray HJ, Lail VJ, Cooperberg PL. Tiny echogenic foci in the liver and kidney in patients with AIDS: Not always due to disseminated *Pneumocystis carinii*. AJR 1992; 158:81–82.

81. Prego V, Glatt AE, Roy V, et al. Comparative yield of blood culture for fungi and mycobacteria, liver biopsy, and bone marrow biopsy in the diagnosis of fever of undetermined origin in human immunodeficiency virus–infected patients. Arch Intern Med 1990; 150:333–336.

82. Gill VJ, Park CH, Stock F, et al. Use of lysis-centrifugation (Isolator) and radiometric (BACTEC) blood culture systems for the detection of mycobacteria. J Clin Microbiol 1985; 22:543–546.

83. Witebsky FG, Keiser JF, Conville PS, et al. Comparison of BACTEC 13A medium and Du Pont Isolator for detection of mycobacteremia. J Clin Microbiol 1988; 26:1501–1505.

84. Stone BL, Cohn DL, Kane MS, et al. Utility of paired blood cultures and smears in diagnosis of disseminated *Mycobacterium avium* complex infections in AIDS patients. J Clin Microbiol 1994; 32:841–842.

85. Ahn CH, McLarty JW, AHN SS, et al. Diagnostic criteria for pulmonary disease caused by *Mycobacterium kansasii* and *Mycobacterium intracellulare*. Am Rev Respir Dis 1982; 125:338–391.

86. Havlik JA JR. Metchock B, Thompson SE III, et al. A prospective evaluation of *Mycobacterium avium* complex colonization of the respiratory and gastrointestinal tracts of persons with human immunodeficiency virus infection. J Infect Dis 1993; 168:1045–1048.

87. Ellner JJ, Goldberger MJ, Parenti DM. *Mycobacterium avium* infection and AIDS: a therapeutic dilemma in rapid evolution. J Infect Dis 1991; 163:1326–1335.

88. Chin DP, Hopewell PC, Yajko DM, et al. *Mycobacterium avium* complex in the respiratory or gastrointestinal tract and the risk of *M. avium* complex bacteremia in patients with human immunodeficiency virus infection. J Infect Dis 1994; 169:289–295.

89. Sumartojo E. When tuberculosis therapy fails: A social behaviorial account of patient adherence. Am Rev Respir Dis 1993; 147:1311–1320.

90. Masur H, Public Health Service task force on the prophylaxis and therapy for *Mycobacterium avium* complex. Recommendations on prophylaxis and therapy for disseminated *Mycobacterium avium* complex disease in patients infected with human immunodeficiency virus. N Engl J Med 1993; 329:898–904.

91. DeCock KM, Soro B, Coulibaly IM, Lucas SB. Tuberculosis and HIV infection in sub-Saharan Africa. JAMA 1992; 268:1581–1587.

92. Chaisson RE, Schecter GF, Theuer CP, et al. Tuberculosis in patients with the acquired immunodeficiency syndrome: Clinical features, response to therapy, and survival. Am Rev Respir Dis 1987; 136:570–574.

93. Horsburgh CR Jr, Selik RM. The epidemiology of disseminated nontuberculous mycobacterial infection in the acquired immunodeficiency syndrome (AIDS). Am Rev Respir Dis 1989; 139:4–7.

94. Carpenter JL, Parks JM. *Mycobacterium kansasii* infections in patients positive for human immunodeficiency virus. Rev Infect Dis 1991; 13:789–796.

95. Bessessen MT, Shlay J, Stone-Venohr B, et al. Disseminated *Mycobacterium genavense* infection: Clinical and microbiologic features and response to therapy. AIDS 1993; 7:1357–1361.

96. Bergman F, Schuermann D, Gruenewald T, Ruf B. Frequency and clinical features of pulmonary infections with *Mycobacterium xenopi*. 8th International Conference on AIDS, Amsterdam, 1992; abstract PuB 7037.

97. Ausina V, Barrio J, Luquin M, et al. *Mycobacterium xenopi* infections in the acquired immunodeficiency syndrome (letter). Ann Intern Med 1988; 109:927–928.

98. Huminer D, Dux S, Samra Z, et al. *Mycobacterium simiae* infection in Israeli patients with AIDS. Clin Infect Dis 1993; 17:508–509.

99. Levy-Frebault V, Pangon B, Bure A, et al. *Mycobacterium simiae* and *Mycobacterium avium–M. intracellulare* mixed infection in acquired immune deficiency syndrome. J Clin Microbiol 1987; 25:154–157.

100. Vandercam B, Gennote AF, Degraux J, et al. Disseminated *Mycobacterium simiae* infection in an African patient with AIDS. 8th International Conference on AIDS, Amsterdam, 1992; abstract PoB 3178.

101. Levine B, Chaisson RE. *Mycobacterium kansasii*: A cause of treatable pulmonary disease associated with advanced human immunodeficiency virus (HIV) infection. Ann Intern Med 1991; 114:861–868.

102. Sherer R, Sable R, Sonnenberg M, et al. Disseminated infection with *Mycobacterium kansasii* in the acquired immunodeficiency syndrome. Ann Intern Med 1986; 105:710–712.

103. Bamberger DM, Driks MR, Gupta MR, et al. *Mycobacterium kansasii* among patients infected with human immunodeficiency virus in Kansas City. Clin Infect Dis 1994; 18:395–400.

104. Fiss E, Brooks GF. Detection of *Mycobacterium kansasii* from a brain lesion and *Mycobacterium avium* from blood of an AIDS patient using PCR and reverse dot blot hybridization. Abstracts of the General Meeting of the American Society of Microbiology, New Orleans, LA, 1992; abstract 175.

105. Hirschel B, Chang HR, Mach N, et al. Fatal infection with a novel, unidentified mycobacterium in a man with the acquired immunodeficiency syndrome. N Engl J Med 1990; 323:109–113.

106. Bottger EC, Teske A, Kirschner P, et al. Disseminated *Mycobacterium genavense* infection in patients with AIDS. Lancet 1992; 340:76–80.

107. Jackson K, Sievers A, Ross BC, Dwyer B. Isolation of fastidious Mycobacterium species from two AIDS patients. J Clin Microbiol 1992; 30:2934–2937.

108. Wald A, Coyle MB, Carlson LC, et al. Infection with a fastidious mycobacterium resembling *Mycobacterium simiae* in seven patients with AIDS. Ann Intern Med 1992; 117:586–589.

109. Gaynor CD, Clark RA, Loontz FP, et al. Disseminated *Mycobacterium genavense* infection in two patients with AIDS. Clin Infect Dis 1994; 18:455–457.

110. Dever LL, Martin JW, Seaworth B, Jorgensen JH. Varied presentations and responses to treatment of infections caused by *Mycobacterium haemophilum* in patients with AIDS. Clin Infect Dis 1992; 14:1195–1200.

111. Rogers PL, Walker RE, Lane HC, et al. Disseminated *Mycobacterium haemophilum* infection in two patients with the acquired immunodeficiency syndrome. Am J Med 1988; 84:640–642.

112. Males BM, West TE, Bartholomew WR. *Mycobacterium haemophilum* infection in a patient with acquired immune deficiency syndrome. J Clin Microbiol 1987; 25:186–189.

113. Delaporte E, Alfandari S, Piette F. *Mycobacterium ulcerans* associated with infection due to the human immunodeficiency virus. Clin Infect Dis 1994; 18:839.

114. Sack JB. Disseminated infection due to *Mycobacterium fortuitum* in a patient with AIDS (letter). Rev Infect Dis 1990; 12:961–963.

115. Eng RHK, Forrester C, Smith SM, Sobel H. *Mycobacterium xenopi* infection in a patient with acquired immunodeficiency syndrome. Chest 1984; 86:145–147.

116. Tecson-Tumang FT, Bright JL. *Mycobacterium xenopi* and the acquired immunodeficiency syndrome (letter). Ann Intern Med 1984; 100:461–462.

117. Chan J, McKitrick JC, Klein RS. *Mycobacterium gordonae* in the acquired immunodeficiency syndrome (letter). Ann Intern Med 1984; 101:400.

118. Barber TW, Craven DE, Farber HW. *Mycobacterium gordonae*: A possible opportunistic respiratory pathogen in patients with advanced human immunodeficiency virus, type 1 infection. Chest 1991; 100:716–720.

119. Bernard E, Michiels JF, Pinier Y, et al. Disseminated infection as a result of *Mycobacterium gordonae* in an AIDS patient (letter). AIDS 1992; 6:1217–1218.
120. Claydon EJ, Coker RJ, Harris JRW. *Mycobacterium malmoense* infection in HIV positive patients. J Infect 1991; 23:191–194.
121. Arbeit RD, Slutsky A, Barber TW, et al. Genetic diversity among strains of *Mycobacterium avium* causing monoclonal and polyclonal bacteremia in patients with AIDS. J Infect Dis 1993; 167:1384–1390.
122. Inderlied CB, Kemper CA, Bermudez LM. The *Mycobacterium avium* complex. Clin Microbiol Rev 1993; 6:266–310.

5

Microbiology and In Vitro Susceptibility Testing

CLARK B. INDERLIED and KEVIN A. NASH

University of Southern California and
Children's Hospital Los Angeles
Los Angeles, California

I. Classification

The *Mycobacterium avium* complex (MAC) is classified as acid-fast, slowly growing bacilli that may produce yellow pigment that often intensifies with exposure to light. Wayne and Sramek (1) recently reviewed the systematics of mycobacteria and proposed the term *potentially pathogenic environmental mycobacteria* for acid-fast bacteria that are capable of causing disease in humans but for which there is little evidence for transmission of disease between humans. This term seems particularly appropriate for MAC, since soil or water is a major environmental reservoir for these mycobacteria, the primary portals of entry leading to colonization and infection in humans are the respiratory and gastrointestinal tracts, and person-to-person transmission has not been described.

The designation "*M. avium* complex" refers to a serological complex consisting of 28 serovars of two species, *M. avium* and *M. intracellulare*, although there is evidence for a third genospecies (2). Taxonomic systematics clearly have shown that *M. scrofulaceum*, a species sometimes included in the *M. avium* complex in the past, is taxonomically distinct (1). Based on phenotypic properties and nucleic acid studies, the *M. avium* species is further divided into three subspecies: *M. avium* subsp. *avium*, *M. avium* subsp. *paratuberculosis*, and *M. avium* subsp. *silvaticum*. With increased evidence for the predominant role of *M. avium* in disseminated disease in patients infected with human immunodeficiency virus (HIV) and with the identification of putative virulence factors, there may be increasing benefit to routinely identifying MAC isolates to the level of species; that is, to distinguish *M. avium* and *M. intracellulare* in order to assist in the choice of antimicrobial agents, aggressiveness of treatment, and overall management of the patient with MAC disease.

A. MAC Serovars

The clinical and epidemiological significance of serovar distinctions is not entirely clear, except to indicate that MAC colonization and infection probably relates to environmental exposure; that is, isolates from patients with MAC disease are most likely to be a serovar commonly found in the patient's environment. The biochemical basis of the serovars is discussed later; however, in brief, serological specificity is conferred by specific oligosaccharide residues in the C-mycoside glycopeptidolipid (GPL) component of the cell wall. The oligosaccharide haptens have been defined for the most common serovars of the MAC strains isolated from patients with acquired immunodeficiency syndrome (AIDS) in the United States; that is, serovars 1, 4, and 8 (3). DNA relatedness studies have led to a consensus that serovars 1 through 6 and 8 through 11 are *M. avium*, whereas serovars 7, 12 through 17, and 19, 20, and 25 are *M. intracellulare* (4). This evidence coupled with DNA homology studies and ribosomal RNA sequence analysis (including AccuProbe* [GenProbe,* San Diego, CA] identification) has led to the conclusion that disseminated MAC disease is caused primarily (90% or greater) by *M. avium*.

B. MAC Plasmids

As with many other bacteria, plasmids and insertion sequences (elements) have been found in MAC. At least two groups have identified plasmids in MAC strains isolated from HIV-infected patients that hybridize to fragments of a small plasmid (pLR7) derived from a serovar 4 strain of MAC (5,6). In

---

*AccuProbe and GenProbe are registered trademarks.

addition, there is some evidence for the association of MAC plasmids with antimicrobial resistance (7,8), catalase activity (9), and virulence in an animal model (10). Despite these observations, there is no clear association between the presence of plasmids and the ability of MAC strains to cause disease in patients with AIDS, since only 30–75% of MAC strains isolated from patients with AIDS carry plasmids (11,12). In this regard, it is noteworthy that Meissner and Falkinham (13) showed on average only 19% of MAC strains isolated from the environment carried plasmids. Furthermore, Hellyer et al. (6) concluded that there was no difference in plasmid profiles for 128 MAC strains from patients with AIDS and those without AIDS, and Morris et al. (12) also concluded that the presence of plasmids did not correlate with the ability to cause MAC disease.

II. Cell Wall Structure

A. Overview

The structural and functional differences between the cell wall of mycobacteria and other rapidly growing bacteria and the mounting evidence for a pivotal role of the cell wall in intrinsic antimicrobial resistance of mycobacteria (and MAC in particular) is the focus of the following discussion. The chemistry and structure of the mycobacterial cell wall has been well described (14) and discussed in other recent reviews (15,16).

Superficially, the cell wall of mycobacteria resembles that of gram-positive bacteria in that there is a relatively thick (20–50 nm) peptidoglycan layer that is exterior to the cytoplasmic membrane. Indeed, mycobacteria are weakly gram positive with a characteristic ''beaded'' appearance when stained with a routine Gram stain. The typical gram-positive cell wall, in addition to peptidoglycan, also contains teichoic acids, which are long chains of glycerol or ribitol. These polymers, usually in the form of lipoteichoic acid, are bound at one end to the cytoplasmic membrane and span the thickness of the cell wall. In some gram-positive bacteria, the teichoic acids are directly bound to the peptidoglycan. Other components that may be present in typically gram-positive bacteria include covalently bound polysaccharides and protein layers (e.g., *Streptococcus* M protein).

Like gram-positive bacteria, mycobacteria have long chain molecules bound to both the cytoplasmic membrane and to peptidoglycan; however, rather than teichoic acid based, these polymers are composed of the lipopoly-saccharides (LPS) lipoarabinomannan and lipoarabinogalactan. The latter is also found in species of *Nocardia*, *Rhodococcus*, and *Corynebacterium* (17).

Perhaps the most distinctive feature of the mycobacterial cell wall is the extremely high lipid content, which may comprise 30–40% of the total cell weight, as in the case of MAC (16). This lipid is predominantly found in two forms, covalently bound, mainly as mycolic acid residues terminating the lipoarabinogalactan and loosely bound or free. The latter material is in the form of glycopeptidolipids (GPL) which appear to reside primarily in the outermost layers of the cell wall and are major mycobacterial antigens. GPL can be further divided into nonspecific (nsGPL) and species specific (ssGPL), which are the antigens used in MAC serovar typing (Fig. 1). In addition, there is evidence that GPL are responsible for the rough and smooth colony variants of mycobacteria grown on solid media (18–20). As with the strongly gram-positive bacteria, mycobacterial cell walls also contain protein molecules which are likely to be associated with the actual synthesis and modification of the wall components.

Like many other pathogenic bacteria, intracellular MAC are able to generate a capsule which by electron microscopy appears as a 50- to 100-nm thick electron-transparent zone (ETZ) surrounding the cell wall (Fig. 2) In common with the cell wall, the capsule appears to be lipid rich and is presumed to be of bacterial origin, since it contains MAC-specific antigens (21). The presence of a capsule almost certainly aids the survival of MAC within macrophages, although these bacteria are also able to inhibit phago-lysosome fusion (22) which is essential to the intracellular bactericidal activity of phagocytic cells.

Fatty acyl - NH - D-Phe - D-aThr - D-Ala - L-Alaninol - O - (3,4,-Me-2-L-Rhamnose)
                                                      I

                                                      O

                                                      I

                 6-d-L-Tal - <u>Serovar-Specific Oligosaccharide</u>

Serovar   Serovar-Specific Oligosaccharides

  1   L-Rhamnose
  2   L-Rhamnose - 2,3,-di-Methyl-L-Fucose
  4   L-Rhamnose - 2-Methyl-L-Fucose - 4-Methyl-L-Rhamnose
  8   L-Rhamnose - 3-Methyl-D-Glucose- 4,6-(1'-Carboxyethylidene)

All sugars are in the pyranose form.

Figure 1   Structure of the ssGPLs from a range of clinically important *M. avium* serovars.

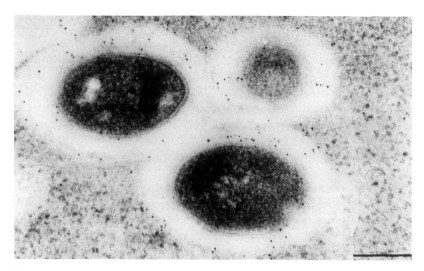

Figure 2   *M. avium* within a macrophage phagocytic vesicle; the electron-transparent capsule is seen speckled with colloidal-gold labeled *M. avium*–specific antibodies, showing, at least partially, the bacterial source of this structure. Bar represents 200 nm. (Source Ref. 16).

Little is known about the biochemical pathways involved in the synthesis and maintenance of the mycobacterial cell wall; however, recently a gene-cluster was identified that encodes for the synthesis of the serovar-specific oligosaccharide component of MAC ssGPL (18). This cluster, designated ser2, was contained within a 22- to 27-kbp chromosome fragment obtained from a MAC serovar 2 strain, and when it was transferred into *M. smegmatis* strain mc^{2}155, enabled the xenogenic expression of serovar 2–specific GPL. In addition, a mycobacterial isomerase was identified that converts ribulose-5-phosphate to arabinose-5-phosphate (24), one of the building blocks of cell wall LPS

The uniqueness of the mycobacterial cell wall and the intragenera differences (e.g., ssGPL) can be used to aid the identification and characterization of members of this genera. For example, tuberculostearic acid (10-methyloctadecanoate), a component of the lipoarabinomannan of *M. tuberculosis*, is also useful as a marker of this species. In fact, analysis of cell wall lipid components is considered a definitive tool in speciation within the genus *Mycobacterium* (25,26).

B. Role in Antimicrobial Resistance

The complexity and high lipid content of the cell has been proposed as a major mechanism for the intrinsic resistance of mycobacteria to many antimicrobial agents (15,16). X-ray analysis of the cell wall of *M. chelonae* suggests that the lipid hydrocarbon chains are oriented predominantly perpendicular to the surface of the bacterium (27). In this orientation, it is likely that the hydrophobic nature of the mycobacterial cell wall would present a formidable barrier to hydrophilic molecules. Furthermore, evidence points to the existence of only one type of porin within the cell membrane of mycobacteria (28), which may further limit the penetration of antimicrobial agents through the cell wall and membrane into the cytoplasm of mycobacteria. There is little biophysical evidence that the mycobacterial cell wall is the permeability barrier to antimicrobial agents; however, Jarlier and Nikaido (29) measured the permeability coefficient for cephalosporins in a β-lactamase–producing strain of *M. chelonae* by studying drug hydrolysis by intact and sonicated bacteria. The permeability coefficient was several orders of magnitude lower (i.e., less permeable) than the permeability coefficient for *Pseudomonas aeruginosa* and *Escherichia coli*. The role of mycobacterial cell wall as the source of intrinsic resistance (impermeability) is underscored by the observation that in cell-free extracts, ribosomes bind antimicrobial agents and ribosome function is inhibited, whereas intact organisms are resistant to the same agents (30).

One of the fascinating as well as perplexing features of MAC isolates is the occurence of colony-type variations. Three variant types are observed: a smooth, opaque, and domed type (SmD); a smooth, transparent, and flat type (SmT); and a rough type. Most clinical isolates of MAC appear as SmT or SmD types (Fig. 3) or as a mixture of the two along with infrequent rough colony variants, although on primary isolation from blood, MAC isolates are often exclusively of the transparent SmT type. The nonpigmented SmT variants are intrinsically more resistant to antimicrobial agents (31–33) and more virulent in animal models of MAC disease than the other types (34–37). Thorel et al. (38) showed that colony variants differ significantly in the expression of cell surface antigens, but they did not ascribe any functional differences to colony variant–specific antigens.

Woodley and David (31) showed that the transparent to opaque transition was not a consequence of mutation and could not be attributed to a plasmid (39), but they showed that the frequency of transition from transparent to opaque is high (1 in 5×10^4 cells), whereas in the opposite direction, the frequency is quite low (1 in 10^6 cells) (31). In contrast, for MAC isolates the mutation rate to resistance for specific drugs or heavy metals

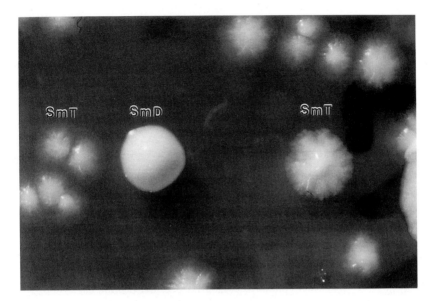

Figure 3 The appearance of SmT and SmD variants of *M. avium* grown on a Middlebrook 7H11 agar-based medium.

ranges from 10^{-5} to 10^{-9} per bacterium per generation. This leads to a potentially confusing situation, since antimicrobial resistance can reflect both colony variant type and mutation. However, our own view is that the antimicrobial resistance associated with colony types is a relative low-level resistance of unknown clinical significance, whereas resistance associated with mutation is a high-level resistance with proven clinical significance (40,41). In general, MAC isolates should be considered potentially very heterogeneous with resistant subpopulations that may range in frequency from 10^{-4} to 1 (42) and that the resistance associated with colony type may be phenotypic or adaptive and expressed to varying degrees with any particular MAC isolate (14,30,32). The implications of these observations for in vitro susceptibility testing are discussed in a later section.

Functional evidence supporting a significant role of the cell wall in drug resistance has been derived from studies of effects of agents known to disrupt the cell wall synthesis and maintenance. Ethambutol is believed to interfere with the modification of D-glucose for use in mycobacterial LPS

(43,44) and even at subinhibitory levels enhances the antimycobacterial activities of agents with cytoplasmic targets such as clarithromycin (45,46), quinolones (47,48) and rifamycins such as KRM-1648 (49,50). Other substances that disrupt the mycobacterial cell wall and enhance the activities of other antimicrobial agents include m-fluorophenylalanine (51), which blocks GPL synthesis, and Tween 80 (52), which may act by increasing the hydrophilicity of the cell wall.

III. Acquired Resistance to Antimicrobial Agents

Although the permeability barrier offered by the MAC cell wall undoubtedly plays a key role in intrinsic drug resistance, acquired resistance in MAC, like in other microorganisms, is likely to involve agent inactivation, target modification, or a modified transport activity (influx or efflux), but there is a dearth of information on the molecular basis of acquired resistance in MAC. There is no evidence that MAC produce aminoglycoside and peptide-inactivating enzymes (30), but there is evidence for the low-level production of β-lactamases (53). In a study of the genetic basis of macrolide resistance, Meier et al. (54) showed that base substitution within the V domain of the 23S ribosomal RNA gene of *M. intracellulare* was linked to clarithromycin resistance. Although the mutation has not been associated with a functional effect in MAC, the mutation is homologous to an erythromycin resistance–associated base substitution within the V domain of *Escherichia coli* 23s rRNA gene (55). Recently, Williams et al. (56) showed that two isolates of MAC that were resistant to rifampin at 40 μg/ml had missense mutations in the *rpoB* gene in positions that correlated with rifampin resistance in *M. tuberculosis*. Two additional rifampin-resistant strains did not have mutations in the *rpoB* gene. At this point in time, it appears that the mechanisms of acquired antimicrobial resistance in MAC are similar to the mechanisms of acquired resistance in *M. tuberculosis*. For examle, in *M. tuberculosis* acquired rifamycin resistance correlates with an altered RNA polymerase (*rpoB* gene) (57); quinolone resistance is a result of altered DNA gyrase genes, *gyrA* and *gyrB* (58); and streptomycin resistance involves either an altered S12 ribosomal protein or altered 16S rRNA gene (59,60). The multiple drug–resistance phenotype in *M. tuberculosis* appears to be a result of the accumulation of mutations rather than the acquisition of a single genetic trait, and one might anticipate that multiple drug resistance in MAC (other than the characteristic intrinsic resistance) will follow the same pattern.

IV. Growth and Physiology

A. Growth

Considerable basic information about the growth and physiology of the MAC is lacking; that is, there is little or no information about anabolic or catabolic enzymatic pathways, energy metabolism, or carbon and nitrogen cycles. Furthermore, there have been few studies directed at understanding transport functions, signal transduction, regulation of macromolecular synthesis, or gene expression. There is limited or sparse information about the biosynthetic pathways, including the enzymatic pathways of cell wall synthesis. By studying partially synchronized cultures of either transparent or opaque colony variants, McCarthy et al. (61) showed that the growth of MAC isolates occurs in three stages. First, cells elongate accompanied by a rapid uptake of fatty acids and protein and DNA content increase but without cell division. Second, cell division occurs by binary fission with a generation time as short as 6 hr. During this stage of growth, protein synthesis continues at a diminished rate. The uptake of fatty acids decreases and intracellular pools of triglycerides are catabolized to supply carbon and energy, and at this stage most cells are in the form of coccobacilli. Third, the culture enters a stage analogous to the stationary growth phase of rapidly growing bacteria. In this stage of growth the cells become a pleomorphic mixture of filaments, rods, and coccobacilli. McCarthy and her colleagues concluded that the cells derived from the opaque variant increase in number during the third stage, since these cells are nutritionally less demanding than the cells derived from the transparent variant type (61). The clinical significance of these largely in vitro observations are unclear; however, the hetergeneity of growth of MAC has compelling implications for in vitro studies of antimicrobial resistance, including routine in vitro susceptibility testing and animal studies of virulence. In addition, there is the intriguing possibility that the heterogeneity of MAC growth reflects a more fundamental property of these fascinating microorganisms, including a prokaryotic differentiation system perhaps driven by a genetic system such as transposition.

B. Physiology

Palmitic and oleic acids are important sources of carbon and energy for the MAC. McCarthy (62) showed that during the first stage of growth there was a rapid uptake of ^{14}C palmitic acid which ceased with the initiation of cell division or fragmentation. Cells of both the transparent and the opaque colony types exhibited a similar response to palmitic acid. Other carbon sources, such as glycerol and glucose, failed to support cell division. During the first part of the growth cycle, exogenous fatty acids are initially incorporated into the triglyceride fraction and then redistributed into other components. By the end of the fission stage of growth, exogenous fatty acid is incorporated into the polar fraction, primarily glycolipids. The triglyceride fraction is metabolized during the cell division phase as the uptake of exogenous fatty acids ceases. Curiously, smooth transparent–type cells produce large numbers of nonviable particles during all phases of growth, and these particles consist in large part of sulfolipids (63). McCarthy also showed that nitrogen metabolism varies depending on the stage of growth within the cell cycle. During elongation, cells are unable to use organic forms of nitrogen such as glutamic acid or glutamine, but they use these amino acids as well as sulfur during periods of rapid cell fission (64). Also, McCarthy (65) showed that MAC preferentially use ammonia and nitrite but not amino acids with the exception of glutamine as a source of nitrogen.

V. Culture and Identification

A. General

Several methods can be used to culture MAC from blood, bone marrow, respiratory secretions, and other specimens; however, the most sensitive laboratory diagnosis requires the use of both solid and liquid media (66–69). The frequency and type of specimens submitted for diagnosis of MAC disease depends on the type of infection and the patient's signs and symptoms. Disseminated disease is rare in immunocompetent patients and in immunodeficient patients with greater than 100 CD4 lymphocytes-mm^3 of blood (70). In HIV-infected patients with <100 CD4 lymphocytes-mm^3 (often <50 CD4), a single blood culture is usually sufficient to diagnose disseminated disease (71,72). However, in patients with a negative blood culture and persistent symptoms consistent with MAC disease, it may be necessary to perform repeated blood cultures. There have been no systematic studies of the effect of antimicrobial therapy on blood cultures; however, the dilution factor inherent in most blood culture systems (especially lysis centrifugation methods) should be sufficient to prevent false-negative cultures caused by carryover of antimicrobial agents. The detection of MAC in blood is significantly improved with the use of a cytolytic agent such as sodium deoxycholate or the commercial lysis-centrifugation system (Isolator*, Wampole Laboratories,

---

*Isolator is a registered trademark.

Cranbury, NJ). This is because MAC in the blood is most likely to be present within the circulating monocytes and macrophages (67,68,73). The presence of MAC in respiratory tract and stool specimens from HIV-infected patients has been somewhat difficult to interpret, and the predictive value of a negative smear or culture is poor. Although the presence of MAC in these specimens predicts disseminated disease, the routine smear and culture of these specimens is unwarranted (74–78). In patients with chronic respiratory tract infections, including those with cystic fibrosis (79), it can be difficult to distinguish colonization from infection based on microbiological evidence alone. Repeated isolation of MAC from a patient with symptomatic respiratory infection is perhaps the most reliable microbiologic indicator of disease without resorting to biopsy (80).

B. Bactec* Cultures

The Bactec system is a broth radiometric culture method in which sterile tissue, blood (concentrated or unconcentrated), or a decontaminated specimen is inoculated into a modified Middlebrook 7H9 liquid medium (Bactec 12B medium) containing radioactively labeled palmitic acid (Bactec TB System) (68,81,82). Alternatively, a larger volume (up to 5 ml) of unconcentrated blood can be inoculated directly into Bactec 13A medium (83,84), which is a medium developed specifically for diagnosing mycobacteremia. In one report, the growth of MAC in Bactec 12B medium was slower and fewer cultures were positive when the blood was collected in an Isolator tube (85).

C. Plate Cultures

For culture on solid media, specimens can be inoculated onto an agar-based medium such as Middlebrook 7H11; an egg-base medium such as Löwenstein-Jensen (68); or the biphasic Septi-Chek* AFB System (Roche Diagnostic Systems, Nutley, NJ), also referred to as the MB-Check* System. The isolation of MAC and certain other nontuberculous mycobacteria on egg-based media may be improved by lowering the pH to <6.5 and adding pyruvate or glycerol (86). In two early reports, the Septi-Chek System proved as sensitive as the Bactec method and more sensitive then conventional culture (87,88). More recent reports support the observation that the Septi-Chek System is as sensitive as Bactec for the detection of both *M. avium* and *M. tuberculosis*, but the time to detection with Bactec is faster (89–91). Agy et

---

*Bactec, Septi-Chek and MB-Check are registered trademarks.

al. (66) compared four blood culture systems for mycobacteria and found that the single most sensitive (94% of 32 positive cultures) system for blood cultures was the Bactec System using Bactec 13A medium. The mean time to detection using Bactec 13A or 12B media was approximately 14 days compared with 21 and 24 days, respectively, using Middlebrook 7H11 agar or a biphasic culture system. In general, positive cultures are detected in 7 to 14 days using the Bactec method, 21–28 days (or longer) using conventional agar- or egg-based media (82) and approximately 20 days using the Septi-Chek AFB System (87).

Quantitative colony counts (cfu/ml) have been used to monitor therapeutic efficacy in clinical trials, but the methods are laborious and should be limited to investigative studies. The Bactec System provides a convenient approximation of the level of the bacteremia, since there is a correlation between the days to a positive Bactec 13A blood culture and the quantitative level of the mycobacteremia (92,93). Bactec blood cultures that were positive in <7 days had >400 CFU/mL whereas those that were positive after ≥12 days of incubation had low levels of bacteremia (<9 CFU/ml). Using blood inoculated with known concentrations of mycobacteria, von Reyn et al. (94) demonstrated that MAC isolates remain viable in the Isolator lysis centrifugation tubes for at least 7 days, and Havlir et al. (93) showed that interlaboratory results using the Isolator culture method were comparable for identical blood specimens processed using the same protocol.

D. Identification

MAC colonies tend to be visible sooner and colony morphology is more apparent on agar-based media such as Middlebrook 7H10, whereas pigment production is enhanced when MAC are grown on egg-based media such as Löwenstein-Jensen medium. It is important to note that when evaluated by colony morphology alone, some MAC colonies may be mistaken for *M. tuberculosis*, and if susceptibility tests are performed on such an isolate, it could be incorrectly reported as a multiple drug–resistant *M. tuberculosis*. The identification of several clinically significant mycobacteria (i.e., *M. tuberculosis*, *M. avium*, *M. intracellulare*, *M. avium* complex, *M. kansasii*, and *M. gordonae*) can be achieved within a few hours, if sufficient growth is available, using nonradioactive (acridinium esters) DNA probes (GenProbe) (95– 99). These acridinium probes that hybridize to species-specific regions of the 16S ribosomal RNA of mycobacteria have been evaluated in a variety of studies and shown to be 95–100% sensitive and specific for culture confirmation (identification) (100–103). For example, Lebrun et al. (104) showed that the acridinium ester–labeled probes from GenProbe using 40 MAC isolates had 100% specificity and 95% sensitivity. By first testing AFB isolates from patients with AIDS with the *M. avium* or MAC probe or highly characteristic colonies with the *M. tuberculosis* probe, the high cost of these probes can be controlled (95,96). Chromatographic analysis of cell wall fatty acids provides a rapid and accurate alternative or adjunct to probe-based identification of MAC (105,106), and conventional biochemical methods of identification can be improved by using a strategy that limits the number of tests (107).

Positive Bactec broth cultures can be concentrated by centrifugation and directly tested with the GenProbe acridinium probes; however, it is prudent to subculture onto a solid medium to confirm the identification, to check for mixed cultures, and to provide an inoculum for susceptibility testing (100,108,109). Peterson et al. (109) showed that by combining the Bactec System with GenProbe indentification, >86% of clinically significant MAC-positive specimens could be reported within 7 days; however, they noted that blood strongly interfered with the chemiluminescent reading of the acridinium assay, and Bactec samples had to be treated with detergent and EDTA and a background control was necessary (110). The use acridinium probes for the direct identification of *M tuberculosis* of MAC is improved if the growth index of the Bactec vial is >400 before testing (100,108).

E. Direct Detection by Stain

The direct examination of blood lymphocytes (buffy coat) (111–113) or auramine-rhodamine staining with fluorescent microscopy of bone marrow aspirates (114) may be of value; however, the predictive value of these techniques is poor and one cannot exclude *M. tuberculosis* or other mycobacteria on the basis of a smear alone. Furthermore, mixed infections can occur and clinicians and laboratory personnel should be alert to the possibility that the presence of MAC on the culture plate may obscure the detection of *M. tuberculosis* (111) or coinfection with *M. simiae* (115). Wiley et al. (116) reported on the use of mixed polyclonal antibodies to three species of mycobacteria to detect microorganisms in tissue, including bone marrow biopsies (Fig. 4). In this study, 32 of 34 cases of proven mycobacterial disease were positive using an immunohistochemical technique. In addition, 8 of 10 specimens that were negative by conventional staining methods were positive using the mixed antibodies method. Using this technique with bone marrow core biopsies from HIV-infected patients, Wiley et al. (117) showed that the immunohistochemical stain was more sensitive than a Kinyoun stain, 90 versus 66%, but neither of these methods was as sensitive as blood culture. They

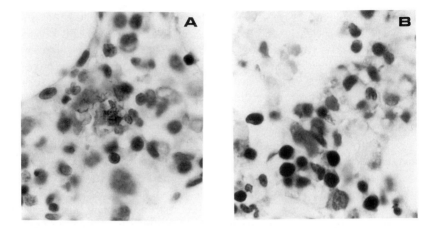

Figure 4   Bone marrow: (A) immunoperoxidase-stained using polyclonal antibodies specific for mycobacteria; (B) Kinyoun-stained.

reported a poor correlation between the level of mycobacteremia and the number of bacilli observed by the immunohistochemical stain; the potential clinical significance of this observation is intriguing. Finally, there is a preliminary report on the detection of MAC antigenuria which showed a low sensitivity (<60%) but good specificity (100%); however, the number of specimens tested was small (118).

F.   Polymerase Chain Reaction Detection of MAC

Hance et al. (119) described one of the first polymerase chain reaction (PCR) assays for mycobacteria, including MAC, based on the amplification of a 383-bp target within the gene encoding the 65-kDa cell surface antigen. Species were identified with probes specific for *M. tuberculosis, M. avium,* or *M. fortuitum,* and the sensitivity of the assay was 10 to 1000 bacilli depending on the method of visualization. Telenti et al. (120) used this same target for a PCR assay with universal primers and showed that strains could be distinguished using two restriction enzymes, BstEII and HaeIII, to generate species-specific restriction products. Two other groups used 65-kDa PCR assays to detect and identify mycobacteria in paraffin-embedded tissues (121,122), and Ghossein et al. (121) showed that formalin-treated tissue that was 7 years old contained amplifiable DNA. Plikaytis et al. (123) identified a 1380-bp target within the highly conserved hsp65 gene which is present in at least 19 different species of mycobacteria. Species identification was based on restriction fragment length polymorphism (RFLP) profiles generated by BstNI or XhoI endonuclease digestion of the amplification product. The validity of the RFLP identities was assessed by using a computer program to normalize and cluster the various profiles.

Kunze et al. (124) described four separate PCR assays for targets within the insertion sequences (IS) IS901, found in certain strains of MAC, and IS901, apparently found in most strains of *M. paratuberculosis*. The four PCR assays were specific for (1) a 1108-bp target within IS901 found in RFLP type A/I strains; (2) the regions upstream and downstream of IS901 that produce a 1742-bp target in RFLP-type A/I or a 300-bp product in strains lacking IS901; (3) at 453-bp target within IS900; and (4) a 574- or 577-bp target that was common to both IS900 and 901. PCR analysis showed that none of the tested MAC strains from patients with AIDS contained IS900 or IS901, whereas all but one isolate from birds contained IS901 and 89% of *M. paratuberculosis* strains contained IS900. RFLP analysis of the MAC strains showed that a certain RFLP type, designated A, commonly infects patients with AIDS; however, these strains do not contain IS elements (125). IS elements have proven to be valuable targets for diagnostic purposes with *M. tuberculosis*, because these elements are frequently found in multiple copies and their distribution can be used to generate strain-specific RFLP patterns, providing the IS elements are relatively stable within the genomic DNA (126).

Boddinghaus et al. (127) described a generic mycobacterial PCR assay based on a target within a 16S ribosomal RNA sequence. Species identification was based on the hybridization of species-specific probes to variable regions within the amplified target. The assay detected as few as 10 tubercle bacilli; however, the assay was not tested with clinical specimens containing MAC. The use of ribosomal RNA as a PCR target has the advantage that each viable bacilli may contain thousands of ribosomes; however, the ribosomal RNA must first be converted to DNA using a reverse transcriptase. The amplification of ribosomal RNA is also the basis of the GenProbe Amplified *M tuberculosis* Direct Test except that the DNA generated by reverse transcription is amplified using RNA polymerase (128). The amplified ribosomal RNA is detected with the conventional GenProbe acridinium probes and the method is applicable to the direct detection of MAC.

VI. Susceptibility Testing

In vitro susceptibility testing of MAC using the methods and interpretive criteria commonly used to test *M. tuberculosis* has little or no value in guiding the initial treatment of patients with MAC disease. This includes both the modified proportion and the Bactec methods using "critical concentrations" of conventional antituberculosis agents (129). At present, in the majority of clinical situations, it is inappropriate to perform in vitro susceptibility tests on initial MAC isolates, but susceptibility testing may be useful if a patient relapses on therapy, especially when therapy includes a macrolide, or if the infection is intractable and the clinical situation is acute or desperate.

A. Conventional Antimycobacterial Agents

Most MAC isolates are intrinsically resistant to isoniazid and all are resistant to pyrazinamide, and many clinicians believe that neither of these drugs has a role in the treatment of MAC disease and should not be tested. MAC isolates are variably susceptible to aminoglycosides (i.e., amikacin, kanamycin, and streptomycin) and rifamycins (e.g., rifampin and rifabutin). In general, the susceptibility patterns of MAC isolates are considerably more variable than those of *M. tuberculosis* (130–133), suggesting the potential importance of susceptibility testing as more antimycobacterial agents are identified with clinically useful activity against MAC. There is some evidence that MAC isolates from patients with AIDS are more resistant to antimicrobial agents than isolates from patients without AIDS (134), but these results have been challenged by other studies (135). If there is a difference between MAC isolates, this may reflect that *M. avium* is much more common in HIV-infected patients than is *M. intracellulare*, and *M. avium*, on average, is more intrinsically resistant. Other agents that might be considered for susceptibility testing include azithromycin, clarithromycin, ethambutol, ciprofloxacin, clofazimine, and cycloserine; however, when and if any or all of these agents should be tested is not entirely clear.

B. Macrolide Testing

In vitro susceptibility testing of the macrolides clarithromycin and azithromycin (azithromycin is an azalide, a subclass of macrolides) against MAC has taken on greater significance with the recent reports showing that these drugs have substantial activity as single agents in the treatment of disseminated and pulmonary MAC disease (40,41,136,137). Interpretive criteria for defining macrolide resistance are presently not available; however, an increase of two or three dilutions in the minimum inhibitory concentration (MIC) for a MAC strain is likely to indicate clinically significant resistance (138,139) (140,141); for clarithromycin, a MIC of >16 μg/ml should be considered resistant. Macrolides are significantly more active at pH 7.2–7.4 than at pH 6.7–6.9, which is the usual pH of growth media for mycobacteria, leading to possible confusion in the interpretation of susceptibility tests. Although raising the pH improves the activity of macrolides, some strains of MAC may grow more slowly at this pH, and one must be concerned that the inhibition of growth is a result of the combined effect of pH and the antimicrobial agent. Nevertheless, to compare test results between macrolides or between MAC isolates, all the tests must be performed at the same pH; that is, perform all the tests at either pH 6.7–6.9 or 7.2–7.4.

C. Areas of Consensus

Although there are no clearly compelling reasons that broth media are preferable to agar media for in vitro susceptibility testing of MAC, Heifets (140) identified three important advantages of a broth medium: (1) several antimycobacterial agents appear to irreversibly bind to agar or the protein components within an agar matrix; (2) agar media tests require longer incubation times to reach a discernible endpoint, which increases the potential for the degradation of unstable agents; and (3) mycobactericidal agents, for unexplained reasons, are less potent in agar, and regrowth may occur over the extended incubation times used with these media. At present there is no standard method for testing MAC; however, there is some consensus on certain aspects of in vitro susceptibility testing of MAC isolates (129,141). As indicated above, a broth medium may be more reliable than an agar medium. Radiometric broth (Bactec 12B medium, pH 6.8) macrodilution or broth microdilution (142) has yielded reproducible results (129,141). Careful attention must be paid to the preparation of the inoculum, especially to avoid the selection of colony-type variants during subculture; only transparent colony types should be tested (31). The inoculum should be between 10^4 and 10^5 for the radiometric broth macrodilution test and approximately 10^5 CFU/ml for the broth microdilution test. Drugs should be tested at 3–5 concentrations in increments of $\log_2$, and activity should be measured as a MIC (μg/ml). The period of incubation should not extend beyond 7 days, and the "no drug" control should not exceed a growth index of 999 in less than 4 days in the Bactec test. Finally, Tween 80 or other surfactants should not be used to disperse clumps of bacilli because of the potential synergistic effect between surfactants and antimicrobial agents (33).

D. Areas of Controversy

The areas of remaining controversy include preparation of the inoculum, the range of drug concentrations to test, reading and interpreting the Bactec results, and the MIC interpretive criteria. Some laboratories advocate the use of "seed" Bactec vials (subcultures of fresh growth) as a source of inoculum, whereas others prefer to prepare a suspension of mycobacteria directly from agar plates in a manner similar to the direct inoculum method advocated for testing fastidious rapidly growing aerobic bacteria (143). Interpretation of the Bactec GI readings follow the recommendations of the manufacturer (144) or are somewhat more restrictive (141). Alternatively, Inderlied (129) described a method of analysis based on a kinetic measurement of growth inhibition and dose-response relationships (Fig. 5). With all of these methods, the MIC is defined as the lowest concentration of drug that inhibits the growth of the microorganism to an extent that is less than a control. A common control is the inoculum diluted 1:100 (99% inhibition), which follows the convention used in testing *M. tuberculosis*. However, the 99% endpoint has not been verified for MAC, and Inderlied (129) has suggested the use of a 1:1000 (99.9%) control, which follows the convention used in testing rapidly growing bacteria.

E. Interpretive Criteria

In the absence of well-established correlations with clinical efficacy and outcome, the choice of MIC interpretive criteria (resistant or susceptible) is problematic. Some workers (141,145) have advocated the use of criteria based on maximum (peak) serum concentrations and the highest MICs for "wild-type" strains of *M. tuberculosis*, whereas others suggest no criteria (144). It is important to recognize that disseminated MAC disease is principally an infection of the blood, macrophages, bone marrow, spleen, and other tissues and that clinical effectiveness is likely to relate to both potent activity and the ability of drugs to accumulate in tissue to levels above the MIC of the infecting microorganism. Clearly, whatever interpretive criteria are used for susceptibility test results, the criteria must relate to meaningful and reliable measure of clinical efficacy.

F. Combination Testing

The treatment of MAC pulmonary infections has been based largely on the assumption that multiple antimycobacterial agents act in a synergistic manner. Zimmer et al. (146) showed that 96% of 49 MAC isolates from patients with pulmonary disease were susceptible to serum concentrations of rifampin and ethambutol and this combination was synergistic. Synergistic activity was defined as a fourfold decrease in the MIC of the combination compared with

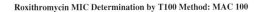

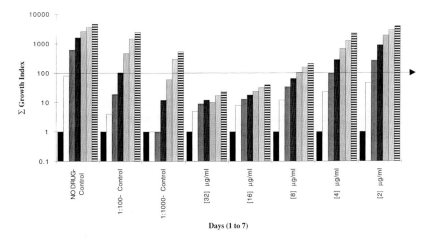

Days (1 to 7)

Figure 5   An example of the T100 method of datum analysis using the Bactec 460 radiometric broth macrodilution method to measure the in vitro susceptibility of a strain of *Mycobacterium avium* (MAC 100) tested against five concentrations of roxithromycin (2–32 μg/mL). Eight Bactec 12B vials were inoculated with 10^4 to 10^5 CFU/ml of MAC 100 and each bar represents the daily cumulative Growth Index (Σ GI) for a vial read for 7 days, thus there are seven Σ GI values for each vial. The first 3 vials are controls and include (1) a no drug control, (2) a 1:100 control, inoculum diluted 1:100, and (3) a 1:1000 control, inoculum diluted 1:1000. Based on the growth kinetics of *M. avium* complex isolates in Bactec 12B medium, Σ GI value of 100 was chosen as a threshold to distinguish growth from no growth. As shown, the undiluted no drug control exceeded the threshold at 3 days, whereas the 1:100 and 1:1000 controls exceed the threshold at 5 and 6 days, respectively. Therefore, the MIC for roxithromycin can be taken as the concentration of drug that prevents growth equal to or less than the 1:100 or 1:1000 controls. However, by examining growth in each vial in a kinetic manner and using the cumulative GI threshold of 100 (time to reach a cumulative GI of 100 or T100), it is clear that the MIC is between 8 and 16 μg/ml, but only slightly more than 8 μg/ml. The graphical representation of the daily Σ GI values is constructed using Excel 3.0 spreadsheet software and Bactec 460 data are automatically downloaded into the spreadsheet using an interface from Argus of Florida, Inc., and software written by K.A. Nash. (Source: Inderlied, C.B. Eur. J. Clin. Microbiol. Infect. Dis. 1994; 13:980–993).

the MIC of each agent alone. Heifets (147) examined two and three drug combinations of rifampin, ethambutol, ethionamide, and streptomycin tested against the MAC using an isobologram analysis of subinhibitory concentrations. Using this agar-based method, all two-drug combinations appeared to be synergistic against the three serovar 8 strains included in this study. Hoffner et al. (148) confirmed the synergistic interaction between ethambutol and rifampin or ethambutol and streptomycin against the MAC using an entirely different broth-based method. Thus, there is precedent for the use of in vitro susceptibility tests to identify synergistic combinations of drugs and such studies have proved to have clinical value in the treatment of MAC pulmonary disease. However, it is unclear how useful such combination testing is in guiding the treatment of disseminated MAC disease. Furthermore, in the treatment of disseminated MAC disease, which almost always occurs in a severely immunocompromised patient, there is heightened concern about both improved efficacy and the prevention of resistance (149). Nevertheless, it is unclear whether in vitro susceptibility testing can be used to predict if a combination drug regimen will prevent drug resistance.

As with the susceptibility testing of single antimycobacterial agents, there are no standard methods or interpretive criteria for testing agents in combination. In addition, in approaching combination testing the objective of the test should be clear. Four methods can be envisioned for measuring the interaction between antimycobacterial agents depending on the objective. A maximum effect or time-kill curve method is more appropriate to determine if there is a synergistic bactericidal interaction. If an minimum bactericidal concentration (MBC) is the endpoint of the assay, an isobologram method can be used to measure synergistic bactericidal activity. A time-kill curve and an emergence of resistance analysis are similar; for example, the time-kill curve analysis may readily reveal subpopulations of resistant organisms but can also provide hints about the mechanism of action of drugs. An emergence of resistance analysis would be specifically designed to measure the synergistic effect of combinations of agents on an already identified resistant subpopulation. The application of interpretive criteria to each of these methods is not uniform. There is some broad appeal for a 99.9% endpoint in time-kill curve measurements (143), but in comparing combinations of agents, a time factor should be included in the criteria. Indeed, in the treatment of MAC disease, the rate of killing may have more clinical significance than the degree of killing. The limits of the maximum effect type of analysis will be set in part by pharmacokinetic features of the component drugs. Criteria for distinguishing significant differences between combinations of agents may not be easily defined.

G. Molecular Methods of Testing

The need to improve the timeliness of mycobacterial drug susceptibility testing has spawned an interest in the use of molecular assays. Telenti et al. (57, 150) showed that rifamycin resistance in *M. tuberculosis* can be identified using PCR and single-strand conformation polymorphism (SSCP) electrophoresis. PCR was used to amplify a target within the gene that encodes for the β-subunit of the RNA polymerase (*rpoB*); the target includes the majority of mutation sites associated with rifampin resistance. Slight differences in the DNA sequence of rifampin-resistant mutants, as compared with rifamycin-sensitive wild-type *M. tuberculosis*, were readily detected by SSCP. Although there appears to be a good correlation between mutant rpoB gene sequences and rifampin resistance, a functional association has not been established for all mutations. Williams et al. (56) used a variation of this approach and showed that direct sequencing of the PCR products of the *rpoB* target permitted a rapid and accurate determination of rifampin resistance with both *M. tuberculosis* and *M. avium*.

A very different approach to the rapid detection of resistance in mycobacteria was developed based on the effect of antimicrobial activity on gene expression (151,152). The gene for firefly luciferase was inserted into an expression vector under the control of the heat-shock protein 60 (hsp60) promoter of *M. tuberculosis*. The chimeric vector was introduced into either *M. tuberculosis* or *M. smegmatis* and constituitive expression of luciferase was detected and quantitated by the light emitted from the enzymatic modification of luciferin in the presence of adenosine triphosphate (ATP). In the presence of antimicrobial agents, susceptible mycobacteria containing the hsp60-luciferase chimera showed reduced luciferase expression, whereas resistant strains appeared relatively unaffected. Although the luciferase assay can be completed in as little as 48 hr, there are a number of important limitations. The hsp60-luciferase chimera needs to be introduced into the mycobacteria, which can be an inefficient procedure and may inadvertently result in the selection of subpopulations. This may not be a serious problem with *M. tuberculosis* isolates; however, with MAC there may be multiple strains or subpopulations present with significantly different susceptibility profiles. It is clear, however, that the incorporation of luciferase or other reporter molecules into a collection of standard *M. tuberculosis* or MAC strains would be of considerable value in drug development studies.

References

1. Wayne LG, Sramek HA. Agents of newly recognized or infrequently encountered mycobacterial diseases. Clin Microbiol Rev 1992; 5:1–25.

2. Wayne LG, Good RC, Krichevsky MI, et al. Fourth report of the cooperative, open-ended study of slowly growing mycobacteria by the International Working Group on Mycobacterial Taxonomy. Int J Syst Bacteriol. 1991; 41:463–472.

3. Rivoire B, Ranchoff BJ, Chatterjee D, et al. Generation of monoclonal antibodies to the specific sugar epitopes of *Mycobacterium avium* complex serovars. Infect Immunity 1989; 57:3147–3158.

4. Saito H, Tomioka H, Sato K, et al. Identification of various serovar strains of *Mycobacterium avium* complex by using DNA probes specific for *Mycobacterium avium* and *Mycobacterium intracellulare*. J Clin Microbiol 1900; 28:1694–1697.

5. Crawford JT, Bates JH. Analysis of plasmids in *Mycobacterium avium-intracellulare* isolates from persons with acquired immunodeficiency syndrome. Amer Rev Respir Dis. 1986; 134:659–661.

6. Hellyer TJ, Brown IN, Dale JW, Easmon CS. Plasmid analysis of *Mycobacterium avium-intracellulare* (MAI) isolated in the United Kingdom from patients with and without AIDS. J. Med Microbiol 1991; 34:225–231.

7. Franzblau SG, Takeda T, Nakamura M. Mycobacterial plasmids: screening and possible relationship to antibiotic resistance in *Mycobacterium avium-Mycobacterium intracellulare*. Microbiol Immunol 1986; 30:903–907.

8. Mizuguchi Y, Fukunaga M, Taniguchi H. Plasmid deoxyribonucleic acid and translucent-to-opaque variation in *Mycobacterium intracellulare* 103. J Bacteriol 1981; 146:656–659.

9. Pethel ML, Falkinham JO III. Plasmid-influenced changes in *Mycobacterium avium* catalase activity. Infect Immun. 1989; 57:1714–1718.

10. Gangadharam PR, Perumal VK, Crawford JT, Bates JH. Association of plasmids and virulence of *Mycobacterium avium* complex. Amer Rev Respir Dis 1988; 137:212–214.

11. Jensen AG, Bebbedsen J, Rosdahl VT. Plasmid profiles of *Mycobacterium avium-intracellulare* isolated from patients with AIDS or cervical lymphadenitis and from environmental samples. Scand J Infect Dis 1989; 21:645–649.

12. Morris SL, Rouse DA, Malik A, et al. Characterization of plasmids extracted from AIDS-associated *Mycobacterium avium* isolates. Tubercle 1990; 71:181–185.

13. Meissner PS, Falkinham III JO. Plasmid DNA profiles as epidemiological markers for clinical and environmental isolates of *Mycobacterium avium, Mycobacterium intracellulare*, and *Mycobacterium scrofulaceum*. J Infect Dis 1986; 153:325–331.

14. McNeil MR, Brennan PJ. Structure, function and biogenesis of the cell envelope of mycobacteria in relation to bacterial physiology, pathogenesis and drug resistance; some thoughts and possibilities arising from recent structural information. Res Microbiol 1991; 142:355–486.

15. Inderlied CB, Kemper CA, Bermudez LEM. The *Mycobacterium avium* complex. Clin Microbiol Rev 1993; 6:266–310.

16. Rastogi N, Barrow WW. Cell envelope constituents and the multifaceted nature of *Mycobacterium avium* pathogenicity and drug resistance. Res Microbiol 1994; 145:243–252.

17. Daffe M, McNeil M, Brennan PJ. Major structural features of the cell wall arabinogalactans of *Mycobacterium, Rhodococcus*, and *Nocardia* spp. Carbohydrate Research 1993; 249:383–398.

18. Belisle JT, Pascopella L, Inamine JM, et al. Isolation and expression of a gene cluster responsible for biosynthesis of the glycopeptidolipid antigens of *Mycobacterium avium*. J Bacteriol 1991; 173:6991–6997.

19. Belisle JT, McNeil MR, Chatterjee D, et al. Expression of the core lipopeptide of the glycopeptidolipid surface antigens in rough mutants of *Mycobacterium avium*. J Biol Chem 1993; 268:10510–10516.

20. Belisle JT, Klaczkiewicz K, Brennan PJ, et al. Rough morphological variants of *Mycobacterium avium*. Characterization of genomic deletions resulting in the loss of glycopeptidolipid expression. J Biol Chem 1993; 268:10517–10523.

21. Rastogi N, Hellio R. Evidence that the capsule around mycobacteria grown in axenic media contains mycobacterial antigens: implications at the level of cell envelope architecture. FEMS Microbiol Letters 1990; 58:161–166.

22. Rastogi N, Bachelet M, Carvalho-de-Sousa JP. Intracellular growth of *Mycobacterium avium* in human macrophages is linked to the increased synthesis of prostaglandin E2 and inhibition of the phagosome-lysosome fusions. FEMS Microbiol Immunol 1992; 4:273–279.

23. Benson CA, Kessler HA, Pottage Jr JC, Trenholme GM. Successful treatment of acquired immunodeficiency syndrome-related *Mycobacterium avium* complex disease (D-MAC) with a multiple drug regimen including amikacin. Arch Intern Med 1991; 151:582–585.

24. Deng LL, Brennan PJ, McNeil M. Implication of arabinose-5-phosphate and the enzyme arabinose-5-phosphate: ribulose-5-phosphate isomerase in biosynthesis of mycobacterial cell wall arabinan and the effects of ethambutol thereon. Frontiers in Mycobacteriology: *M. avium*, the Modern Epidemic, Vail, 1992.

25. Glickman SE, Kilburn JO, Butler WR, Ramos LS. Rapid identification of mycolic acid patterns of mycobacteria by high-performance liquid chromatography using pattern recognition software and a Mycobacterium library. J Clin Microbiol 1994; 32: 740–745.

26. Thibert L, Lapierre S. Routine application of high-performance liquid chromatography for identification of mycobacteria. J Clin Microbiol 1993; 31: 1759–1763.

27. Nikaido H, Kim SH, Rosenberg EY. Physical organization of lipids in the cell wall of *Mycobacterium chelonae*. Mol Microbiol 1993; 8:1025–1030.

28. Trias J, Benz R. Characterization of the channel formed by the mycobacterial porin in lipid bilayer membranes. Demonstration of voltage gating and of negative point charges at the channel mouth. J Biol Chem 1993; 268:6234–6240.

29. Jarlier V, Nikaido H. Permeability barrier to hydrophilic solutes in *Mycobacterium chelonei*. J Bacteriol 1990; 172:1418–1423.

30. Mizuguchi Y, Udou T, Yamada T. Mechanism of antibiotic resistance in *Mycobacterium intracellulare*. Micobiol Immunol 1983; 27:425–431.

31. Woodley CL, David HL. Effect of temperature on the rate of the transparent to opaque colony type transition in *Mycobacterium avium*. Antimicrob Agents Chemother 1976; 9:113–119.

32. Rastogi N, Frehel C, Ryter A, et al. Multiple drug resistance in *Mycobacterium avium*: Is the wall architecture responsible for the exclusion of antimicrobial agents? Antimicrob Agents Chemother 1981; 20:666–677.

33. Saito H, Tomioka H. Susceptibilities of transparent, opaque, and rough colonial variants of *Mycobacterium avium* complex to various fatty acids. Antimicrob Agents Chemother 1988; 32:400–402.

34. Schaefer WB, Davis CL, Cohn ML. Pathogenicity of transparent, opaque and rough variants of *Mycobacterium avium* in chickens and mice. Amer Rev Respir Dis 1970; 102:499–506.

35. Rulong S, Aguas AP, da Silva PP, Silva MT. Intramacrophagic *Mycobacterium avium* bacilli are coated by a multiple lamellar structure: freeze fracture analysis of infected mouse liver. Infect Immun 1991; 59:3895–3902.

36. Meylan PR, Richman DD, Kornbluth RS. Characterization and growth in human macrophages of *Mycobacterium avium* complex strains isolated from the blood of patients with acquired immunodeficiency syndrome. Infect Immun 1990; 58:2564–2568.

37. Crowle AJ, Tsang AY, Vatter AE, May MH. Comparison of 15 laboratory and patient-derived strains of *Mycobacterium avium* for ability to infect and multiply in cultured human macrophages. J Clin Microbiol 1986; 24:812–821.

38. Thorel MF, David HL. Specific surface antigens of SmT variants of *Mycobacterium avium*. Infect Immun 1984; 43:438–439.

39. David HL. Response of mycobacteria to ultraviolet light radiation. Amer Rev Respir Dis 1973; 108:1175–1185.

40. Dautzenberg B, Saint MT, Meyohas MC, et al. Clarithromycin and other antimicrobial agents in the treatment of disseminated *Mycobacterium avium* infections in patients with acquired immunodeficiency syndrome. Arch Intern Med. 1993; 153:368–372.

41. Husson RN, Ross LA, Sandelli S, et al. Orally-administered clarithromycin for the treatment of systemic *Mycobacterium avium* complex infection in children with acquired-immunodeficiency-syndrome. J Pediatr 1994; 124:807–814.

42. David HL. Basis for lack of drug susceptibility of atypical mycobacteria. Rev Infect Dis 1981; 3:878–884.

43. Silve G, Valero-Guillen P, Quemard A, et al. Ethambutol inhibition of glucose metabolism in mycobacteria: a possible target of the drug. Antimicrob Agents Chemother 1993; 37:1536–1538.

44. Takayama K, Kilburn JO. Inhibition of synthesis of arabinogalactan by ethambutol in *Mycobacterium smegmatis*. Antimicrob Agents Chemother 1989; 33: 1493–1499.

45. Rastogi N, Labrousse V. Extracellular and intracellular activities of clarithromycin used alone and in association with ethambutol and rifampin against *Mycobacterium avium* complex. Antimicrob Agents Chemother 1991; 35: 462–470.

46. Stauffer F, Dörtbudak O, Lahnok E. In vitro testing of clarithromycin in combination with ethambutol and rifampin against *Mycobacterium avium* complex. Infect 1991; 19:343–345.

47. Rastogi N, Labrousse V, Goh KS, De SJP. Antimycobacterial spectrum of sparfloxacin and its activities alone and in association with other drugs against *Mycobacterium avium* complex growing extracellularly and intracellularly in murine and human macrophages. Antimicrob Agents Chemother 1991; 35: 2473–2480.

48. Hoffner SE, Kratz M, Olsson-Liljequist B, et al. In-vitro synergistic activity between ethambutol and fluorinated quinolones against *Mycobacterium avium* complex. J Antimicrob Chemother 1989; 24:317–324.

49. Inderlied CB, Barbara-Burnham L, Wu M, et al. Activities of the benzoxazinorifamycin KRM-1648 and ethambutol against mycobacterium avium complex in-vitro and in macrophages. Antimicrob Agents Chemother 1994; 38: 1838–1843.

50. Bermudez LE, Kolonoski P, Young LS, Inderlied CB. Activity of KRM-1648 alone or in combination with ethambutol or clarithromycin against *Mycobacterium avium* in beige mouse model of disseminated infection. Antimicrob Agents Chemother 1994; 38:1844–1848.

51. Rastogi N, Goh KS, David HL. Enhancement of drug susceptibility of *Mycobacterium avium* by inhibitors of cell envelope synthesis. Antimicrob Agents Chemother 1990; 34:759–764.

52. Yamori S, Tsukamura M. Paradoxical effect of Tween 80 between the susceptibility to rifampicin and streptomycin and the susceptibility to ethambutol and sulfadimethoxine in the *Mycobacterium avium-Mycobacterium intracellulare* complex. Microbiol Immunol 1991; 35:921–926.

53. Mizuguchi Y, Ogawa M, Udou T. Morphological changes induced by β-lactam antibiotics in *Mycobacterium avium-intracellulare* complex. Antimicrob Agents Chemother 1985; 27:541–547.

54. Meier A, Kirschner P, Springer B, et al. Identification of mutations in 23S rRNA gene of clarithromycin-resistant *Mycobacterium intracellulare*. Antimicrob Agents Chemother 1994; 38:381–384.

55. Ettayebi M, Prasad SM, Morgan EA. Chloramphenicol-erythromycin resistance mutations in a 23s rRNA gene of Escherichia coli. J Bacteriol 1985; 162: 551–557.

56. Williams DL, Waguespack C, Eisenach K, et al. Characterization of rifampin resistance in pathogenic mycobacteria. Antimicrob Agents Chemother 1994; 38:2380–2386.

57. Telenti A, Imboden P, Marchesi F, et al. Detection of rifampicin-resistance mutations in *Mycobacterium tuberculosis*. Lancet 1993; 341:647–650.

58. Takiff HE, Salazar L, Guerrero C, et al. Cloning and nucleotide-sequence of *Mycobacterium tuberculosis* gyra and gyrb genes and detection of quinolone resistance mutations. Antimicrob Agents Chemother 1994; 38:773–780.

59. Meier A, Kirschner P, Bange FC, et al. Genetic alterations in streptomycin-resistant *Mycobacterium tuberculosis*: mapping of mutations conferring resistance. Antimicrob Agents Chemother 1994; 38:228–233.

60. Honore N, Cole ST. Molecular basis of rifampin resistance in *Mycobacterium leprae*. Antimicrob Agents Chemother 1993; 37:414–418.

61. McCarthy C, Ashbaugh P. Factors that affect the cell cycle of *Mycobacterium avium*. Rev Infect Dis 1981; 3:914–925.

62. McCarthy C. Effect of palmitic acid utilization on cell division in *Mycobacterium avium*. Infect Immun 1974; 9:363–372.

63. McCarthy C. Synthesis and release of sulfolipid by *Mycobacterium avium* during growth and cell division. Infect Immun 1976; 14:1241–1252.

64. McCarthy C. Ammonium ion requirement for the cell cycle of *Mycobacterium avium*. Infect Immun 1978; 19:304–311.

65. McFadden JJ, Butcher PD, Chiodini R, Hermon-Taylor J. Crohn's disease-isolated mycobacteria are identical to *Mycobacterium paratuberculosis*, as determined by DNA probes that distinguish between mycobacterial species. J Clin Microbiol 1987; 25:796–801.

66. Agy MB, Wallis CK, Plorde JJ, et al. Evaluation of four mycobacterial blood culture media: Bactec 13A, Isolator/Bactec 12B, Isolator/Middlebrook agar and a biphasic medium. Diag Microbiol Infect Dis 1989; 12:303–308.

67. Gill VJ, Park CH, Stock F, et al. Use of lysis-centrifugation (Isolator) and radiometric (BACTEC) blood culture systems for the detection of mycobacteria. J Clin Microbiol 1985; 22:543–546.

68. Kiehn TE, Cammarata R. Laboratory diagnosis of mycobacterial infections in patients with acquired immunodeficiency syndrome. J Clin Microbiol 1986; 24:708–711.

69. Salfinger M, Stoll EW, Piot D, Heifets L. Comparison of three methods for recovery of *Mycobacterium avium* complex from blood specimens. J Clin Microbiol 1988; 26:1225–1226.

70. Nightingale SD, Byrd LT, Southern PM, et al. Incidence of *Mycobacterium avium-intracellulare* complex bacteremia in human immunodeficiency virus-positive patients. J Infect Dis 1992; 165:1082–1085.

71. Stone BL, Cohn DL, Kane MS, et al. Utility of paired blood cultures and smears in diagnosis of disseminated *Mycobacterium avium* complex infections in AIDS patients. J Clin Microbiol 1994; 32:841–842.

72. Yagupsky P, Menegus MA. Cumulative positivity rates of multiple blood cultures for *Mycobacterium avium-intracellulare* and Cryptococcus neoformans in patients with the acquired immunodeficiency syndrome. Arch Path Lab Med 1990; 114:923–925.

73. Young LS, Inderlied CB, Berlin OG, Gottlieb MS. Mycobacterial infections in AIDS patients, with an emphasis on the *Mycobacterium avium* complex. Rev Infect Dis 1986; 8:1024–1033.

74. Poropatich CO, Labriola AM, Tuazon CU. Acid-fast smear and culture of respiratory secretions, bone marrow, and stools as predictors of disseminated *Mycobacterium avium* complex infection. J Clin Microbiol 1987; 25:929–930.

75. Morris A, Reller LB, Salfinger M, et al. Mycobacteria in stool specimens: the nonvalue of smears for predicting culture results. J Clin Microbiol 1993; 31: 1385–1387.

76. Horsburgh CR Jr, Metchock BG, McGowan JE, Thompson SE. Clinical implications of recovery of *Mycobacterium avium* complex from the stool or respiratory tract of HIV infected individuals. AIDS 1992; 6:512–514.

77. Chin DP, Hopewell PC, Yajko DM, et al. *Mycobacterium avium* complex in the respiratory or gastrointestinal tract and the risk of *M. avium* complex bacteremia in patients with human immunodeficiency virus infection. J Infect Dis 1994; 169:289–295.

78. Havlik JA Jr, Metchock B, Thompson SE3, et al. A prospective evaluation of *Mycobacterium avium* complex colonization of the respiratory and gastrointestinal tracts of persons with human immunodeficiency virus infection. J Infect Dis 1993; 168:1045–1048.

79. Kilby JM, Gilligan PH, Yankaskas JR, et al. Nontuberculous mycobacteria in adult patients with cystic fibrosis. Chest 1992; 102:70–75.

80. Marchevsky A, Damsker B, Gribetz A, et al. The spectrum of pathology of nontuberculous mycobacterial infections in open-lung biopsy specimens. Amer J Clin Pathol 1982; 78:695–700.

81. Hoffner SE. Improved detection of *Mycobacterium avium* complex with the Bactec radiometric system. Diag Microbiol Infect Dis 1988; 10:1–6

82. Kirihara JM, Hillier SL, Coyle MB. Improved detection times for *Mycobacterium avium* complex and *Mycobacterium tuberculosis* with the BACTEC radiometric system. J Clin Micobiol 1985; 22:841–845.

83. Kiehn TE, Cammarata R. Comparative recoveries of *Mycobacterium avium-M. intracellulare* from Isolator lysis-centrifugation and BACTEC 13A blood culture systems. J Clin Microbiol 1988; 26:760–761.

84. Strand CL, Epstein C, Verzosa S, et al. Evaluation of a new blood culture medium for mycobacteria. Amer J Clin Path 1989; 91:316–318.

85. Wasilauskas B, Morrell R Jr. Inhibitory effect of the Isolator blood culture system on growth of *Mycobacterium avium-M. intracellulare* in BACTEC 12B bottles. J Clin Microbiol 1994; 32:654–657.

86. Katila ML, Mattila J. Enhanced isolation of MOTT on egg media of low pH. APMIS 1991; 99:803–807.

87. Isenberg HD, D'Amato RF, Heifets L, et al. Collaborative feasibility study of biphasic system (Roche Septi-Chek AFB) for the rapid detection and isolation of mycobacteria. J Clin Microbiol 1991; 29:1719–1722.

88. D'Amato RF, Isenberg HD, Hochstein L, et al. Evaluation of the Roche Septi-Chek AFB system for recovery of mycobacteria. J Clin Microbiol 1991; 29: 2906–2908.

89. Piersimoni C, Morbiducci V, De-Sio G, Scalise G. Comparative evaluation of the MB-Check system for recovery of mycobacteria from clinical specimens. Eur J Clin Microbiol Infect Dis 1992; 11:1174–1177.

90. Hoffner SE, Haile M, Källenius G. A biphasic system for primary isolation of mycobacteria compared to solid medium and broth culture. J Med Microbiol 1992; 37:332–334.

91. Abe C, Hosojima S, Fukasawa Y, et al. Comparison of MB-Check, BACTEC, and egg-based media for recovery of mycobacteria. J Clin Microbiol 1992; 30: 878–881.

92. Havlir DV, Keyes L, Davis C. Measurement of *Mycobacterium avium* bacteremia; quantitative Isolator lysis centrifugation versus BACTEC 13A blood culture systems. Program Abstr. 31st Intersci Conf Antimicrob Agents Chemother, Chicago, 1991.

93. Havlir D, Kemper CA, Deresinski SC. Reproducibility of lysis-centrifugation cultures for quantification of *Mycobacterium avium* complex bacteremia. J Clin Microbiol 1993; 31:1794–1798.

94. von Reyn CF, Hennigan S, Niemczyk S, Jacobs NJ. Effect of delays in processing on the survival of *Mycobacterium avium- M. intracellulare* in the Isolator blood culture system. J Clin Microbiol 1991; 29:1211–1214.

95. Drake TA, Herron RM, Hindler JA, et al. DNA probe reactivity of *Mycobacterium avium* complex isolates from patients without AIDS. Diag Microbiol Infect Dis 1988; 11:125–128.

96. Gonzalez R, Hanna BA. Evaluation of GenProbe DNA hybridization systems for the identification of *Mycobacterium tuberculosis* and *Mycobacterium avium-intracellulare*. Diag Microbiol Infect Dis 1987; 8:69–77.

97. Lim SD, Todd J, Lopez J, et al. Genotypic identification of pathogenic mycobacterium species by using a nonradioactive oligonucleotide probe. J Clin Microbiol 1991; 29:1276–1278.

98. Picken RN, Plotch SJ, Wang Z, et al. DNA probes for *Mycobacteria. i.* Isolation of DNA probes for the identification of *Mycobacterium tuberculosis* complex and for mycobacteria other than tuberculosis (MOTT). Mol Cell Probes 1988; 2:111–124.

99. Sherman I, Harrington N, Rothrock A, George H. Use of a cutoff range in identifying mycobacteria by the GenProbe Rapid Diagnostic System. J Clin Microbiol 1989; 27:241–244.

100. Body BA, Warren NG, Spicer A, et al. Use of Gen-Probe and Bactec for rapid isolation and identification of mycobacteria. Correlation of probe results with growth index. Amer J Clin Pathol 1990; 93:415–420.

101. Goto M, Oka S. Okuzumi K, et al. Evaluation of acridinium-ester–labeled DNA probes for identification of *Mycobacterium tuberculosis* and *Mycobacterium avium-Mycobacterium intracellulare* complex in culture. J Clin Microbiol 1991; 29:2473–2476.

102. Lumb R, Lanser JA, Lim IS. Rapid identification of mycobacteria by GenProbe Accuprobe system. Pathology 1993; 25:313–315.

103. Musial CE, Tice LS, Stockman L, Roberts GD. Identification of mycobacteria from culture by using the GenProbe Rapid Diagnostic System for *Mycobacterium avium* complex and *Mycobacterium tuberculosis* complex. J Clin Microbiol 1988; 26:2120–2123.

104. Lebrun L, Espinasse F, Poveda JD, Vincent-Levy-Frebault V. Evaluation of nonradioactive DNA probes for identification of mycobacteria. J Clin Microbiol 1992; 30:2476–2478.

105. Fourche J, Capdepuy M, Maugein J, Le MF. Analysis of cellular fatty acids and proteins by capillary gas chromatography and sodium dodecyl sulphate polyacrylamide gel electrophoresis to differentiate *Mycobacterium avium*, *Mycobacterium intracellulare* and *Mycobacterium scrofulaceum* (MAIS) complex species. J Chromatography 1990; 532:209–216.

106. Woods GL. Disease due to the *Mycobacterium avium* complex in patients infected with human immunodeficiency virus: diagnosis and susceptibility testing. Clin Infect Dis 1994; 18:S227–S232.

107. Wayne LG. The "atypical" mycobacteria: recognition and disease association. CRC Crit Rev Microbiol 1985; 12:185–222.

108. Chapin-Robertson K, Dahlberg S, Waycott S, et al. Detection and identification of Mycobacterium directly from BACTEC bottles by using a DNA-rRNA probe. Diag Microbiol Infect Dis 1993; 17:203–207.

109. Peterson EM, Lu R, Floyd C, et al. Direct identification of *Mycobacterium tuberculosis*, *Mycobacterium avium*, and *Mycobacterium intracellulare* from amplified primary cultures in BACTEC media using DNA probes. J Clin Microbiol 1989; 27:1543–1547.

110. Evans KD, Nakasone AS, Sutherland PA, et al. Identification of *Mycobacterium tuberculosis* and *Mycobacterium avium-intracellulare* directly from primary BACTEC cultures by using acridinium-ester-labeled DNA probes. J Clin Microbil 1992; 30:2427–2431.

111. Eng RHK, Bishburg E, Smith SM, Mangia A. Diagnosis of mycobacterium bacteremia in patients with acquired immunodeficiency syndrome by direct examination of blood films. J Clin Microbiol 1989; 27:768–769.

112. Godwin JC, Stopeck A, Chang VT, Godwin TA. Mycobacteremia in acquired immune deficiency syndrome: rapid diagnosis based on inclusions in the peripheral blood smear. Amer J Clin Path 1991; 95:369–375.

113. Nussbaum JM, Dealist C, Lewis W, Heseltine PNR. Rapid diagnosis by buffy coat smear of disseminated *Mycobacterium avium* complex infection in patients with acquired immunodeficiency syndrome. J Clin Microbiol 1990; 28:631–632.

114. Uribe-Botero G, Prichard JG, Kapalowitz HJ. Bone marrow in HIV infection. A comparison of fluorescent staining and cultures in the detection of mycobacteria. Amer J Clin Path 1989; 91:313–315.

115. Torres RA, Nord J, Feldman R, et al. Disseminated mixed *Mycobacterium simiae-Mycobacterium avium* complex infection in acquired immunodeficiency syndrome. J Infect Dis 1991; 164:432–433.

116. Wiley EL, Mulhollan TJ, Beck B, et al. Polyclonal antibodies raised against Bacillus Calmette-Guerin, *Mycobacterium duvalii*, and *Mycobacterium paratuberculosis* used to detect mycobacteria in tissue with the use of immunohistochemical techniques. Amer J Clin Path 1990; 94:307–312.

117. Wiley EL, Perry A, Nightingale SD, Lawrence J. Detection of *Mycobacterium avium-intracellulare* complex in bone marrow specimens of patients with acquired immunodeficiency syndrome. Amer J Clin Path 1994; 101:446–451.

118. Sippola AA, Gillespie SL, Daniel TM. Diagnosis of *Mycobacterium avium* disease in AIDS patients by detection of *M. avium* antigenuria. Clin Res 1992; 40:695A.

119. Hance AJ, Grandchamp B, Levy FV, et al. Detection and identification of mycobacteria by amplification of mycobacterial DNA. Mol Microbiol 1989; 3: 843–849.

120. Telenti A, Marchesi F, Balz M, et al. Rapid identification of mycobacteria to the species level by polymerase chain-reaction and restriction enzyme analysis. J Clin Microbiol 1993; 31:175–178.

121. Ghossein RA, Ross DG, Salomon RN, Rabson AR. Rapid detection and species identification of mycobacteria in paraffin-embedded tissues by polymerase chain reaction. Diag Mol Path 1992; 1:185–191.

122. Perosio PM, Frank TS. Detection and species identification of mycobacteria in paraffin sections of lung biopsy specimens by the polymerase chain reaction. Amer J Clin Path 1993; 100:643–647.

123. Plikaytis BB, Plikaytis BD, Yakrus MA, et al. Differentiation of slowly growing mycobacterium species, including *Mycobacterium tuberculosis*, by gene amplification and restriction fragment length polymorphism analysis. J Clin Microbiol 1992; 30:1815–1822.

124. Kunze ZM, Portaels F, McFadden JJ. Biologically distinct subtypes of *Mycobacterium avium* differ in possession of insertion sequence IS901. J Clin Microbiol 1992; 30:2366–2372.

125. McFadden JJ, Kunze ZM, Portaels F, et al. Epidemiological and genetic markers, virulence factors and intracellular growth of *Mycobacterium avium* in AIDS. Res Microbiol 1992; 143:423–430.

126. Eisenach KD, Cave MD, Bates JH, Crawford JT. Polymerase chain reaction amplification of a repetitive DNA sequence specific for *Mycobacterium tuberculosis*. J Infect Dis 1990; 161:977–981.

127. Boddinghaus B, Rogall T, Flohr T, et al. Detection and identification of mycobacteria by amplification of rRNA. J Clin Microbiol 1990; 28:1751–1759.

128. Jonas V, Alden MJ, Curry JI, et al. Detection and identification of *Mycobacterium tuberculosis* directly from sputum sediments by amplifications of rRNA. J Clin Microbiol 1993; 31:2410–2416.
129. Inderlied CB. Antimycobacterial agents: in vitro susceptibility testing, spectrums of activity, mechanisms of action and resistance, and assays for activity in biological fluids. In: Lorian V, eds. Antibotics in Laboratory Medicine. Baltimore: Williams & Wilkins, 1991:134–197.
130. Heifets L, Iseman M, Lindholm-Levy P. Ethambutol MICs and MBCs for *Mycobacterium avium* complex and *Mycobacterium tuberculosis*. Antimicrob Agents Chemother 1986; 30:927–932.
131. Heifets L. MIC as a quantitative measurement of the susceptibility of *Mycobacterium avium* strains to seven antituberculosis drugs. Antimicrob Agents Chemother 1988; 32:1131–1136.
132. Inderlied CB, Young LS, Yamada JK. Determination of in vitro susceptibility of *Mycobacterium avium* complex isolates to antimicrobial agents by various methods. Antimicrob Agents Chemother 1987; 31:1697–1702.
133. Tsukamura M, Miyachi T. Correlations among naturally occurring resistances to antituberculosis drugs in *Mycobacterium avium* complex strains. Am Rev Respir Dis 1989; 139:1033–1035.
134. Horsburgh CR Jr, Cohn DL, Roberts RB, et al. *Mycobacterium avium-M. intracellulare* isolates from patients with or without acquired immunodeficiency syndrome. Antimicrob Agents Chemother 1986; 30:955–957.
135. Heifets L, Lindholm-Levy P. Comparison of bactericidal activities of streptomycin, amikacin, kanamycin, and capreomycin against *Mycobacterium avium* and *M. tuberculosis*. Antimicrob Agents Chemother 1989; 33:1298–1301.
136. Benson CA. Treatment of disseminated disease due to the *Mycobacterium avium* complex in patients with AIDS. Clin Infect Dis 1994; 18:S237–S242.
137. Wallace RJ Jr, Brown BA, Griffith DE, et al. Initial clarithromycin monotherapy for *Mycobacterium avium–intracellulare* complex lung disease. Amer J Respir Crit Care Med 1994; 149:1335–1341.
138. Heifets LB, Lindholm-Levy PJ, Comstock RD. Clarithromycin minimal inhibitory and bactericidal concentrations against *Mycobacterium avium*. Am Rev Respir Dis 1992; 145:856–858.
139. Heifets L, Mor N, Vanderkolk J. *Mycobacterium avium* strains resistant to clarithromycin and azithromycin. Antimicrob Agents Chemother 1993; 37:2364–2370.
140. Heifets L. Qualitative and quantitative drug-susceptibility tests in mycobacteriology. Amer Rev Respir Dis 1988; 137:1217–1222.
141. Siddiqi SH, Heifets LB, Cynamon MH, et al. Rapid broth macrodilution method for determination of MICs for *Mycobacterium avium* isolates. J Clin Microbiol 1993; 31:2332–2338.
142. Yajko DM, Nassos PS, Hadley WK. Broth microdilution testing of susceptibilities to 30 antimicrobial agents of *Mycobacterium avium* strains from pa-

tients with acquired immune deficiency syndrome. Antimicrob Agents Chemother 1987; 31:1579–1584.

143. National Committee for Clinical Laboratory Standards. Methods for Determining Bactericidal Activity of Antimicrobial Agents (M26-P). Villanova, PA: National Committee for Clinical Laboratory Standards, 1987,

144. Siddiqi SH. Radiometric (Bactec) tests for slowly growing mycobacteria. In: Isenberg HD, ed. Clinical Microbiology Procedures Handbook. Washington, DC: American Society for Microbiology, 1992: 5.14.1–5.14.25.

145. Heifets LB, Iseman MD. Choice of antimicrobial agents for *M. avium* disease based on quantitative tests of drug susceptibility. N Engl J Med 1990; 323: 419–420.

146. Zimmer BL, DeYoung DR, Roberts GD. In vitro synergistic activity of ethambutol, isoniazid, kanamycin, rifampin, and streptomycin against *Mycobacterium avium-intracellulare* complex. Antimicrob Agents Chemother 1982; 22:148–150.

147. Heifets LB. Synergistic effect of rifampin, streptomycin, ethionamide, and ethambutol on *Mycobacterium intracellulare*. Amer Rev Respir Dis 1982; 125: 43–48.

148. Hoffner SE, Svenson SB, Källenius G. Synergistic effects of antimycobacterial drug combinations of *Mycobacterium avium* complex determined radiometrically in liquid medium. Eur J Clin Microbiol 1987; 6:530–555.

149. Hoffner SE, Heurlin N, Petrini B, et al. *Mycobacterium avium* complex develop resistance to synergistically active-drug combinations during infection. Eur Respir J 1994; 7:247–250.

150. Telenti A, Imboden P, Marchesi F, et al. Direct automated detection of rifampin-resistant *Mycobacterium tuberculosis* by polymerase chain-reaction and single-strand conformation polymorphism analysis. Antimicrob Agents Chemother 1993; 37:2054–2058.

151. Jacobs WR Jr, Barletta RG, Udani R, et al. Rapid assessment of drug susceptibilities of *Mycobacterium tuberculosis* by means of luciferase reporter phages. Science 1993; 260:819–822.

152. Cooksey RC, Crawford JT, Jacobs WR Jr, Shinnick TM. A rapid method for screening antimicrobial agents for activities against a strain of *Mycobacterium tuberculosis* expressing firefly luciferase. Antimicrob Agents Chemother 1993; 37:1348–1352.

6

Animal Models in Anti-*Mycobacterium avium*-Complex Drug Development

LOWELL S. YOUNG and LUIZ E. BERMUDEZ

Kuzell Institute for Arthritis and Infectious Diseases
California Pacific Medical Center Research Institute
San Francisco, California

I. Introduction

The advent of the acquired immunodeficiency syndrome (AIDS) pandemic has led a number of investigators to evaluate the chemotherapy of opportunistic infection in suitable animal models. Many of the opportunistic pathogens encountered in AIDS were uncommonly observed in immunosuppressed patients prior to 1975. This is particularly true of organisms such as *Pneumocystis carinii* and those that belong to the *Mycobacterium avium* complex (MAC).

The long duration of immunosuppression before the onset of MAC disease is a factor which underscores the difficulty of finding a suitable animal test system for evaluating *M. avium* chemotherapy. MAC organisms are slow growing, and thus we have a problem of finding a suitable animal system that is susceptible to MAC and where further manipulations in pathological conditions might be analogous to what is seen in patients with AIDS.

141

An animal model is one that faithfully seeks to duplicate the abnormality that is seen in humans and on exposure to an infectious agent leads to disease by an identical pathogenetic mechanism. An animal test system, however imperfect, allows the investigator to derive knowledge from the study of in vivo infection. As we shall see, no ideal animal model of MAC disease exists. Intuitively, we could hypothesize that a higher mammal infected (i.e., primate) with a retroviral infection that acts in a manner analogous to human immunodeficiency virus 1 (HIV-1) and has a similar chronic effect on the immune system with a long period of clinical latency would be the most appropriate candidate. However, to develop such a model would not be easy and the constraints of time over which period the immune system would be suppressed would be a major factor limiting the development of such an experimental system.

One can easily list the characteristics of a desirable animal model. These characteristics would include:

1. Ease of manipulation.
2. Affordable.
3. Highly reproducible.
4. Mimic pathological changes observed in human disease
5. When drugs are administered in vivo they have similar pharmacokinetics, toxicities and interactions as in human subjects.
6. The animal has an immunological disorder predisposing to infection that parallels human disease states.

Some might question point number 6. Providing that the host can be infected with resultant similar pathogenic changes, it may not be obligatory to have a similar immunological defect.

Another important point to consider is the interaction between the host and the parasite. Although the emphasis on the mammalian host for MAC is obvious, one should not forget that there are two elements to any experimental infection: a susceptible host and a virulent challenge organism. Although much of the literature has emphasized the search for suitable animals to be challenged by routes that mimic human disease, we should not forget that in the search for a fairly reliable system for evaluating chemotherapy the role of the organism is as important as the susceptible host.

It has long been appreciated that MAC organisms assume different morphotypes when grown on agar and that organism growing in smooth transparent colonies are more virulent than organisms from opaque colonies (1). It is important to note when employing MAC organisms in animal testing, if one continually cultures MAC organisms in vitro, and initially smooth

Table 1 Some Therapeutic Agents Found to Be Active Against MAC in Vivo (Approximate Chronology)

Drugs	Mouse strain	Investigators
Rifabutin	Beige	Gangadharam et al., 1987 (5)
Rifabutin	Thymectomized mice	Orme, 1988 (10)
Clofazimine	Beige	Gangadharam et al., 1987 (5)
Ethambutol	Beige	Gangadharam et al., 1987 (5)
Amikacin	Beige	Gangadharam et al., 1988 (33)
Amikacin	Beige	Bertram et al., 1986 (8)
Liposome amikacin	Beige	Duzgunes et al., 1988 (35)
Liposome amikacin	Beige	Cynamon et al., 1988 (36)
Clarithromycin	Beige	Fernandez et al., 1989 (42)
Azithromycin, liposome amikacin	Beige	Bermudez et al., 1990 (34)
Paromomycin	Beige	Kanyok et al., 1994 (39)
Clarithromycin	Beige	Ji et al., 1991 (32)
Streptomycin	Beige	Gangadharam et al., 1991 (54)
Liposome streptomycin	Beige	Gangadharam et al., 1991 (54)
Liposome streptomycin	Beige	Duzgunes et al., 1991 (55)
KRM 1648	Beige	Tomioka et al., 1992 (29)
Gangamycin/Azaquinone	Beige	Gangadharam et al., 1993
KRM 1648	Beige	Bermudez et al., 1994 (24)
Liposome gentamicin	Beige	Bermudez et al., 1990 (34)
Bay Y 3118	Beige	Bermudez et al., 1994 (submitted)
Sparfloxacin	Beige	Bermudez et al., 1992 (submitted)

transparent form will revert to a smooth opaque and less virulent morphotype (i.e., the LD_{50} of these opaque forms increases, so more organisms are needed to achieve lethality or sustained bacteremia). In addition, one should also employ serovars of MAC that are similar to what is encountered in pulmonary or AIDS-associated disease depending on what the goal of the study is. Last, one should remember that the dissociants of virulent strains (originally smooth opaque colonies assuming the ''ground glass'' morphotype) generally are more antibiotic susceptible and less virulent in animals (2,3).

II. Specific Experimental Test Systems

A. Beige Mouse

Collins was the first to show that mice could be infected with MAC (4). However, in his mice, the progression of disease was extremely slow, making them unsuitable for chemotherapeutic studies. The murine species that subsequently has been utilized most often to evaluate drug efficacy and host immune response against MAC has been the beige mouse (C57/BL6 bg$^+$/bg$^+$), which is a test system first described by Gangadharam and colleagues (5). Despite their susceptibility to infection, these mice are easy to handle and do not require special caging or protective isolation. For establishment of infection, it is not necessary to use specific antibodies against membrane antigens for depletion of cell populations or to use immunosuppressive drugs. Beige mice are susceptible to MAC infection and depending on the MAC

Table 2 Some Murine/Rodent Species that Have Been Used to Study Experimental Infections

Mouse strain	Investigators
Balb/c	Tomioka 1992 (29)
C57BL/6	Collins et al., 1987 (4)
C57 bg$^+$/bg$^+$	Gangadharam, et al., 1983 (5)
CD4$^+$ T cell deficient	Furney et al., 1990 (11)
Cyclosporine	Sheldon Brown et al., (13)
Hens	Meissner, 1981 (17)
MAIDS	Orme, 1988 (10)
SCID	Appelberg et al., 1994 (16)
Thymectomized	Orme, 1988 (10)
Nude	Ji et al., 1992 (15)

strain used in them to establish bacteremia (which can be quantitated), the tissue level of infection is usually consistent and predictable. The nature of the immunodeficiency in beige mice has not been fully defined but is believed to be both a defect in natural killer (NK) cells and T helper lymphocyte function. The beige mouse is considered the murine equivalent to the Chédiak-Higashi syndrome in humans, in which abnormalities of the degranulation of lysosomes and migration of neutrophils are observed. Although neutrophils from beige mice show these abnormalities, apparently macrophages have no functional difference from the macrophages of C57BL/6 black mice (6,7). The fact that beige mice are direct descendants of C57BL/6 mice, considered to be the best murine model available for *M. tuberculosis* infections, and that they have deficiencies in immune functions similar to those observed in patients with AIDS, makes them attractive (7). Infection of beige mice with transparent morphotypes of *M. avium* usually leads to the development of disseminated disease with large numbers of bacteria being isolated from blood, spleen, liver, and lungs (8).

To establish the baseline infection, beige mice (6–8 weeks old, average weight 20 g) are inoculated intravenously, by tail vein injection, with approximately 3×10^7 colony-forming units (CFU) of MAC strain 101 (or other known virulent clinical strains) in 0.1 ml of saline. After 1 week, blood specimens are drawn from the tail vein and 0.05 ml of blood is inoculated into Bactec 12B vials. The quantity of bacteria, expressed as CFU/ml, is determined by T100 analysis first described by Inderlied and colleagues (9). In the protocol most commonly followed in our laboratory, drug therapy is initiated after the initial blood culture is determined to be positive and continued for 28 days. One day after the last dose of antimicrobial(s), mice are bled a second time for quantitative culture and then killed by cervical dis-

Table 3 Agents Shown to Be Active Against MAC in Vivo

Drug	Animal	Treatment	Prophylaxis	Reference
Clarithromycin	Mouse	Yes	Yes	26, 44, 45
Azithromycin	Mouse/rat	Yes	Yes	47, 49
Rifabutin	Mouse	Yes	No	26, 30
KRM 1648	Mouse/rabbit	Yes	Not tested	27, 33, 34
Amikacin	Mouse	Yes	Not tested	35, 51
Ethambutol	Mouse	Yes	Not tested	26, 54

Not all experimental studies are listed: We have indicated initial reports but where there is duplication of the experimental methods and/or vehicles may have different significance.

location. Animals are then transferred to an externally vented biocontainment hood. Liver and spleen are dissected, weighed, and homogenized with sterile glass homogenizers in 5 ml of 7H9 broth containing 20% glycerol. Serial dilutions of the organ homogenates are made in 7H9 broth and plated onto Middlebrook 7H11 agar plates in duplicate. Plates are incubated at 37°C for 7–10 days, after which numbers of colonies are counted. The CFU/g of tissue is calculated as follows:

$$\text{CFU/g tissue} = \frac{\text{average number of CFU/plate} \times \text{dilution factor} \times 5 \text{ ml}}{\text{organ weight}}$$

For purposes of statistical analysis, we compare pretreatment bacteremia and organ burden with that quantitated 28 days later.

B. Other Rodent Models

Thymectomized and CD4⁺ T Cell–Depleted Mice

Both mouse models are based on the observation that $CD4^+$ T lymphocytes are important to the mechanisms of host defense against MAC.

Mice are thymectomized at 4 weeks of age and 1 week later given anti-CD4 monoclonal antibody (approximately 250 μg) intravenously (IV). $CD4^+$ T cells are enumerated by either fluorescent microscopy or flow cytometer analysis. According to data obtained by Orme and colleagues (10), this mouse system contains fewer T cells bearing the CD4 marker than any other animal host available. The number of CD4 T cells is usually reduced by approximately 90%. T-cell responsiveness to mitogens such as phytohemaglutinin and concanavalin A is severely reduced, usually barely above background control responses (10). Infection with *M. avium* strains are markedly exacerbated by direction depletion of CD4 T cells as determined by the number of bacteria in organs.

C57/BL6 black mice have also been depleted of T lymphocytes by the use of anti-Thy 1.2, $L3T4^+$, and $Lyt2^+$ monoclonal antibody (11). The use of anti-Thy 1.2 antibody resulted in enhanced growth of MAC in spleen and lung, but use of $L3T4^+$ (anti-CD4) or $Lyt2^+$ (anti-CD8) by themselves did not greatly abate the expression of the immunity in the recipient.

Major problems in applying these T cell–deficient mice to the screen of anti-MAC activity of antimicrobials is that it is a very expensive model and also it requires close monitoring of the number of lymphocytes. Nonetheless, there is always the possibility that at any moment during the course of infection, the number of T cells in antibody-treated mice would not fall into the same consistent range, therefore making interpretation of data difficult.

C. MAIDS Model

In the MAIDS model, C57/BL6 mice are infected with the LP-BPM5 retrovirus and develop an immunodeficiency that is similar to the one found in patients with AIDS (10). Although $CD4^+$ T cells are normal in number, they show signs of prominent functional deficits 6 weeks after infection with LP-BM5 virus. Enhanced susceptibility to a series of infectious agents has been shown with the MAIDS model, such as cytomegalovirus, *Toxoplasma gondii*, *Trypanosoma cruzi*, *Cryptosporidium parvum*, and *Listeria monocytogenes* (12). Studies by Orme and colleagues showed that MAIDS mice infected with MAC had a marked enhancement of MAC replication with an average of 0.5 log to 1 log greater number of organisms in spleen and liver than beige mice.

We have used the same system and determined that MAIDS mice have greater mortality than beige mice at 4 weeks after infection. The MAIDS mouse can be infected with smaller numbers of bacteria and reflect a number of the abnormalities observed in patients with AIDS.

Nonetheless, the mechanisms responsible for these effects have not been explored in depth. Although the MAIDS mouse seems close to the ideal animal model, for purposes of drug screening in vivo against MAC, it is expensive. Furthermore, a drawback of the MAIDS model is that viruses present in mixtures of LP-BM5 have been shown to include a complex of replication-competent and replication-defective viruses (12).

D. Rates Immunosuppressed with Cyclosporin A

A new rodent system susceptible to disseminated MAC infection has recently been described in Sprague-Dawley rats immunosuppressed with cyclosporin A (13). Rats are immunosuppressed with the administration of 20 mg/kg of body weight by cyclosporin A twice a week and 40 mg/kg once a week. MAC infection can be established in the model, but the number of bacteria in spleen or liver do not increase. An increase in the number of organisms was reported in the lung.

An obvious deficiency of this model as a model to screen anti-MAC antimicrobials is that cyclosporin A has been reported to have pharmacokinetic interactions with a number of drugs, including rifamycins and macrolides (14). Furthermore, rifamycins may induce increased hepatic metabolism of cyclosporin A, thus causing reversal of the immunological deficiency.

E. SCID and Nude Mouse Models

Recent studies comparing the growth of MAC in SCID and nude mice demonstrated that although those models can be extremely useful for immunological studies, the observations do not suggest that they are better than the beige mouse for evaluation of an anti-MAC therapy (15,16).

Since SCID mice still have natural killer cells, we have found them in preliminary experiments to be less susceptible than beige mice to MAC infection. We are now working with another genetic variant, SCID-beige mice.

F. Oral Infection System (Beige Mouse)

In this model of MAC infection, C57/BL6 beige mice are given 1×10^4 bacteria orally every other day for 10 days (total five doses, 5×10^4 bacteria). After 4 weeks, 100% of the animals developed disseminated disease and approximately 30–40% had bacteremia (17). The presence of bacteremia has been shown to be dependent on the MAC strain used.

This alternative model to intravenously or intraperitoneally infected rodents offers a series of advantages in studying the activity of antimicrobial agents against MAC in vivo. First, it is an attempt to mimic MAC infection in patients with AIDS, patients in which evidence indicates that the gastrointestinal route is likely to be the most common manner of acquiring MAC (18,19). Second, the animal model is suitable for investigating the prophylactic use of oral antimicrobials against MAC. Third, the presence of large numbers of organisms in the gut and appendix, resembling the human infection, could allow for the better evaluation of therapeutic efficacy of certain antimicrobials. Finally, the use of the gut model of infection allows for the evaluation of possible cofactors in MAC infection, such as other concurrent infections and the ingestion of ethanol or substances of abuse.

III. Evaluation of Anti-MAC Activity Therapy Using a Rodent Test System

In contrast to *Mycobacterium tuberculosis*, MAC is resistant to most of the available antituberculosis antimicrobials. Through an enormous effort, treatment regimens with significant activity against MAC infections have been established. Successful treatment of established infections probably requires combination therapy with two or more effective antimicrobials. Investigators should use a transparent morphotype of a MAC strain belonging to serovars commonly found in AIDS patients; that is 1, 4, and 8.

A. Ethambutol

Ethambutol is a dextro-2-2'-(ethylenedimino)-di-1-butahol-dihydrochloride with a high degree of antituberculous activity. A recent analysis demonstrated that only 7% of the MAC isolates tested were susceptible to 5 μg/ml of ethambutol per milliliter, but 76% of the isolates were susceptible to 10 μg/ml (1). Although these results suggest that ethambutol is not a very active agent, recent studies demonstrated that ethambutol potentiates the anti-MAC activity of other compounds (20). A recent animal study by Gosey and colleagues (21) showed that ethambutol used as a single agent (100 mg/kg/day) for 9 weeks reduced the bacterial load in the spleen by approximately 1.0 $\log_{10}$. Furthermore, Kemper and colleagues (22) showed that ethambutol used as a single dose in humans (15 mg/kg/day) reduced MAC bacteremia by 0.6 $\log_{10}$ CFU/ml after 4 weeks in patients with AIDS.

In our own experience with beige mice, treatment of MAC infection with ethambutol at 100 mg/kg/day was associated with 0.6 $\log_{10}$, 0.65 $\log_{10}$, and 0.56 $\log_{10}$ reduction in bacteremia, and CFU/g in liver and spleen, respectively, at 4 weeks of therapy. Combination of ethambutol with clarithromycin or with clarithromycin and clofazimine was shown to be superior to clarithromycin alone (23). Unfortunately, these results cannot be interpreted because of the absence of necessary controls in the study, such as a group of mice receiving ethambutol alone and a group of mice receiving the combination of ethambutol and clofazimine.

In a separate report of ethambutol used at 100 mg/kg/day for 4 weeks in combination with KRM 1648, a new benzoxazinorifamycin, was not significantly better than KRM 1648 alone (24).

B. Rifabutin

Rifabutin is an ansamycin derived from rifamycin-S, and has significantly better in vitro activity against MAC compared with rifampin (25). Rifabutin is concentrated in tissues 5–10 times the serum level (25). Strains of MAC that are highly resistant to rifampin are also resistant to rifabutin.

Several studies evaluated the efficacy of rifabutin against MAC strains in the beige mouse model. Rifabutin administered in combination with clarithromycin at 20 mg/kg/day for 10 days was significantly more active than clarithromycin alone in one study (23). However, again, the lack of control group treated with rifabutin alone makes the results difficult to interpret.

In another study by Lazard and colleagues (26) using beige mice, rifabutin administered at 40 mg/kg/day was as effective as clarithromycin (50 mg/kg/day) in the spleen and in the lung after 15 and 21 days of treatment. Treatment of disseminated MAC infection with rifabutin was also reported using two other animal test systems. In one study, rifabutin was administered at 40 mg/kg/day to thymectomized, CD4[+] T cell–deficient mice for 120 days (27). It was shown that the load of bacteria in liver and spleen could be significantly decreased and in some cases sterilized by the treatment. However, the investigators did not follow the animals long enough to make sure that they had achieved sterilization.

Rifabutin was also used in cyclosporin-treated rats to treat MAC infection (13). In this model, rifabutin at 20 mg/kg/day for 68 days showed greater activity than azithromycin and rifapentine, achieving reduction in bacterial load of 2–4 log_{10} in the spleen, liver, and lung. However, those results are difficult to interpret because rifabutin can in theory increase the metabolism of cyclosporin A in the liver; therefore, diminishing the degree of immunosuppression in this model and consequently making the rats more resistant to MAC infection.

C. KRM 1648

KRM 1648, a new benzoxazinorifamycin, exhibited strong activity against mycobacteria, especially MAC (28), with minimal inhibitory concentration (MIC) severalfold smaller than rifampin MIC's.

KRM 1648 has recently been evaluated in two animal species, the beige mouse and in rabbits. In both models, KRM 1648 has been shown to be bactericidal against *M. avium* and *M. intracellulare* strains (29,30).

We have evaluated three concentrations of KRM 1648: 10, 20, and 40 mg/kg/day. Although 10 mg/kg/day during 4 weeks did not result in significant reduction of bacteremia and bacterial load in spleen and liver, both 20 and 40 mg/kg resulted in significant reduction of infection, with reductions of 0.4–0.7 log_{10} in bacterial load (26).

Combination of KRM 1648 (40 mg/kg/day) with ethambutol (100 mg/kg/day) was not significantly better than KRM 1648 alone.

D. Clofazimine

Clofazimine is an iminophenazine red dye with a long elimination half-life. The elimination of the drug from fatty tissues as well as macrophages takes approximately 70 days (31). The drug has been shown to be active in vitro against most of the MAC strains. In the beige mouse test system, one study has shown modest inhibitory activity at 20 mg/kg/day. Our own unpublished experience has shown that clofazimine has bacteriostatic activity in MAC-infected beige mice treated for 4 weeks, and that it was equally effective in liver and spleen. However, all the in vivo studies using clofazimine to treat MAC infection present two major problems: (1) It is possible that the period of therapy used in the studies published thus far has been insufficient for maximal concentration of the clofazimine in tissues; and (2) because clofazimine achieves high concentrations in tissues and has a long elimination period, organs harvested from mice that received clofazimine would contain a high concentration of the drug. Therefore, it is very plausible that a ''carryover'' effect (the presence of clofazimine still in inhibitory concentrations on the agar plates) would be very difficult to avoid, making the drug appear more efficacious than it is in reality (32). Further studies are needed in animals to address these specific issues.

E. Amikacin

Amikacin, a semisynthetic aminoglycoside antibiotic derived from kanamycin, is one of the most bactericidal agents against MAC both in vitro as well as in beige mice (9,33). It was initially shown by Gangadharam and colleagues that amikacin when administered at a dose of 50 mg/kg/day was active against MAC strains in beige mice (33). Administration of amikacin resulted in 1.2–2.6 $\log_{10}$ reduction in CFU/g spleen and liver after 4 weeks of therapy.

Amikacin as long-term therapy in humans, however, has two major drawbacks. First, it is not absorbed from the gastrointestinal tract, therefore requiring parenteral administration, and second, it has substantial nephrotoxicity and ototoxicity. Because of its toxicity, amikacin as well as other aminoglycosides with less activity against MAC, such as gentamicin and streptomycin, have been encapsulated within liposomes. Liposomes are lipid preparations that can encapsulate antibiotics (with both hydrophobic and hydrophilic) properties under specific conditions. Theoretically, liposomes can deliver high concentrations of antimicrobial agents to intracellular locations following phagocytosis or endocytosis, with activity directed toward intracellular pathogens. Theoretically, antimicrobials encapsulated in liposomes could be administered at lower doses and reduce the risk of dose-related side effects. Liposome encapsulation has enhanced the activity of amikacin, gentamicin, and streptomycin against MAC in beige mice (34–38).

F. Paromomycin

Paromomycin is an aminosidine, which is an oligosaccharide aminoglycoside. The activity of paromomycin against MAC was recently examined in beige mice (39). Disseminated MAC infection was treated with paromomycin at a concentrations of 100 and 200 mg/kg/day for 8 weeks. Paromomycin significantly reduced mortality and the number of viable bacteria in lung, liver, and spleen. Paromomycin at 200 mg/kg/day was significantly more active than paromomycin at 100 mg/kg/day in liver and spleen after 4 weeks of therapy.

Comparison with amikacin (50 mg/kg/day) showed that paromomycin at 200 mg/kg/day was equally effective at 8 weeks; however, amikacin was significantly more active at 4 weeks.

G. Clarithromycin

Clarithromycin is a macrolide with activity in vitro and in vivo against MAC. Clarithromycin is similar in structure to erythromycin (40) and concentrates to high levels in tissues and macrophages. Clarithromycin differs by a single substitution of a methyl group for a 6-hydroxyl group in the 14-membered ring of erythromycin. Clarithromycin is metabolized in the liver to 14-OH-clarithromycin, which is biologically active against several microorganisms and partially active against MAC. Clarithromycin inhibited more than 90% of MAC strains at concentrations therapeutically achievable in humans (41). Clarithromycin achieved a peak level in serum of 2.5 μg/ml. This was first described by Fernandes and colleagues (42) and the results were later confirmed by several groups (23,26,43) in C57/BL6 mice after a dose of 50 mg/kg.

In beige mice infected with MAC, treatment with clarithromycin at 200 mg/kg/day resulted in a significant reduction in the number of bacteria in liver, spleen, and blood (43). Klemens and colleagues had examined the efficacy of regimens in which clarithromycin was combined with other anti-MAC drugs such as amikacin, clofazimine, ethambutol, rifampin, rifabutin, and temafloxacin, observing additive effects with combinations of clarithromycin and clofazimine and clarithromycin and rifabutin (23). However, no definitive conclusions can be drawn from these results owing to the absence of appropriate control groups treated with single antibiotics. Several other groups, including our own, have evaluated the efficacy of clarithromycin in beige mice and these studies have shown consistent in vivo activity against MAC.

Most recently, we have examined the prophylactic activity of clarithromycin against MAC using the oral route of infection in beige mice (43). Clarithromycin was given at 200 mg/kg/day daily for 10 days (period of administration of oral MAC). After 8 weeks, it was observed that prophylaxis with clarithromycin resulted in significant reduction in the number of viable organisms in blood, liver, and spleen. Combination with dapsone, a drug used commonly in patients with AIDS as prophylaxis of *Pneumocystis carinii* pneumonia, did not enhance the prophylactic effect of clarithromycin.

H. Azithromycin

Azithromycin, an azalide, has an additional nitrogen in the erythromycin ring structure, resulting in a 15-member macrolide derivative. The drug has a prolonged half-life (68 hr in humans) and achieves tissue concentrations as high as 2000 μg/g (44). In vitro activity of azithromycin is modest with MICs ranging from 32- to 64-fold above peak serum levels in humans.

In beige mice, azithromycin (200 mg/kg/day) had significant activity against MAC, resulting in a decrease of mortality compared with control mice and reduction of 1.5 $\log_{10}$ of the bacteria load in spleen and 2.0 $\log_{10}$ in liver after 4 weeks of treatment (45). Cynamon and Klemens (46) reported on a comparative study using clarithromycin (200 mg/kg/day) and azithromycin (both at 100 and 200 mg/kg/day). They observed that azithromycin at 200 mg/kg/day had comparable activity with clarithromycin (200 mg/kg/day), whereas at a dose of 100 mg/kg/day azithromycin was less active.

Azithromycin also has been evaluated in combination with clofazimine, ciprofloxacin, and ethambutol. None of these combinations were associated with significant reduction in bacterial load in liver, spleen, and lung compared with azithromycin alone (46). The acivity of azithromycin was also examined in cyclosporin A–treated rats. In this model, azithromycin administered at 100 mg/kg/day was associated with sterilization of blood after 68 days of therapy and a decrease of approximately 2.0 $\log_{10}$ in the number of viable bacteria recovered from liver, spleen, and lung after 68 days of therapy.

When used as a prophylactic agent, administration of azithromycin at 100 mg/kg three times a week for 2 months to cyclosporin A–treated rats resulted in approximately 2.5–3.0 $\log_{10}$ fewer bacteria in spleen, liver, and lung (13). In orally infected beige mice, azithromycin given at 200 mg/kg for 10 days (during the period of infection) was associated with an average of 0.6–1.2 $\log_{10}$ fewer MAC in spleen and liver after 8 weeks (47).

I. Ciprofloxacin

Ciprofloxacin and the other quinolones (ofloxacin, levofloxacin, sparfloxacin) have varied in vitro activities against MAC (48). Only 30% of MAC isolates were susceptible to 2 μg/ml of ciprofloxacin. Administration of ciprofloxacin at 40 mg/kg/day for 4 weeks did not result in significant reduction of bacteremia or bacteria per gram of spleen and liver (49).

Combination of ciprofloxacin with amikacin and imipenem was not significantly better than amikacin alone (49).

J. Bay Y 3118

Bay Y 3118 is a novel fluoroquinolone with a broad spectrum of antibacterial activity in vitro. Bay Y 3118 has been shown to be active against MAC in vitro, with MIC_{90} of 1 μg/ml (50). Beige mice infected with MAC received Bay Y 3118 at 10 mg/kg/day. Treatment with Bay Y 3118 resulted in inhibition of growth of MAC (bacteriostatic activity) in the liver and spleen. It was also associated with reduction of 0.5 log_{10} in bacteremia after 4 weeks of treatment.

K. Sparfloxacin

Sparfloxacin is a fluoroquinolone with activity in vitro against 30–50% of the tested MAC strains (51). In one study, treatment of disseminated infection in beige mice with sparfloxacin (50 mg/kg/day) for 21 days resulted in a modest (0.3 log) reduction of the number of bacteria in the spleen and a reduction of 0.5 log of the number of bacteria in the lung. In our own experience, treatment of beige mice with sparfloxacin was associated with a modest reduction in viable bacteria in liver and spleen (an average of 0.2–0.3 log_{10}) compared with untreated controls. Combination of sparfloxacin with ethambutol both (50 and 100 mg/kg) did not result in increased anti-MAC activity compared with ethambutol alone (52). In addition, combination of sparfloxacin with clarithromycin (200 mg/kg/day) was also not better than clarithromycin alone.

IV. Limitations of Animal Models or Animal Test Systems

From a pragmatic viewpoint, most of the animal test systems studied in the last decade have been small rodents. The underlying reasons are clear: Statistically valid studies require large numbers of experimental subjects and small rodents cost much less than larger species such as primates. They are relatively easy to handle, and blood and tissues for microbial quantitation are readily processed by conventional techniques. However, any in vivo assessment of therapeutic or prophylactic activity must also recognize the inherent limitations of the test system. Probably the most significant limiting factor relates to drug pharmacokinetics. In general rodents "turn over" drugs much faster than humans. This rapid turnover makes it difficult precisely to approximate human pharmacokinetics. Since the effect of pharmacological agents (and antibiotics in particular) on microorganisms is related to the time of exposure of the organism to the drug, a significant difference in pharmacokinetics could well lead to erroneous assessments of in vivo drug activity. A number of reviews (53) have focused on so-called "correction factors" that are necessary to approximate drug doses for various animal species that will approximate those achieved in humans. However, even such approximations have their limitations. For rodents, a dose of drug some 8–10 times larger than what is administered to humans may be necessary to obtain "peak" serum levels that are comparable to what have been observed in human pharmacokinetic studies. One can easily concede, however, that peak serum levels may be transient and rodents are relatively hypermetabolic relative to humans. Therefore, short-lived "peak" serum levels may well be accompanied by a decay in serum concentrations that will be considerably more rapid than what is seen in humans. A related approach to measure "area under the curve" for drug levels and obtain a pharmacokinetic profile in rodents that approximates what is observed in humans. When this is done for mice, a figure of 8- 10-fold larger doses also seems to apply in selecting the appropriate dose for use in the animal test system. There probably is no substitute for actually conducting pharmacokinetic studies in animals so as to obtain the "best fit" of a drug pharmacokinetic profile using as a standard for comparison those pharmacokinetic measurements that are obtained for the same drug in average-sized humans. It must be acknowledged that pharmacokinetic profiles or area under the curve estimations may miss significant species variations in the handling of different medications. Clearly, single-drug pharmacokinetic profiles may not permit us to anticipate drug interactions. For combination therapy studies, there may well be differences in human versus murine pharmacokinetics, and if there are species differences in the handling of one or more components of a drug combination, it is obvious that some of the experimental results could be misleading. The effect of drug on hepatic metabolism of other compounds must also be taken into consideration. Furthermore, because most rodents are usually quite resistant to the toxic effects of drugs commonly used in humans, it may be necessary to use very large doses of drugs in order to screen for toxicity. Taken together, all of these limitations could lead to misleading conclusions about the potential efficacy and toxicity of a therapeutic agent under study.

V. How Can Animal Models Be Useful in Anti-MAC Drug Development—Concluding Perspective

Clearly, if an experimental animal model perfectly mimicked what occurs in humans, physician-scientists could have substantial confidence in extrapolating the results of experimental studies to human therapy. In other words, if an animal model were truly ideal, it should consistently predict the results of human therapy, and one might argue that the potential benefits could lead to the substantial reduction in the human clinical data that are required for drug approval. Rarely (if ever), however, is this the case. The experience with MAC infection is that the various animal test systems provide useful information but that in the final analysis they can only set the stage for a human clinical study. One cannot assume that drug effects in the animal system automatically predict either efficacious results or warn of potential problems. For example, the limitations of experimental test systems in predicting what may be encountered in human therapy are the drug interactions that have been observed with clarithromycin, fluconazole, and rifabutin. In experimental animals (probably because they are resistant to toxic side effects such as uveitis), our combination studies with clarithromycin and rifabutin failed to anticipate this complication which has been noted in the human clinical studies. Because an animal test system deals or may reflect such factors as tissue accumulation, it can point out or identify a potentially useful drug where the in vitro screen might provide somewhat negative results. Perhaps the best example of this is with the new macrolides or azalides. Although in vitro studies do suggest some activity of agents such as clarithromycin based on calculations of achievable serum levels and MICs, where serum levels have failed to predict efficacy has been with even more highly tissue concentrated drugs like azithromycin. Successful treatment of experimental animals was observed by ourselves and others with azithromycin (45). In both mice and humans, the peak serum levels of azithromycin are far lower than the MICs for most MAC strains. Thus, one of the principal advantages of the beige mouse system such as we have employed has been to provide in vivo data that reflect tissue drug activity and most likely intracellular drug activity.

Overall, the beige mouse model has proven to be the most useful test system for assessing anti-MAC drug effects. Looking back on the compounds that have been screened thus far in our laboratory, we believe that virtually every agent shown to be therapeutically and prophylactically useful in humans has been identified in the beige mouse system. Clearly, we have not taken drugs that have been totally unpromising in in vitro studies and then subjected them to clinical investigation using the beige mouse system (it would be impractical, expensive, and difficult to justify to funding agencies). Where there has been a suggestion of effect in beige mice, the subsequent human clinical studies have provided some basis for efficacy.

We believe that the beige mouse model has been sufficiently modified so as to assess both treatment and prophylaxis. Based on limited experience thus far, the effect of nontraditional antibacterial substances such as cytokines or immunomodulators have also been evaluated and their combination effects determined. In dealing with drugs of different classes, such as two totally different antibiotics or an antibiotic plus an immunomodulator, the animal test systems might well provide us information that reflects the dynamic serum or tissue levels of drugs in vivo that cannot be obtained just by a test tube study. Emergence of resistance and combination drug effects are two areas where we also believe the use of the beige mouse system has provided important information. For instance, in vitro studies have suggested that ethambutol, of all of the traditional antimycobacterial agents, has a potentiating effect on many other compounds such as macrolides, azalides, quinolones, rifamycins, and aminoglycosides. This effect has been seen in a single human clinical trial with ethambutol monotherapy, and although modest, the results were statistically significant (24). Although not dramatic, ethambutol both in vitro and in vivo appears to enhance the effect of other active agents, and this has been confirmed in beige mouse experiments (46).

We believe that the use of animal models such as those which we and others have worked with represents a logical progression in the preclinical investigation of any potentially effective agent against MAC. The beginnings must include in vitro test screening with all of the novel variations that have been widely used. In addition, we feel that the step which should follow in vitro screening is assessment in an in vitro test system using cultured human or murine macrophages. In such a manner, we can evaluate intracellular concentration and static/cidal effects, which are important considerations when we recognize that MAC organisms are intracellular pathogens. If an agent proves sufficiently promising in the in vitro screen as well as the macrophage test system, then experimental studies such as we have described using the beige mouse appear both logical and justified. A decade of human experimentation supports the finding that this logical progression of experimental steps can identify therapeutically and prophylactically useful compounds.

Thus, such experiments should set the stage for carefully designed human clinical studies if a drug continues to show promise when this logical sequence of experimental studies is performed.

This work was supported by the National Institutes of Health contract number NO1-A1-25140.

References

1. Inderlied C, Kemper CA, Bermudez LE. The *Mycobacterium avium* complex. Clin Microbiol Rev 1993; 6:266–310.
2. Rastogi N, Frehel C, Ryter A, et al. Multiple drug resistance in *Mycobacterium avium*: Is the wall architecture responsible for the exclusion of antimicrobial agents? Antimicrob Agents Chemother 1981; 20:666–677.
3. Schaefer WB, Davis CL, Cohn ML. Pathogenicity of transparent, opaque and rough variants of *Mycobacterium avium* in chickens and mice. Am Rev Respir Dis 1970; 102:499–506.
4. Collins FM. Acquired resistance to mycobacterial infections. Adv Tuberc Res 1972; 18:1–30.
5. Gangadharam PR, Pratt PF, Davidson PT. Experimental infections with *Mycobacterium intracellulare*. Rev Infect Dis 1981; 3:973–978.
6. Bermudez LE, Young LS. Phagocytosis and intracellular killing of *Mycobacterium avium* complex by human and murine macrophages. Braz J Med Biol Res 1987; 20:191–200.
7. Gangadharam PRJ, Perumal VK, Jariam BT, et al. Virulence of *Mycobacterium avium* complex strains from AIDS patients: relationship with characteristics of the parasite and host. Microb Pathog 1989; 7:263–278.
8. Bertram MA, Inderlied CB, Yadegar S, et al. Confirmation of the beige mouse model for study of disseminated infection with *Mycobacterium avium* complex. J Infect Dis 1986; 154:194–195.
9. Inderlied CB, Young LS, Yamada JK. Determination of in vitro susceptibility of *Mycobacterium avium* complex isolates to antimicrobial agents by various methods. Antimicrob Agents Chemother 1987; 31:1697–1702.
10. Orme IM, Furney SK, Roberts AD. Dissemination of enteric *Mycobacterium avium* infections in mice rendered immunodeficient by thymectomy in CD4 depletion or by prior infection with murine AIDS retrovirus. Infect Immun 1992; 60:4747–4753.
11. Hubbard RD, Flory CM, Collis FM. T-cell immune response in *Mycobacterium avium*-infected mice. Infect Immun 1992; 60:150–153.
12. Morse HC III, Chattopadhyay SK, Makino M, et al. Retrovirus-induced immunodeficiency in the mouse: MAIDS as a model for AIDS. AIDS 1992; 6:607–621.

13. Brown ST, Edwards FF, Bernard EM, et al. Azithromycin, rifabutin and rifapentine for treatment and prophylaxis of *Mycobacterium avium* complex in rats treated with cyclosporin. Antimicrob Agents Chemother 1993; 37:398–402.
14. Scott JP, Higgenbottom TW. Adverse reactions and interactions of cyclosporine. Med Toxicol 1988; 3:107–127.
15. Ji B, Lounis N, Tuffot-Pernot C, Grosset J. Susceptibility of immunocompetent beige and nude mice to *Mycobacterium avium* infection and response to clarithromycin. In: Program and abstracts of 31st Interscience Conference on Antimicrobial Agents and Chemotherapy. Abstract no. 291, Washington DC, 1991.
16. Appelberg R, Castro AG, Pedrosa J, et al. Role of gamma interferon and tumor necrosis factor alpha during T-cell–independent and dependent phases of *Mycobacterium avium* infection. Infect Immun 1994; 62:3962–3971.
17. Bermudez LE, Petrofsky M, Kolonoski P, Young LS. An animal model of *Mycobacterium avium* complex disseminated infection after colonization of the intestinal tract. J Infect Dis 1992; 165:75–79.
18. Gray JR, Rabeneck L. Atypical mycobacterial infection of the gastrointestinal tract in AIDS patients. Am J Gastroenterol 1989; 84:1521–1525.
19. Klatt EC, Jensen DF, Meyer PR. Pathology of *Mycobacterium avium-intracellulare* infection in acquired immunodeficiency syndrome. Hum Pathol 1987; 18: 709–714.
20. Rastogi N, Goh KS, David HL. Enhancement of drug susceptibility of *Mycobacterium avium* by inhibitors of cell envelope synthesis. Antimicrob Agents Chemother 1990; 34:759–764.
21. Gosey L, Vigen W, Dempsey W, et al. A dose-ranging study of selected antimycobacterial agents in beige mice with disseminated *Mycobacterium avium* complex infection. In: Program and abstracts of 8th Interscience Conference on AIDS. Abstract no. PoB 3181, Berlin, 1992.
22. Kemper, CA, Tze-Chiang M, Nussbaum J, et al. Treatment of *Mycobacterium avium* complex bacteremia in AIDS with a four-drug oral regimen: rifampin, ethambutol, clofazimine, and ciprofloxacin. Ann Intern Med 1992; 116:466–472.
23. Klemens SP, DeStefano MS, Cynamon MH. Activity of clarithromycin against *Mycobacterium avium* complex infection in beige mice. Antimicrob Agents Chemother 1992; 11:2413–2417.
24. Bermudez LE, Kolonoski P, Young LS, Inderlied CB. Activity of KRM 1648 alone or in combination with ethambutol or clarithromycin against *Mycobacterium avium* complex in the beige mouse. Antimicrob Agents Chemother 1994; 38:1844–1848.
25. Saito H, Sato K, Tomioka H. Comparative in vitro and in vivo activity of rifabutin and rifampin against *Mycobacterium avium* complex. Tubercle 1991; 69: 187–192.
26. Lazard T, Perronne C, Grosset J, et al. Clarithomycin, minocycline, and rifabutin treatments before and after infection of C57BL/6 mice with *Mycobacterium avium*. Antimicrob Agents Chemother 1993; 8:1690–1692.

27. Furnery SK, Roberts AD, Orme IM. Effect of rifabutin on disseminated My-cobacterium avium infections in thymectomized, CD4 T-cell deficient mice. Antimicrob Agents Chemother 1990; 9:1629–1632.

28. Inderlied CB, Barbara-Burnham L, Wu M, et al. Activity of Benzoxazinorifa-mycin-KRM 1648 against *Mycobacterium avium* complex in the beige mouse. Antimicrob Agents Chemother 1994; 38:1838–1843.

29. Tomioka H, Saito H, Sato K, et al. Chemotherapeutic efficacy of a newly synthesized benzoxazinorifamycin, KRM 1648, against *Mycobacterium avium* complex induced in mice. Antimicrob Agents Chemother 1992; 36:387–393.

30. Emori M, Saito H, Sato K, et al. Therapeutic efficacy of the benzoxazinorifa-mycin, KRM-1648, against experimental *Mycobacterium avium* infection induced in rabbits. Antimicrob Agents Chemother 1993; 37:722–728.

31. Garrelts JC. Clofazimine: a review of its use in leprosy and *Mycobacterium avium* complex infection. Ann Pharmacol 1991; 25:525–531.

32. Ji B, Lounis N, Truffot-Pernot C, Grosset J. Effectiveness of various antimicro-bial agents against *Mycobacterium avium* complex in the beige mouse model. Antimicrob Agents Chemother 1994; 38:2521–2529.

33. Gangadharam PRJ, Mehuchamy PK, Podapti NR, et al. In vivo activity of ami-kacin alone or in combination with clofazimine or rifabutin or both against acute experimental *Mycobacterium avium* complex infection in beige mice. Antimi-crob Agents Chemother 1988; 32:1400–1403.

34. Bermudez LE, Yau-Young AO, Lin JP, et al. Treatment of disseminated *Myco-bacterium avium* complex infection of beige mice with liposome-encapsulated aminoglycosides. J Infect Dis 1990; 161:1262–1268.

35. Duzgunes N, Ashtekar DR, Flasher DL, et al. Treatment of *Mycobacterium avium-intracellulare* complex infection in beige mice with free and liposome-encapsulated streptomycin: role liposome type and duration of treatment. J Infect Dis 1991; 164:143–151.

36. Cynamon MH, Swenson CE, Palmer GS, Ginsberg RS. Liposome-encapsulated amikacin therapy of *Mycobacterium avium* complex infection in beige mice. Antimicrob Agents Chemother 1989; 33:1179–1184.

37. Duzgunes N, Perumal V, Kesavalu L, et al. Enhanced effect of liposome-encap-sulated amikacin on *Mycobacterium avium-Mycobacterium intracellulare* com-plex infection in beige mice. Antimicrob Agents Chemother 1988; 32:1404–1411.

38. Klemens SP, Cynamon H, Swenson CE, Ginsberg RS. Liposome encapsulated gentamicin therapy of *Mycobacterium avium* complex infection in beige mice. Antimicrob Agents Chemother 1990; 34:967–970.

39. Kanyok TP, Reddy MV, Chinnaswamy J, et al. In vivo activity of paromomycin against susceptible and multi-drug resistant *M. tuberculosis* and *M. avium* com-plex strains. Antimicrob Agents Chemother 1994; 38:170–173.

40. Piscitelli SC, Danziger LH, Rodvold KA. Clarithromycin and azithromycin: new macrolides antibiotics. Clin Pharmacol 1992; 11:137–152.

41. Heifets L, Mor N, Vanderkolk J. *Mycobacterium avium* strains resistant to clarithromycin and azithromycin. Antimicrob Agents Chemother 1993; 37:2364–2370.
42. Fernandes PB, Hardy DJ, McDaniel D, et al. In vitro and in vivo activities of clarithromycin against *Mycobacterium avium.* Antimicrob Agents Chemother 1989; 33:1531–1536.
43. Bermudez LE, Inderlied CB, Kolonoski P, et al. Clarithromycin, dapsone and their combination to treat or prevent disseminated *Mycobacterium avium* complex in beige mice. Antimicrob Agents Chemother 1994; 38:
44. Girard AE, Girard D, Englisn AR, et al. Pharmacokinetic and in vivo studies with azithromycin (CP-62, 993), a new macrolide with an extended half life and excellent tissue distribution. Antimicrob Agents Chemother 1987; 31:1948–1954.
45. Inderlied CB, Kolonoski PT, Wu M, Young LS. In vitro and in vivo activity of azithromycin (CP 62, 993) against the *Mycobacterium avium* complex. J Infect Dis 1989; 159:994–997.
46. Cynamon MH, Klemens SP. Activity of azithromycin against *Mycobacterium avium* infection in beige mice. Antimicrob Agents Chemother 1992; 36:1611–1618.
47. Bermudez LE, Petrofsky M, Inderlied CB, Young LS. Prophylactic efficacy of azithromycin and rifabutin against *Mycobacterium avium* complex infection in beige mice. J Antimicrob Chemother 1995; in press.
48. Leysen DC, Haemers A, Pattyn SR. Mycobacteria and the new quinolones. Antimicrob Agents Chemother 1989; 33:1–5.
49. Inderlied CB, Kolonski PT, Wu M, Young LS. Amikacin, ciprofloxacin and imipenem treatment for disseminated *Mycobacterium avium* complex infection of beige mice. Antimicrob Agents Chemother 1989; 33:176–180.
50. Bermudez LE, Wu M, Barbara-Burnham L, et al. Anti-*M. avium* effect of Bay Y 3118 in vitro and in vivo. In: Program and abstracts of 34th Interscience Conference on Antimicrobial Agents and Chemotherapy. Abstract no. B28, Orlando, FL, 1994.
51. Perronne C, Gikas, A. Truffot-Pernot C, et al. Activities of sparfloxacin, azithromycin, temafloxacin, and refapentine compared with that of clarithromycin against multiplication of *Mycobacterium avium* complex within human macrophages. Antimicrob Agents Chemother 1991; 35:1356–1359.
52. Perronne C, Cohen Y, Truffot-Pernot C, et al. Sparfloxacin, ethambutol, and cortisol receptor inhibitor RU-40 555 treatment for disseminated *Mycobacterium avium* complex infection of normal C57BL/6 mice. Antimicrob Agents Chemother 1992; 11:2408–2412.
53. National Cancer Institute. Monograph on animal models. Chemotherapy 1967; Vol. 16.
54. Gangadharam PRJ., Ashtekar DR, Glori N, et al. Chemotherapeutic potential of free and liposome encapsulated streptomycin against experimental *Mycobacterium avium*-complex infections in beige mice. J. Antimicrob Chemother 1991; 28:425–435.
55. Duzgunes N, Perumal VK, Kesavalu L, et al. Treatment of *M. avium intracellulare*-complex infection in beige mice with free and liposome encapsulated streptomycin. J Infect Dis 1991; 164:143–151.

7

Pathogenesis of *Mycobacterium avium*–Complex Infection in Humans: Interactions of Monocytes and *Mycobacterium avium*

HIROE SHIRATSUCHI
and JERROLD J. ELLNER

Case Western Reserve University
Cleveland, Ohio

JOHN L. JOHNSON

Case Western Reserve University
and University Hospitals of Cleveland
Cleveland, Ohio

I. Pathogenicity of *M. avium*

M. avium isolates have traditionally been grouped by seroagglutination. Serogroup differences are due to variations in the haptenic oligosaccharide of the surface glycopeptidolipid (GPL) layer of the mycobacterium. Most isolates recovered from patients with acquired immunodeficiency syndrome (AIDS) are from a small number of serogroups—1, 4, and 8 (1). This is poorly understood given the widespread presence of the organism in nature. In addition to serogroup restriction, *M. avium* isolates from patients with AIDS differ from non-AIDS isolates in plasmid content and antimicrobial resistance (2–4). Patients with AIDS may be infected with multiple *M. avium* strains at the same time; Arbeit et al. demonstrated that some patients with AIDS with disseminated *M. avium* infection were infected with at least two distinct *M. avium* strains using pulsed-field gel electrophoresis (5).

 M. avium is predominatly an intracellular pathogen; most organisms are situated within macrophages in affected tissues. The capacity of microorganisms to replicate intracellularly in vitro is an important correlate of virulence. *M. avium* grown on solid media exhibits two distinct colonial morphologies. Smooth, flat, and transparent (SmT) morphotypes are associated with increased capacity for intracellular *M. avium* growth as compared with smooth, domed, and opaque (SmD) appearing colonies (6,7). Fresh clinical isolates from patients with AIDS usually exhibit SmT colony morphotype and are highly virulent for intracellular growth in human monocyte–derived macrophages (8). We also have confirmed that the factor most consistently related to *M. avium* virulence for intracellular growth in human monocytes is the colonial morphotype (SmT vs SmD) (Fig. 1) (9). *M. avium* of SmD mor-

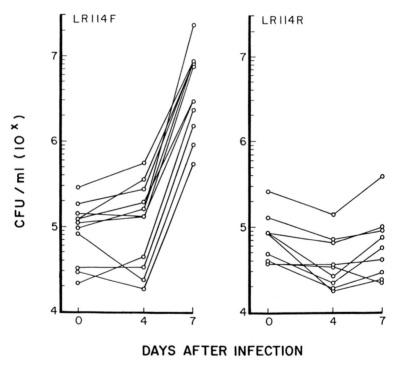

DAYS AFTER INFECTION

Figure 1 Growth curves of two different colonial morphotypes of *M. avium* strains in human monocytes. Each point represents the mean colony-forming units (CFU) of *M. avium* per milliliter of monocyte lysates from 12 subjects for strain LR114F (SmT; flat, transparent strain) and 10 subjects for strain LR114R (SmD; domed, opaque) at each time point. (Adapted from Ref. 9, Copyright 1990 by The University of Chicago. All rights reserved.)

photype are phagocytosed more efficiently but replicate more slowly within human monocytes than isogeneic SmT morphotypes of the same *M. avium* strains (9).

After serial passage in in vitro culture, the SmT colonial morphotype is transformed into the SmD morphotype and loses the capacity to replicate intracellularly in mice, chickens, and humans (6,7,9). Mechanisms underlying the transition from SmT to SmD colonial morphology are not well understood but may involve quantitative or qualitative alterations in the mycobacterial cell wall glycopeptidolipid (GPL). Quantitative and qualitative differences in GPL expression have been described in studies of *M. avium* strains with differing colonial morphology (10). All *M. avium* organisms possess a common singly glycosylated GPL moiety. Serotypic differences between strains are due to individual variations in GPL via multiglycosylation at the threonine substituent of a conserved lipopeptide core (11,12). Purified GPL may itself have important immunomodulating properties. Modulation of mononuclear phagocyte effector functions by these mycobacterial cell wall components may contribute significantly to *M. avium* pathogenicity. GPL from *M. avium* serogroup 4 inhibits mitogenesis of murine splenic lymphocytes (13). *M. avium* GPL also inhibited the killing of *Candida albicans* by bovine macrophages and mitogen-induced lymphocyte proliferation (13–15). GPL and related substances may also be important in the intracellular survival of the pathogen.

II. Phagocytosis of *M. avium* by Human Mononuclear Phagocytes

Serum complement C′3 and its receptors have crucial roles in the initial attachment and ingestion of intracellular pathogens by phagocytic cells (16,17). Complement receptor (CR) 1, CR3, and CR4 expressed on mononuclear phagocytes (18) are important in the binding and phagocytosis of *M. leprae* and *M. tuberculosis* (19–22). Alveolar macrophages, tissue macrophages, and monocyte-derived macrophages express more CR4 receptors than do freshly isolated circulating monocytes (18). CR4 binding, therefore, is more important in mycobacterial phagocytosis by macrophages than monocytes (21,22). CR1 and CR3 may be more important in phagocytosis by freshly isolated monocytes. We have demonstrated the importance of alternate complement pathway activation and deposition of C′3 in *M. avium* phagocytosis and indentified a synergistic role for CR1 and CR3 receptors in *M. avium* uptake by freshly isolated peripheral blood monocytes (Fig. 2). Prein-

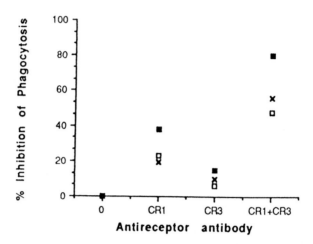

Figure 2 Effect of anticomplement receptor antibodies on *M. avium* phagocytosis by human monocytes. Data from three independent experiments using monocytes from three healthy subjects are shown. Monocytes were preincubated in the presence or absence of monoclonal anti-CR1 or anti-CR3 antibody alone or a combination of both antibodies for 30 min prior to infection with *M. avium* previously stained with Lucifer yellow and opsonized with unheated human serum. Uptake of *M. avium* by monocytes was analyzed by flow cytometry. Data are expressed as the mean fluorescent intensity of monocytes under each condition.

cubation with anti-CR1 or anti-CR3 antibody alone decreased *M. avium* uptake by 20–40% and 10–20%, respectively, whereas incubation with both antibodies decreased phagocytosis by 50–80%. CR3, fibronectin, and mannosyl-fucosyl receptors also are important for *M. avium* uptake (23).

   Preincubation with heated or cobra venom factor–depleted serum decreases *M. avium* attachment or phagocytosis (24). Selective pretreatment with EGTA and magnesium chloride results in levels of *M. avium* phagocytosis comparable to incubation with normal serum; in contrast, preincubation with EDTA or heat-inactivated serum decreases *M. avium* uptake, suggesting that the alternate complement pathway is essential for *M. avium* phagocytosis (24). Recently, *M. avium* has been demonstrated to bind to extracellular matrix proteins of eukaryotic cells, including fibronection, laminin, and collagen I, through a β_1-integrin protein on the mycobacterial cell surface (25); these bacterial surface constituents also may play an important role in the initial adherence of the pathogen to basement membrane proteins in host tissues.

Antibodies against mycobacterial components may also directly modulate phagocytosis. Natural antibodies against *M. leprae* in sera from nonimmune hosts have been shown to enhance complement fixation and attachment of mycobacteria to phagocytic cells (26). Antibodies against GPL of *M. avium* have been detected in 2.4% of normal individuals, and 44% of homosexual men positive for human immunodeficiency virus (HIV) and 33% of HIV-negative homosexual men (27). These antibodies may enhance attachment via Fc receptors and ingestion of bacteria by host phagocytes.

Circulating and locally produced cytokines have critical roles in host defenses against many opportunistic pathogens. Certain cytokines such as interferon-γ (INF-γ), granulocyte-macrophage colony-stimulating factor (GM-CSF), macrophage-colony stimulating factor (MCSF), and transforming growth factor-β (TGF-β) decrease *M. avium* phagocytosis in a dose-dependent manner (28) (Table 1). These effects are evident using *M. avium* strains of both flat, transparent (SmT), and domed, opaque (SmD) colony morphotypes. Pretreatment with IFN-γ for 2 days inhibited *M. avium* phagocytosis by monocytes from healthy subjects and patients with AIDS (9,29). This effect may be due to downregulation of surface C′3 receptor expression by monocytes after stimulation with IFN-γ. IFN-γ has been shown to decrease C3bR expression (30) and binding of C3b and C3bi on human peripheral

Table 1 Effect of Cytokines on *M. avium* Phagocytosis by Human Monocytes

		AFB/100 Monocytes	
	n	LR114 SmT	86m2096
Control	4	44 ± 15	566 ± 145
GM-CSF	4	19 ± 7	297 ± 122
Control	5	66 ± 12	554 ± 150[a]
M-CSF	5	61 ± 31	408 ± 147[a]
Control	5	40 ± 9	453 ± 155[b]
TGF-β	5	24 ± 3	252 ± 135[b]

Plastic adherent monocytes were precultured in the presence or absence of recombinant human GM-CSF 1000 U/ml, M-CSF 1:1000 dilution, or TGF-β 0.03 ng/ml for 2 days prior to infection with *M. avium* (10^7 bacteria/ml). *M. avium* strain LR114F is a virulent strain with flat, transparent colony morphology; 86m2096 is an AIDS-associated clinical isolate with flat colony morphology. After infection, monocytes were fixed with methanol and stained by Kinyoun's modified acid-fast staining method. Data are expressed as the mean ± SE of the number of acid-fast bacilli (AFB) counted by light microscopy per 100 monocytes.
[a]*P* < 0.02, paired *t*-test.
[b]*P* < 0.05, paired *t*-test.

monocytes (31). These interactions may be important in limiting the uptake of a pathogen that is poorly killed in the intracellular environment.

After phagocytosis, *M. avium* replicates inside nonacidic phagosomes of macrophages (32). Failure of phagosomes to acidify and inhibition of phagosome-lysosome fusion via inhibition of proton-ATPase (33) may enhance mycobacterial survival within phagocytic cells. On electron microscopy, intracellular organisms are enclosed in membrane-bound phagosomes and are surrounded by a multilamellar electron-translucent zone (ETZ) which resembles GPL (34,35). The ETZ may represent a barrier preventing intracellular killing of the organisms and therefore may be a potential mycobacterial virulence factor.

III. Cytokine Modulation of *M. avium* Growth

Macrophages activated by cytokines express potent antimicrobial and tumoricidal activities. Body fluids and infected tissues also contain increased amounts of cytokine mediators that have important biological activities leading to enhancement or suppression of intracellular and extracellular *M. avium* growth. Results of in vitro studies on the effects of cytokines on mycobacterial killing have been controversial. Differing results in these studies probably reflect several factors influencing *M. avium* growth in in vitro culture systems, including strain-to-strain and donor-to-donor differences in the virulence of *M. avium* (9,36), species-to-species differences in host innate resistance to *M. avium*, and differences in culture conditions, especially the duration of cell culture prior to *M. avium* infection (37,38). *M. avium*–infected macrophages become more permissive to intracellular mycobacterial replication after longer periods in culture (39).

Cytokines differ in functional activities, targets, and their interactions with other cytokines. Certain cytokines may act synergistically with other cytokines to activate monocytes (40), may stimulate monocytes to produce other cytokines (41–45), or modulate surface cytokine receptor expression on target cells (46,47). Other cytokines exhibit macrophage-activating factor (MAF)–like activity against certain targets (48–56).

The results of studies assessing cytokine effects on *M. avium* growth in human mononuclear phagocytes have been controversial with different investigators describing different or no effects of the same cytokine (Table 2). This complex literature will be summarized in this section.

IFN-γ, the prototypical cytokine with MAF activity, inhibits the replication of *Leishmania* species (64,65) and other pathogens (66,67). IFN-γ

Table 2 Effects of Cytokines on *M. avium* Growth in Human Mononuclear Phagocytes

Cytokine	Intracellular *M. avium* growth		
	inhibit (Ref.)	enhance (Ref.)	no effect (Ref.)
IL-1α		+ (57)	
IL-1β			+ (57)
IL-2			+ (57)
IL-4			+ (57)
IL-6		+ (57,58)	
TNF-α	+ (57–60)		
TGF-β		+ (61)	
IFN-γ	+ (9,29,57,61)	+ (38)	+ (38)
IL-3		+ (57)	
M-CSF		+ (57)	+ (62)
GM-CSF	+ (52,63)		+ (57)
IFN-γ + M-CSF	+ (62)		

enhances intracellular growth inhibition of *M. tuberculosis* by murine macrophages (68). Rook et al. reported significant donor-to-donor variability of the effect of IFN-γ on intracellular growth of *M. tuberculosis* in human macrophages; IFN-γ increased *M. tuberculosis* growth in some donors' macrophages but significantly decreased growth in others (69). Previously we demonstrated that, after *M. avium* infection, coculturing monocytes with IFN-γ decreased intracellular growth in human monocytes from healthy subjects and patients with AIDS (9,29); further enhancement of intracellular growth inhibitory activity was observed when indomethacin was added to these cultures (Fig. 3) (57). After infection with *M. avium*, coculturing monocytes with prostaglandin E_2 (PGE_2) increased intracellular *M. avium* growth in human monocytes (unpublished observation). Bone marrow macrophages from mice chronically infected with *M. tuberculosis* exhibit increased PGE_2 production (70) which inhibits macrophage activation by IFN-γ (71). IFN-γ has been used successfully in the treatment of patients with chronic granulomatous diseases (72), leprosy (73), visceral leishmaniasis (74), and other serious intracellular infections. IFN-γ has also been evaluated as an adjunct to drug therapy in patients with disseminated *M. avium* infection. In a recent report, Holland et al. demonstrated the efficacy of chronic subcutaneous IFN-γ in-

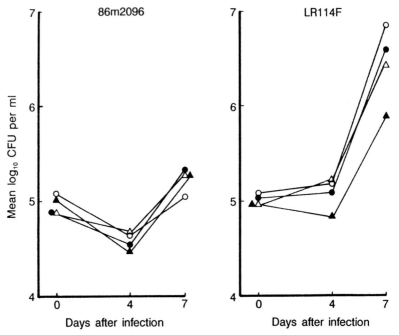

Figure 3   Effect of IFN-γ alone and in combination with indomethacin (IM) on the intracellular growth of *M. avium* in cultured monocytes. Two-day precultured monocytes were infected with two strains of *M. avium*. After infection, monocytes were cultured continuously in the presence of IFN-γ 300 U/ml final concentration (●----●), IM 1 μg/ml (△----△), IFN-γ 300 U/ml + IM 1 μg/ml (▲----▲), or without added IFN or IM (○----○). Data are shown as the mean CFU/ml of *M. avium* in monocyte lysates from three donors at each time point. The combination of IFN-γ and IM decreased intracellular *M. avium* growth at 7 days in culture by 10-fold (*P*<0.01, paired *t*-test compared with control culture). This growth inhibitory effect exceeded the effect of either IFN-γ or IM alone. Growth inhibition in the presence of IFN + IM was apparent only in experiments using the more virulent LR114F (SmT) *M. avium* strain. (From Ref. 57, Copyright 1991, The Journal of Immunology.)

jection combined with antimycobacterial chemotherapy in non-HIV–infected patients with refractory disseminated *M. avium* disease (75).

Bermudez and Young (59) reported that interleukin-2 (IL-2) alone did not inhibit *M. avium* growth in 7-day precultured human monocyte-derived macrophages, but the combination of TNF-α and IL-2 decreased intracellular *M. avium* growth when the macrophages were pretreated with these cytokines for 2 days before infection. Schnittman et al. (76) also have reported that TNF-α had moderate inhibitory activity affecting intracellular *M. avium* growth.

Colony-stimulating factors (CSFs), including IL-3, MCSF, and GM-CSF, exhibit MAF activity against *Trypanosoma cruzi* (54), *Listeria monocytogenes* (77), and other important human intracellular pathogens. GM-CSF inhibited intracellular *M. avium* replication in human monocyte/macrophages (63,78); however, IL-3 and MCSF increased intracellular *M. avium* growth when the CSFs were added to monocyte cultures after infection with a virulent *M. avium* strain (57) (Table 3). Rose et al. have reported that the combination of MCSF and IFN-γ, but not MCSF or IFN-γ alone, inhibits intracellular growth of *M. avium* in human alveolar macrophages (62). CSFs do not directly affect mycobacterial growth in tissue culture medium alone and, therefore, probably modulate intracellular *M. avium* growth via indirect mechanisms on target cell populations.

Other cytokines, including IL-2 and IL-4, produced predominantly by T lymphocytes, also have MAF activity. Recombinant IL-2 directly activates peripheral blood monocytes to produce IL-1 (41) and augments the cytotoxicity of human monocytes against tumor cells (49). Intraperitoneal administration of recombinant human IL-2 limits *M. lepraemurium* and *M. bovis* BCG (bacille Calmette-Guérin) replication in mice (79). According to studies

Table 3 Effect of Colony-Stimulating Factors on the Growth of *M. avium* Strain LR114F (SmT) in Human Monocytes

	Mean CFU *M. avium* ml ($\times 10^5$) in monocyte lysate		
	Day 0	Day 4	Day 7
Control	2.15 ± 0.54[a]	3.06 ± 1.14	33.2 ± 11.8
IL-3 100 U/ml	2.56 ± 0.60	3.07 ± 1.10	79.5 ± 30.4[b]
Control	1.09 ± 0.24	1.25 ± 0.32	41.7 ± 29.9
M-CSF (1:3000)	1.27 ± 0.42	1.66 ± 0.67	64.8 ± 32.8[c]
Control	1.19 ± 0.36	1.36 ± 0.44	16.4 ± 7.51
GM-CSF 5000 U/ml	1.40 ± 0.46	1.70 ± 0.32	36.4 ± 28.0

[a]Data shown are the mean ± SE *M. avium* CFU/ml in monocyte lysates harvested 0, 4, and 7 days after infection with *M. avium*. Data are from studies using monocytes from four to six healthy donors.
[b]$P < 0.01$ compared with control (−) culture.
[c]$P < 0.02$ compared with control (−) culture.
Source: Ref. 57, Copyright 1991, The Journal of Immunology.

by Schnittman (76) and Bermudez (59), however, IL-2 alone does not inhibit intracellular *M. avium* growth in human monocytes in vitro. IL-4 (51,52), and IL-6 stimulate colony formation and differentiation by mouse hemopoietic stem cells (80) and augment human NK cell activity (81). Coculture of human monocytes in vitro in the presence of IL-1β, IL-2, or IL-4 resulted in minimal inhibition of intracellular *M. avium* growth with marked donor-to donor variation (57). On the other hand, IL-1α and IL-6 consistently increased intracellular *M. avium* growth in human monocytes when added to cultures after infection (Table 4).

IL-10 and TGF-β are immunosuppressive cytokines that decrease the antigen-presenting capacity of monocytes secondarily resulting in inhibition of lymphocyte proliferation and decreased IL-1, TNF-α, and IL-6 production by lipopolysaccharide (LPS)−activated human monocytes (82,83). TGF-β and IL-10 enhanced intracellular *M. avium* growth in human and murine macrophages, respectively, and induction of TGF-β production by human monocyte-derived macrophages was associated with increased *M. avium* replication (61,84). Alterations in the dynamic local balance of these mycobacterial growth inhibitory and growth enhancing factors, therefore, may lead to increased intracellular replication of this pathogen.

In addition to blocking the effects of certain MAFs, cytokines also may directly augment intracellular *M. avium* growth (57,58). Recently, IL-1, IL-2, and IL-6 have been reported to possess bacterial growth factor activity. Certain bacteria have cytokine receptor−like molecules on their surface. Vir-

Table 4   Effect of Cytokines on the Growth of *M. avium* in Human Monocytes[a]

| | Mean CFU/ml in monocyte lysate ($\times 10^4$) | | |
	Day 0	Day 4	Day 7
Control	20.3 ± 5.7[b]	9.9 ± 3.1	19.0 ± 4.3
IL-1α 10 U/ml	19.3 ± 5.1	10.7 ± 3.5	84.2 ± 35.8[c]
IL-1β 10 U/ml	19.6 ± 5.4	9.8 ± 3.3	21.6 ± 5.9
Control	11.3 ± 4.9	1.6 ± 0.6	7.2 ± 2.3
IL-6 5 U/ml	10.0 ± 5.1	2.7 ± 0.6[d]	26.7 ± 4.1[d]

[a]Two-day precultured monocytes were infected with *M. avium* strain 86m2096. After infection, monocytes were continuously cultured with or without cytokines.
[b]Data shown are the mean $\pm$ SE of mean CFU/ml in monocyte lysates from five donors for each condition.
[c]$P < 0.01$.
[d]$P < 0.05$ compared with control $(-)$ culture.

ulent strains of *Escherichia coli* bind IL-1, IL-1 receptor antagonist, IL-2, and GM-CSF (85,86). Pathogenic gram-negative bacteria, including *Shigella flexneri, Salmonella typhimurium,* and *E. coli,* possess TNF-α receptors; pretreatment of bacteria with TNF-α enhances uptake of these bacteria by human and murine macrophages (87). Interestingly, the proinflammatory cytokines IL-1α and IL-6 promote *M. avium* replication in cell free medium (57). *M. avium* express surface IL-6 receptors (61). IL-6 also downregulates TNF receptor expression on human macrophages, which may alter the mycobactericidal effects of TNF-α (88). Clearly, both direct and indirect effects of cytokines may alter intracellular killing of *M. avium* by mononuclear phagocytes.

IV. Relationship of *M. avium* Colony Morphology and Cytokine Induction

Infection of human mononuclear phagocytes with *M. avium* induces expression of several cytokines by the infected tissues including IL-1, IL-6, IL-10, GM-CSF, TNF-α and TGF-β (61,78,84,89,90). Previously, we have demonstrated that different strains and different colonial morphotypes of the same *M. avium* strain show striking differences in their ability to grow within human monocytes (9). Differential induction of growth-enhancing or growth-inhibitory cytokines by different strains or colonial morphotypes may underlie these differences in *M. avium* virulence. Michelini-Norris et al. demonstrated that the more virulent SmT morphotype stimulated monocytes to express less extracellular IL-1 and IL-6 and less membrane-associated IL-1 than the avirulent SmD morphotype of the same *M. avium* strain (91). Using a different *M. avium* strain, we also studied the induction of immunoreactive and bioactive cytokine expression by fresh human monocytes stimulated with isogeneic strains of *M. avium.* Stimulation with the SmD morphotype resulted in greater expression of TNF-α and IL-1 activity than the SmT morphotype; IL-6 production was comparable after stimulation with either colonial type (Table 5) (90). TNF-α production by *M. avium*–infected monocytes from patients AIDS and healthy individuals was comparable; however, monocytes from patients with AIDS released lower concentrations of IL-1 into culture supernatant after infection with *M. avium* (92). IL-6 and TNF-α production by *M. avium*–stimulated monocytes differs among healthy donors; high levels of expression of these cytokines is correlated with the ability of monocytes to limit intracellular *M. avium* growth (36). Levels of TNF-α and IL-1– specific mRNA induced by stimulation with SmT and SmD morphotypes of

Table 5 Cytokine Production in Culture Supernatants of Monocytes Cocultured with *M. avium*[a]

	n	IL-1α (pg/ml)	IL-1β (ng/ml)	IL-6 (ng/ml)	TNF-α (ng/ml)
Control	7	0	0	0.8 ± 0.5	0
LPS	4	543 ± 224	16.6 ± 2.0	70.8 ± 11.3	10.4 ± 1.4
SmT	7	47 ± 16[b]	1.7 ± 0.5[c]	42.3 ± 8.9	1.5 ± 0.4[c]
SmD	7	140 ± 32[b]	4.0 ± 0.9[c]	49.2 ± 7.7	2.7 ± 0.5[c]

[a]Monocytes obtained from healthy donors were cultured at 10^6/ml in 24-well tissue culture plates with or without the SmT or SmD strains of *M. avium* (10^7 bacteria/ml), or LPS 10 μg/ml for 24 hr. Culture supernatants were harvested, and cytokine concentrations were determined by the ELISA method. Data are expressed as mean ± SE of cytokine concentrations in culture supernatants.
[b]$P < 0.05$, paired *t*-test.
[c]$P < 0.01$, paired *t*-test.
Source: Ref. 90; Copyright 1993, The Journal of Immunology.

M. avium were similar, suggesting that the observed differences in cytokine expression were related to posttranslational events (90).

Similar observations have been reported by Furney et al. using mouse macrophages (93). Clinical isolates of *M. avium* were separated into two categories based on their ability to replicate in murine bone marrow–derived macrophages. Virulent strains exhibited predominantly smooth-transparent colonial morphotype, whereas strains with smooth-domed colonial morphology were relatively avirulent. TNF-α levels in culture supernatants of *M. avium*–infected macrophages harvested at 24 hr after infection were higher after infection with avirulent strains. Virulent *M. avium* strains also induced more TGF-β expression than avirulent strains (61).

It is possible that the rapid induction of cytokine expression after infection with SmD strains activates the infected phagocyte or adjacent cells in an autocrine or paracrine manner, thereby augmenting local monocyte mycobactericidal activity. Induction of cytokine expression by phagocytic cells is probably mediated, at least in part, by mycobacterial surface components. Differences in expression of differing surface glycolipid components of SmD and SmT morphotypes of *M. avium* may ultimately account for differential triggering of cytokine expression. GPL from avirulent SmD morphotypes of *M. avium* induced more IL-1β and TNF-α expression than GPL from virulent SmT morphotypes (S. Shiratsuchi et al., unpublished data); these observations parallel those from experiments using intact *M. avium*.

V. Interaction of HIV-1 and *M. avium* Infection in Human Monocytes

Disseminated *M. avium* infection in patients with AIDS is characterized by a continuous high-grade bacteremia and enormous tissue burdens of the organism. At the time of initial diagnosis, an average of 500 colony-forming units (CFU)/μl are present in the bloodstream (94). Involved viscera are filled with phagocytes engorged with acid-fast bacilli; tissue macrophages in patients with AIDS with disseminated *M. avium* infection have been found to be as high as 10^9 to 10^{10} AFB/g tissue (95).

Studies of the pathogenesis of this extraordinarily exuberant intracellular mycobacterial growth have focused on the adequacy of phagocytic cell effector functions against mycobacteria, the appropriateness of activation of the macrophage by other cells and cytokines, and innate characteristics of the microbe itself. Earlier studies generated conflicting data regarding whether mononuclear phagocytes of patients with AIDS were intrinsically more permissive to intracellular *M. avium* growth. Effector functions of monocytes from patients with AIDS were intact when tested against certain intracellular pathogens (96,97), although cytokine production and Fc and C3 receptor–mediated phagocytosis were defective (97,98). Phagocytosis of latex beads (99) and *Aspergillus fumigatus* and *Cryptococcus neoformans* (96) by monocytes from patients with AIDS was normal; however, monocyte chemotaxis to several chemoattractants, including lymphocyte-derived chemotactic factor and N-formyl-methionyl-leucyl-phenylalanine, was deficient (99). The general capacity of monocytes for oxidative burst generation assessed by nitroblue tetrazolium reduction was depressed in patients with early asymptomatic HIV infection and worsened in later stages of the disease (100).

We and others demonstrated preserved effector cell function of monocytes obtained from patients with AIDS against in vitro *M. avium* infection (29,76). In contrast, Crowle et al. reported that monocyte-derived macrophages of patients with AIDS exhibited enhanced intracellular *M. avium* growth (101). As noted earlier, some of the disparities in these results may be due to differences in conditions and length of culture and in the virulence of *M. avium* strains used in the studies.

Considerable controversy exists regarding whether HIV or specific viral constituents or products directly impair host immune defenses against opportunistic pathogens or whether the increased occurrence of these infections is due to indirect secondary effects of HIV mediated by progressive depletion of the CD4 helper T-cell population.

More recent work has focused on potential direct or indirect effects of HIV or its components on *M. avium* growth. Using endpoint dilution viral cultures, Sierra-Madero et al. have demonstrated that HIV titers of monocytes and alveolar macrophages are significantly lower than circulating lymphocytes (102). Levels of HIV infection of circulating monocytes are low (102 −104); however, macrophage-associated HIV antigens are readily demonstrable in lymph nodes, brain, and alveolar macrophages (105). In vitro monocyte survival in patients with AIDS is decreased and directly correlated with progressive HIV-related immunosuppression (106).

HIV coinfection could conceivably influence intracellular *M. avium* replication at several levels. Concomitant infection of monocytes with mycobacteria and HIV could directly enhance *M. avium* growth or HIV could have indirect effects on mycobacterial parasitism through its effects on other cells or by induction of cytokine expression and the creation of a local tissue milieu conducive to the growth of *M. avium*. Viral products might also directly promote *M. avium* growth.

We have studied human monocyte effector functions against *M. avium* in patients with AIDS using an in vitro *M. avium* infection model. In studies utilizing 2-day precultured monocytes from patients with AIDS, phagocytosis of *M. avium* by monocytes did not differ among healthy subjects, patients with AIDS, or patients with AIDS and prior known disseminated *M. avium* infection (29,76). Intracellular *M. avium* growth inhibition at 7 days in culture was comparable between patients with AIDS and healthy donors for all four strains (AIDS) and non-AIDS−associated isolates) tested (Fig. 4) (29). Decreased *M. avium* uptake and a modest augmentation of intracellular growth inhibition occurred after stimulation in vitro with IFN-γ, similar to effects previously noted in healthy subjects (29). Schnittman *et al.* also have reported similar capacity of monocytes from patients with AIDS to limit *M. avium* growth in vitro (76).

In contrast, using 7-day precultured monocyte-derived macrophages, Crowle et al. found that monocytes from patients with AIDS were highly permissive to *M. avium* growth and that sera from patients with AIDS lacked a factor which inhibits intracellular growth of *M. avium* (107). *M. avium*, but not *M. intracellulare*, strains replicated more rapidly in monocytes from patients with AIDS than healthy subjects (101). Selectively increased susceptibility to *M. avium* infection may help to explain the higher incidence of *M. avium* disease in HIV-infected patients than that due to the closely related *M. intracellulare* species (101).

Dual infection of human monocyte-derived macrophages with HIV and *M. avium* did not alter intracellular mycobacterial growth in short-term cul-

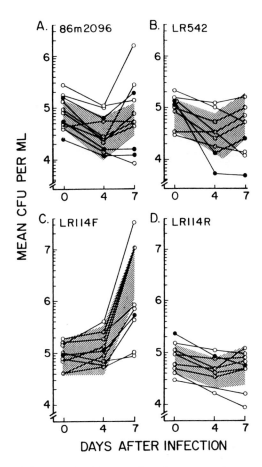

Figure 4 Intracellular growth of four strains of *M. avium* in monocytes from 11 patients with AIDS and healthy subjects. *M. avium* growth curves in monocyte lysates from patients with AIDS but without known prior *M. avium* infection (○) and from patients with AIDS and prior known disseminated *M. avium* infection (●) are shown. Shaded areas present the mean ±1 standard deviation of CFU of *M. avium* in monocyte lysates of 13 healthy subjects. (From Ref. 29, Copyright 1991, Infection and Immunity.)

ture (108), but increased permissiveness of HIV-1–infected macrophages for intracellular *M. avium* growth was present after 14 days of culture (39). Rapid intracellular *M. avium* replication has been reported at early time points when human monocyte-derived macrophages were chronically infected with HIV-1 before infection with *M. avium* (110). Dual infection with HIV-1 and *M. avium* also decreased macrophage viability (109). In vitro infection of monocytes with HIV may not, however, accurately reflect conditions in the tissues of patients with AIDS. HIV infection of monocytes and tissue macrophages in patients with AIDS is quantitatively lower than that of T cells (102,110). Therefore, the effects of HIV-1 infection on mononuclear phagocyte effector functions against *M. avium* are likely to be indirect. Constituents and by-products of HIV-1 might enhance the pathogenicity of AIDS-associated opportunistic infectious agents by interfering with host defense mechanisms.

Viral proteins are abundant in many tissues in AIDS and local effects of these proteins might adversely affect macrophage function directly or by altering the local balance of MAF and mycobacterial growth-enhancing mediators. Several investigators have shown that HIV-1 infection and HIV envelope protein gp120 activate human monocytes to express cytokines (111–113). Earlier reports demonstrated that live or killed HIV and recombinant gp 120 induced IL-1β, IL-6, and TNF production by monocytes (112–114); subsequent studies using LPS-free reagents did not reproduce these effects (115). The source of gp120 also may be relevant as stimulation of monocytes with native, but not recombinant, gp120 increased cytokine production; this effect could be blocked by soluble CD4 (110).

Using an in vitro human monocyte infection model, we examined the effect of HIV-1 proteins, including envelope protein gp120, transmembrane protein p121, and core proteins (p24 and gag5), on monocyte phagocytosis and intracellular growth inhibition of *M. avium*. Monocytes obtained from HIV-negative healthy subjects were pretreated with recombinant HIV-1 proteins for 2 days and then infected with *M. avium*. Pretreatment with gp120 inhibited *M. avium* phagocytosis (Table 6) (116). Despite inhibition of phagocytosis, HIV envelope protein gp120 enhanced intracellular growth of six strains of *M. avium* in human monocytes from healthy subjects (Fig. 5) (116,117). Core proteins p24 and gag5 and transmembrane protein p121 neither inhibited *M. avium* phagocytosis nor increased intracellular growth of *M. avium* (116). HIV-1 gp120 binds specifically to CD4 receptors (118,119). Although monocytes-macrophages express much lower numbers of CD4 receptors than peripheral blood T lymphocytes, binding of gp120 to human monocytes has been demonstrated (120). The effects of gp120 on *M. avium* phagocytosis and intracellular growth appear to be mediated through specific

Table 6 Effect of HIV-1 Proteins on Phagocytosis of *M. avium* by Human Monoctyes

	n	% monocytes infected	AFB/100 monocytes
Control	7	40.0 ± 2.5	138 ± 17
gp120	7	28.8 ± 3.8[a]	97 ± 19[a]
Control	3	41.5 ± 7.6	137 ± 34
gag5	3	39.9 ± 7.8	133 ± 31
Control	4	35.7 ± 4.5	114 ± 19
p121	4	35.0 ± 4.3	122 ± 23

Monocytes obtained from healthy subjects were precultured with or without recombinant HIV-1 gp120 (0.2 µg/ml), gag5 (0.2 µg/ml), or p121 (0.2 µg/ml) for 2 days before infection. Data are expressed as the mean ± SE of the percentage of monocytes infected with ≥1 AFB or the number of AFB/100 monocytes.
[a]$P < 0.001$ compared with control (paired t-test).
Source: Ref. 116, reproduced from the Journal of Clinical Investigation, 1994, 93:885-891, by copyright permission of American Society for Clinical Investigation.

interactions of gp120 and CD4 receptors with monocytes. Soluble CD4 and OKT4A, but not OKT4 alone, abrogated the effects of gp120 on *M. avium* phagocytosis (Fig. 6) (116,117). Soluble CD4 also neutralized the capacity of gp120 to increase intracellular *M. avium* growth. In a preliminary report, Wagner *et al.* demonstrated that HIV-1 gp120 reduced the phagocytosis and enhanced the intracellular growth of *Cryptococcus neoformans*, another common opportunistic pathogen in patients with AIDS, by alveolar macrophages (121). It is not yet clear whether the effects of gp120 on effector function against *M. avium* and *C. neoformans* are similarly mediated.

The source of serum used for monocyte culture markedly affects intracellular *M. avium* replication. Sera from patients with AIDS appear to lack an inhibitory factor contained in normal sera that limits intrcellular *M. avium* growth. Increased intracellular *M. avium* growth occurred when monocytes from healthy subjects were cultured using sera from patients with AIDS (107). Incubation of *M. avium* in tissue culture medium with sera from patients with AIDS in the absence of monocytes did not, however, alter *M. avium* growth patterns (101), suggesting that the sera do not contain a factor that directly promotes *M. avium* growth. The nature of this serum-inhibitory activity is presently unknown.

Sera from patients with AIDS also contain high levels of IL-6, a *M. avium* growth-enhancing factor (122), and soluble TNF receptors (123), which bind circulating TNF-α and inhibit TNF-α binding to tissue macro-

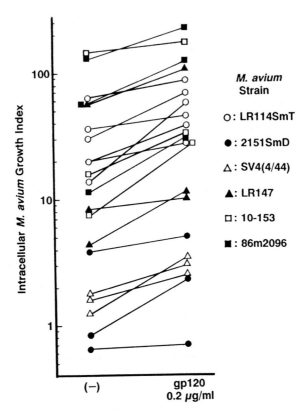

Figure 5   Effect of gp120 pretreatment on intracellular growth of various *M. avium* strains in human monocytes. Monocytes obtained from healthy HIV-negative donors were precultured with or without gp120 0.2μg/ml for 2 days and then infected with 2 avirulent (2151SmD and SV4[4/44]) and four virulent *M. avium* strains (LR114SmT, LR147, 10-153, and 86m2096). After infection, monocytes were cultured with medium alone for 7 days. Samples were harvested at day 0 (immediately after infection) and 7 days after infection. The number of *M. avium* organisms in each sample was assessed by CFU assay. Data are expressed as mean ±SE of a growth index (GI) calculated as CFU in day 7 monocyte lysate divided by CFU in day 0 monocyte lysate. Pretreatment with gp120 enhanced intracellular growth of *M. avium* strains LR114SmT and 10-153 (*P*<0.05 compared with control culture) (paired *t*-test). (From Ref. 117, Copyright 1994, Editions Scientifiques Elsevier.)

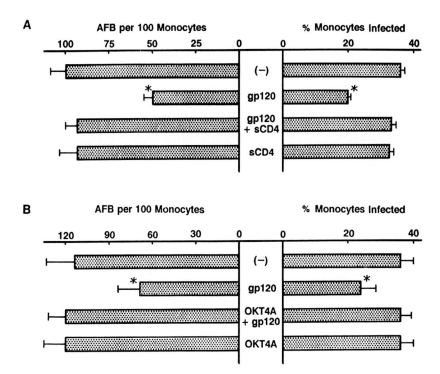

Figure 6 Neutralization of the effects of gp120 on monocyte phagocytosis of *M avium* by sCD4 or monoclonal OKT4A antibody. Phagocytosis of *M. avium* was assayed by counting AFB by light microscopy. A, gp120 (0.2 μg/ml, final concentration) was preincubated with recombinant sCD4 (0.2 μg/ml) at room temperature for 30 min before addition to monocyte cultures. Monocytes from three subjects were cultured with medium alone, gp120 0.2μg/ml, sCD4 0.2μg/ml, or gp120 preincubated with sCD4 for 2 days and then infected with *M. avium* strain LR1114SmT. Data are expressed as the mean ±SE monocytes ingesting ≥1AFB or the number of AFB/100 monocytes in three independent experiments using monocytes from healthy subjects. *: *P*<0.02 compared with control culture, or sCD4 + gp120, or sCD4 alone; paired *t*-test. B, Monocytes obtained from four healthy subjects were preincubated with monoclonal antibody OKT4A (1:200 dilution) at 37°C for 60 min prior to addition of gp120 to monocyte culture. OKT4A pretreated or untreated monocytes were cultured with or without gp120 0.2 μg/ml for 2 days and then infected with *M. avium* strain LR114SmT. Data are expressed as mean ±SE of monocytes ingesting ≥1 AFB or the number of AFB/100 monocytes in four independent experiments using monocytes from healthy subjects. *:*P*<0.01 compared with control culture or OKT4A + gp120 or OKT4A alone; paired *t*-test. (From Ref. 116, reproduced from the Journal of Clinical Investigation, 1994, 93:885–891, by copyright permission of American Society for Clinical Investigation.)

phages (124,125). Spontaneous production of high levels of TNF-α and IL-6 by peripheral monocytes (122,126) and IL-6 and GM-CSF by alveolar macrophages has been demonstrated in patients with AIDS (127,128). Peripheral blood mononuclear cells (PBMC) from HIV-1–infected subjects also exhibit increased TGF-β production compared with normal donors after stimulation with mycobacterial antigens such as *M. tuberculosis* purified protein derivative (PPD) (129). TNF-α production by *M. avium*–infected monocytes from patients with AIDS and healthy individuals was comparable; however, monocytes from patients with AIDS released lower concentrations of IL-1 into culture supernatants after *M. avium* infection than monocytes from healthy subjects (92). Newman et al. reported that chronically HIV-infected human monocyte-derived macrophages exhibited prolonged cytokine mRNA expression and produced more TNF-α, IL-1, and IL-6 after LPS stimulation in vitro (109). In our recent study, pretreatment of human monocytes with gp120 synergistically augmented production of proinflammatory cytokines IL-1, TNF-α, and IL-6 when monocytes were infected with *M. avium* (Table 7) (116,117). Induction of these and other cytokines by HIV-1 proteins may have a net effect of enhancing intracellular mycobacterial growth.

Clearly, HIV infection alters host responses to *M. avium* infection. It also is conceivable that *M. avium* infection may alter the course of HIV infection, presumably by induction of cytokines. Lymphocytes and other cells

Table 7 Effect of gp120 on Induction of Cytokine Expression by Human Monocytes

	IL-1α (pg/ml)	IL-1β (pg/ml)	TNF-α (pg/ml)	IL-6 (ng/ml)
Control	3 ± 1	221 ± 60	112 ± 85	2.1 ± 0.9
gp120	17 ± 8	398 ± 124	159 ± 69	4.4 ± 2.7
M. avium	23 ± 4	553 ± 147	1708 ± 624	40.7 ± 9.4
gp120 + *M. avium*	81 ± 22[a]	1634 ± 397[a]	3535 ± 886[b]	63.2 ± 11.6[b]

Monocytes from healthy subjects were precultured with or without gp120 (1 µg/ml) for 2 days and then stimulated with *M. avium* strain LR114 SmT for another 24 hr. Cytokine activities in culture supernatants were assayed by ELISA. Data presented are the mean ± SE of cytokine concentrations from four to five independent experiments using monocytes obtained from four to five individual subjects.
[a]$P < 0.05$.
[b]$P < 0.01$ compared to cultures stimulated with *M. avium* alone (paired *t*-test).
Source: Ref. 116, reproduced from the Journal of Clinical Investigation, 1994, 93:885–891, by copyright permission of American Society for Clinical Investigation.

capable of harboring HIV are exposed to cytokines in the circulation and at the tissue level. HIV infection of quiescent T cells results in incomplete HIV replication; cellular activation is required for complete transcription of retroviral RNA (130). TNF-α, IL-1β, and IL-6 have been shown to augment HIV replication in vitro in HIV-infected cells (131–134), leading to further depression of host immune defenses in a potential vicious cycle. Cytokine induction due to *M. avium* infection could, therefore, theoretically accelerate the course of HIV infection.

In addition to the alterations in cytokine expression by gp120-treated cells, HIV-1 products may impair other aspects of mononuclear phagocyte defense against intracellular pathogens. Macrophage phagosome-lysosome fusion is another important intermediate step in the killing of intracellular pathogens such as mycobacteria. Inhibition of phagosome-lysosome fusion occurs after phagocytosis by murine bone marrow–derived macrophages of virulent strains of *M. avium* and correlates with increased capacity for rapid intracellular mycobacterial replication (34). Estevez et al. have shown that gp120 inhibits macrophage phagosome-lysosome fusion after phagocytosis of opsonized zymosan particles (135), providing another potential basis for its action on intracellular *M. avium* growth.

VI. Animal Models of *M. avium* Infection

The beige mouse (C57BL/6J/bg/bg), a mutant of C57B1/6J, is a murine model of the Chédiak-Higashi syndrome in humans and has a similar immune defect. The beige mouse is highly susceptible to mycobacterial infection and has been used as an animal model of disseminated *M. avium* infection (136,137). After intravenous inoculation with 10^6 to 10^7 CFU of SmT *M. avium*, widespread infection is demonstrable within 2 weeks. Bacterial counts in liver and spleen range from 10^6 to 10^9 CFU/g of tissue, and the mortality in infected animals may reach 50% 4 weeks following infection with highly virulent *M. avium* strains.

The route of *M. avium* challenge may be an important factor for the development of disseminated disease. Beige mice developed disseminated *M. avium* infection more efficiently after intrarectal than oral challenge (137). Bermudez et al. also demonstrated that oral inoculation results in disseminated *M. avium* infection throughout the gastrointestinal tract in the beige mouse model (138). This may reflect a similar disease process in humans in that *M. avium* has been recovered from both respiratory secretions and stool in patients with AIDS prior to the development of disseminated *M. avium* disease (139).

Orme et al. have developed other animal models of disseminated *M. avium* infection utilizing C57BL/6J and beige mice (C57BL/6J bg/bg) infected with murine AIDS retroviruses (LP-Bm5 or Du5H) or immunosuppressed by neonatal thymectomy and CD4 depletion with anti-CD3 antibody and complement (140). Disseminated disease with exuberant intracellular *M. avium* growth in the liver and spleen following intravenous or enteric *M. avium* challenge has been demonstrated using these models.

An additional animal model of disseminated *M. avium* infection utilizing cyclosporine-treated rats has recently been described by Brown et al. (141). Cyclosporine suppresses T-cell–mediated immune responses and is used clinically to prevent organ rejection in patients with solid organ transplants. Disseminated *M. avium* infection developed in rats treated with daily subcutaneous cyclosporine injections after intravenous challenge with 10^8 CFU of *M. avium*. Splenic burdens of *M. avium* ranged from 10^6 to 10^7 CFU/g tissue. Tissue burdens of *M. avium* decreased and *M. avium*–infected rats were cured spontaneously after cessation of cyclosporine treatment. Histopathological changes in infected tissues were similar to those in patients with AIDS with disseminated *M. avium* infection; numerous AFB and poorly formed granulomata are present in the spleens of cyclosporine-treated rats with disseminated *M. avium* infection. Unlike disseminated *M. avium* infection in patients with AIDS, mycobacteremia was intermittent rather than continuous.

VII. Conclusions

Despite the numerous studies of host–*M. avium* interactions described above, it is not yet clear why the incidence of disseminated *M. avium* infection in patients with AIDS is greatly increased compared with other immunocompromised hosts such as patients with cancer undergoing intensive cytoreductive or immunosuppressive chemotherapy and what factors lead to the unprecedented tissue burdens of *M. avium* in patients with AIDS. Disseminated *M. avium* infection occurs in cyclosporine-treated rats challenged with *M. avium* (141); however, disseminated *M. avium* infection is rare in patients receiving organ transplants treated with cyclosporine, alkylating agents, and corticosteroids. Mechanisms and factors leading to *M. avium* survival and intracellular multiplication in human mononuclear phagocytes are incompletely understood.

As discussed, certain cytokines modulate *M. avium* uptake by phagocytes and have complex and bidirectional effects on intracellular growth of *M. avium* in human phagocytes. Cytokines have important roles in the regulation of local inflammation and granuloma formation, and they also modulate production of other cytokines. *M. avium* infection also generates cytokine induction by mononuclear phagocytes. SmD strains (relatively avirulent) rapidly trigger cytokine production in infected macrophages; these cytokines may enhance bactericidal activity and act as chemoattractants to recruit other mononuclear phagocytes, leading to granuloma formation. SmT strains, which induce less cytokines, may not activate these host defense mechanisms. Evidence demonstrating bidirectional effects of cytokines on intracellular *M. avium* growth suggest that a complex local balance of mycobacterial growth-inhibiting and growth-enhancing factors may modulate *M. avium* virulence.

Direct and indirect interactions between *M. avium*, HIV, and viral proteins such as gp120 are worthy of further study in attempts to elucidate the pathophysiological mechanisms underlying uncontrolled intracellular *M. avium* growth and disseminated infection in HIV-infected individuals. Whether or not cytokine production induced by *M. avium* or other mycobacteria increases HIV replication in otherwise latently infected cells and accelerates the natural history of HIV infection is another important question.

Future studies in these areas should provide new insights into the pathogenesis of disseminated *M. avium* in patients with AIDS and the mechanisms whereby mycobacterial surface components, viral products, and induction of host cytokines contribute to successful parasitism. It is hoped that this knowledge will lead to the inception and application of new therapeutic approaches against this important opportunistic pathogen.

References

1. Kiehn TE, Edwards FF, Brannon P, et al. Infections caused by *Mycobacterium avium* complex in immunocompromised patients: Diagnosis by blood culture and fecal examination, antimicrobial susceptibility tests, and morphological and seroagglutination characteristics. J Clin Microbiol 1985; 21:168–173.
2. Crawford JT, Bates JH. Analysis of plasmids in *Mycobacterium avium–intracellulare* isolates from persons with acquired immunodeficiency syndrome. Am Rev Respir Dis 1986; 134:659–661.
3. Gangadharam PRJ, Perumal VK, Crawford JT, Bates JH. Association of plasmids and virulence of *Mycobacterium avium* complex. Am Rev Respir Dis 1988; 137:212–214.

4. Horsburgh CR Jr, Cohn DL, Roberts RB, et al. *Mycobacterium avium–M. intracellulare* isolates from patients with or without acquired immunodeficiency syndrome. Antimicrob Agents Chemother 1986; 30:955–957.

5. Arbeit RD, Slutsky A, Barber TW, et al. Genetic diversity among strains of *Mycobacterium avium* causing monoclonal and polyclonal bacteremia in patients with AIDS. J Infect Dis 1993; 167:1384–1390.

6. Dunbar FP, Pejovic I, Cacciatore R, et al. *Mycobacterium intracellulare* maintenance of pathogenicity in relationship to lyophilization and colony form. Scand J Respir Dis 1968; 49:153–162.

7. Schaefer WB, Davis CL, Cohn ML. Pathogenicity of transparent, opaque, and rough variants of *Mycobacterium avium* in chickens and mice. Am Rev Respir Dis 1970; 102:499–506.

8. Meylan PR, Richman DD, Kornbluth RS. Characterization and growth in human macrophages of *Mycobacterium avium* complex strains isolated from the blood of patients with acquired immunodeficiency syndrome. Infect Immun 1990; 58:2564–2568.

9. Shiratsuchi H, Johnson JL, Toba H, Ellner JJ. Strain- and donor-related differences in the interaction of *Mycobacterium avium* with human monocytes and its modulation by interferon-γ. J Infect Dis 1990; 162:932–938.

10. Belisle J, Brennan PJ. Molecular basis of colony morphology in *Mycobacterium avium*. Res Microbiol 1994; 143:237–242.

11. Brennan PJ, Goren MB. Structural studies on the type-specific antigens and lipids of *Mycobacterium avium–Mycobacterium intracellulare–Mycobacterium scrofulaceum* serocomplex. J Biol Chem 1979; 254:4205–4211.

12. Camphausen RT, Jones RL, Brennan PJ. Structure and relevance of the oligosaccharide hapten of *Mycobacterium avium* serotype 2. J Bacteriol 1986; 168:660–667.

13. Brownback PE, Barrow WW. Modified lymphocyte response to mitogens after intraperitoneal injection of glycopeptidolipid antigens from *Mycobacterium avium* complex. Infect Immun 1988; 56:1044–1050.

14. Hines ME II, Jaynes JM, Borker SA, et al. Isolation and partial characterization of glycolipid fractions from *Mycobacterium avium* serovar 2 (*Mycobaacterium paratuberculosis* 18) that inhibit activated macrophages. Infect Immun 1993; 61:1–7.

15. Tassell SK, Pourshafie M, Wright EL, et al. Modified lymphocyte response to mitogen induced by the lipopeptide fragment derived from *Mycobacterium avium* serovar-specific glycopeptidolipids. Infect Immun 1992; 60:706–711.

16. Mosser DM, Edelson P. The mouse macrophage receptor for C3bi (CR3) is a major mechanism in the phagocytosis of *Leishmania promastigotis*. J Immunol 1985; 135:2785–2789.

17. Wilson ME, Pearson RD. Roles of CR3 and mannose receptors in the attachment and ingestion of *Leishmania donovani* by human mononuclear phagocytes. Infect Immun 1988; 56:363–369.

18. Myones BL, Dalzell JG, Hogg N, Ross GD. Neutrophil and monocyte cell surface p150,95 has iC3b-receptor (CD4) activity resembling CR3. J Clin Invest 1988; 82:640–651.

19. Schlesinger LS, Horwitz MA. Phagocytosis of leprosy bacilli is mediated by complement receptors CR1 and CR3 on human monocytes and complement component C3 in serum. J Clin Invest 1990; 85:1304–1314.

20. Schlesinger LS, Bellinger-Kawahara CG, Payne NR, Horwitz MA. Phagocytosis of *Mycobacterium tuberculosis* is mediated by human monocyte complement receptors and complement component C3. J Immunol 1990; 144:2771–2780.

21. Schlesinger LS, Horwitz MA. Phagocytosis of *Mycobacterium leprae* by human monocyte-derived macrophages is mediated by complement receptor CR1 (CD35), CR3 (CD11b/CD18), and CR4 (CD11c/CD18) and IFN-γ activation inhibits complement receptor function and phagocytosis of this bacaterium. J Immunol 1991; 147:1983–1994.

22. Hirsch CS, Ellner JJ, Russell DG, Rich EA. Complement receptor-mediated uptake and tumor necrosis factor-α-mediated growth inhibition of *Mycobacterium tuberculosis* by human alveolar macrophage. J Immunol 1994; 152: 743–753.

23. Bermudez LE, Young LS, Enkel H. Interaction of *Mycobacterium avium* complex with human macrophages: Roles of membrane receptors and serum proteins. Infect Immun 1991; 59:1697–1702.

24. Swartz RP, Naai D, Vogel CW, Yeager H Jr. Differences in uptake of mycobacteria by human monocytes: a role for complement. Infect Immun 1988; 56: 2223–2227.

25. Rao SP, Gehlsen KR, Catanzaro A. Identification of a β₁ integrin on *Mycobacterium avium–Mycobacterium intracellulare*. Infect Immun 1992; 60: 3652–3657.

26. Schlesinger LS, Horwitz MA. A role for natural antibody in the pathogenesis of leprosy: Antibody in nonimmune serum mediates C3 fixation to *Mycobacterium leprae* surface and hence phagocytosis by human mononuclear phagocytes. Infect Immun 1994; 62:280–289.

27. Lee B, Chatterjee D, Bozic CM, et al. Prevalence of serum antibody to the type-specific glycopeptidolipid antigens of *Mycobacterium avium* in human immunodeficiency virus-positive and -negative individuals. J Clin Microbiol 1991; 29:1026–1029.

28. Toba H, Crawford JT, Ellner JJ. Pathogenicity of *Mycobacterium avium* for human monocytes: absence of macrophage-activating factor activity of gamma interferon. Infect Immun 1989; 57:239–244.

29. Johnson JL, Shiratsuchi H, Toba H, Ellner JJ. Preservation of monocyte effector functions against *Mycobacterium avium–M. intracellulare* in patients with AIDS. Infect Immun 1991; 59:3639–3645.

30. Esparza I, Fox RI, Schreiber RD. Interferon-γ–dependent modulation of C3b receptors (CR1) on human peripheral blood monocytes. J Immunol 1986; 136: 1360–1365.

31. Wright SD, Detmers PA, Jong MTC, Meyer BC. Interferon-γ depresses binding of ligand by C3b and C3bi receptors on cultured human monocytes, an effect reversed by fibronection. J Exp Med 1986; 163:1245–1259.

32. Crowle AJ, Dahl R, Ross E, May MH. Evidence that vesicles containing living virulent *Mycobacterium tuberculosis* or *Mycobacterium avium* in cultured human macrophages are not acidic. Infect Immun 1991; 59:1823–1831.

33. Sturgill-Koszycki S, Schlesinger PH, Chakraborty P, et al. Lack of acidification in *Mycobacterium* phagosomes produced by exclusion of the vesicular proton-ATPase. Science 1994; 263:678–681.

34. Frehel C, deChastellier C, Lang T, Rastogi N. Evidence for inhibition of fusion of lysosomal and prelysosomal compartments with phagosomes in macrophages infected with pathogenic *Mycobacterium avium*. Infect Immun 1986; 52:252–262.

35. Rulong S, Aguas AP, daSilva PP, Silva MT. Intramacrophagic *Mycobacterium avium* bacilli are coated by a multiple lamellar structure: freeze fracture analysis of infected mouse liver. Infect Immun 1991; 59:3895–3902.

36. Newman GW, Gan HX, McCarthy PL, Remold HG. Survival of human macrophages infected with *Mycobacterium avium intracellulare* correlates with increased production of tumor necrosis factor-α and IL-6. J Immunol 1991; 147: 3942–3948.

37. Douvas GS, Berger EM, Repine JE, Crowle AJ. Natural mycobacteriostatic activity in human monocyte-derived adherent cells. Am Rev Respir Dis 1986; 134:44–48.

38. Blanchard DK, Michelini-Norris MB, Djeu JY. Interferon decreases the growth inhibition of *Mycobacterium avium–intracellulare* complex by fresh human monocytes but not by culture-derived macrophages. J Infect Dis 1991; 164: 152–157.

39. Källenius G, Koivula T, Rydgård KJ, et al. Human immunodeficiency virus type 1 enhances intracellular growth of *Mycobacterium avium* in human macrophages. Infect Immun 1992; 60:2453–2458.

40. Belosevic M, Davis CE, Meltzer MS, Nacy CA. Regulation of activated macrophage antimicrobial activities: Identification of lymphokines that cooperate with IFN-γ for induction of resistance to infection. J Immunol 1988; 141: 890–896.

41. Numerof RP, Aronson FR, Mier JW. IL-2 stimulates the production of IL-1α and IL-1β by human peripheral blood mononuclear cells. J Immunol 1988; 141:4250–4257.

42. Zucali JR, Dinarello CA, Oblon DJ, et al. Interleukin 1 stimulates fibroblasts to produce granulocyte-macrophage colony-stimulating activity and prostaglandin E_2. J Clin Invest 1986; 77:1857–1863.

43. Oster W, Lindemann A, Horn S, et al. Tumor necrosis factor (TNF)–alpha but not TNF-beta induces secretion of colony stimulating factor for macrophages (CSF-1) by human monocytes. Blood 1987; 70:1700–1703.

44. Sisson SD, Dinarello CA. Production of interleukin-1α, interleukin-β, and tumor necrosis factor by human mononuclear cells stimulated with granulocyte-macrophage colony stimulating factor. Blood 1988; 72:1368–1374.
45. Lindemann A, Riedel D, Oster W, et al. Granulocyte/macrophage colony-stimulating factor induces interleukin 1 production by human polymorphonuclear neutrophils. J Immunol 1988; 140:837–839.
46. Hancock WW, Pleau ME, Kobzik L. Recombinant granulocyte-macrophage colony-stimulating factor down-regulates expression of IL-2 receptor on human mononuclear phagocytes by induction of prostaglandin E. J Immunol 1988; 140:3021–3025.
47. Ruggiero V, Tavernier J, Fiers W, Baglioni C. Induction of the synthesis of tumor necrosis factor receptors by interferon-γ. J Immunol 1986; 136:2445–2450.
48. Kurtz RS, Roll JT, Czuprynski CJ. Recombinant human interleukin 1α enhances anti-Listeria resistance in both genetically resistant and susceptible strains of mice. Immunol Lett 1988; 18:289–292.
49. Malkovsky M, Loveland B, North M, et al. Recombinant interleukin-2 directory augments the cytotoxicity of human monocytes. Nature 1987; 325:262–266.
50. Philip R, Epstein LB. Tumor necrosis factor as immunomodulator and mediator of monocyte cytotoxicity induced by itself, γ-interferon and interleukin-1. Nature 1986; 323:86–89.
51. Velde AA, Klomp JPG, Yard BA, et al. Modulation of phenotypic and functional properties of human peripheral blood monocytes by IL-4. J Immunol 1988; 140:1548–1554.
52. Zlotnik A, Fischer M, Roehm N, Zipori D. Evidence for effects of interleukin 4 (B cell stimulatory factor 1) on macrophages: enhancement of antigen presenting ability of bone marrow-derived macrophages. J Immunol 1987; 138:4275–4279.
53. Weisbart RH, Gasson JC, Golde DW. Colony-stimulating factor and host defence. Ann Internal Med 1989; 110:297–303.
54. Reed SG, Nathan CF, Pihl DL, et al. Recombinant granulocyte/macrophage colony-stimulating factor activates macrophages to inhibit *Trypanosoma cruzi* and release hydrogen peroxide. Comparison with interferon-γ. J Exp Med 1987; 166:1735–1746.
55. Handman E, Burgess AW. Stimulation by ganulocyte-macrophage colony-stimulating factor of *Leishmania tropica* killing by macrophages. J Immunol 1979; 122:1134–1137.
56. Wing EJ, Ampel NM, Waheed A, Shadduck RK. Macrophage colony-stimulating factor (M-CSF) enhances the capacity of murine macrophages to secrete oxygen reduction products. J Immunol 1985; 135:2052–2056.
57. Shiratsuchi H, Johnson JL, Ellner JJ. Bidirectional effects of cytokines on the growth of *Mycobacterium avium* within human monocytes. J Immunol 1991; 146:3165–3170.

58. Denis M, Gregg EO. Recombinant tumor necrosis factor-alpha decreases whereas recombinant interleukin-6 increases growth of a virulent strain of *Mycobacterium avium* in human macrophages. Immunology 1990; 71:139–141.

59. Bermudez LEM, Young LS. Tumor necrosis factor, alone or in combination with IL-2, but not IFN-γ, is associated with macrophage killing of *Mycobacterium avium* complex. J Immunol 1998; 140:3006–3013.

60. Hoy J, Mijch A, Sandland M, et al. Quadruple-drug therapy for *Mycobacterium avium–intracellulare* bacteremia in AIDS patients. J Infect DIs 1990: 161: 801–805.

61. Bermudez LE. Production of transforming growth factor-β by Mycobacterium avium–infected human macrophages is associated with unresponsiveness to IFN-γ. J Immunol 1993; 150:1838–1845.

62. Rose RM, Fuglestad JM, Remington L. Growth inhibition of *Mycobacterium avium* complex in human alveolar macrophages by the combination of recombinant macrophage colony-stimulating factor and interferon-gamma. Am J Respir Cell Mol Biol 1991; 248–254.

63. Bermudez LEM, Young LS. Recombinant granulocyte-macrophage colony-stimulating factor activates human macrophages to inhibit growth or kill *Mycobacterium avium* complex. J Leukocyte Biol 1990; 48:67–73.

64. Douvas GS, Looker DL, Vatter AE, Crowle AJ. Gamma interferon activates human macrophages to become tumoricidal and leishmanicidal but enhances replication of macrophage-associated mycobacteria. Infect Immun 1985; 50: 1–8.

65. Passwell JH, Shor R, Shoham J. The enhancing effect of interferon-β and -γ on the killing of *Leishmania tropica major* in human mononuclear phagocytes in vitro. J Immunol 1986; 136:3062–3066.

66. Rothermel CD, Rubin BY, Murray HW. γ-Interferon is the factor in lymphokine that activates human macrophages to inhibit intracellular *Chlamydia psittaci* replication. J Immunol 1983; 131:2542–2544.

67. Bhardwaj N, Nash TW, Horwitz MA. Interferon-γ-activated human monocytes inhibit the intracellular multiplication of *Legionella pneumophila*. J Immunol 1986; 137:2662–2669.

68. Flesch I, Kaufmann SHE. Mycobacterial growth inhibition by interferon-γ–activated macrophages and differential susceptibility among strains of *Mycobacterium tuberculosis*. J Immunol 1987; 138:4408–4413.

69. Rook AW, Steele J, Ainsworth M, Champion BR. Activation of macrophages to inhibit proliferation of *Mycobacterium tuberculosis*: comparison of the effects of recombinant gamma-interferon on human monocytes and murine peritoneal macrophages. Immunology 1986; 59:333–338.

70. Edwards CK III, Hedegaard H, Zlotnick A. et al. Chronic infection due to *Mycobacterium intracellulare* in mice: Association with macrophage release of prostaglandin E_2 and reversal by injection of indomethacin, muramyl dipeptide, or interferon-γ. J Immunol 1986; 136:1820–1827.

71. Sibley LD, Krahenbuhl JL. Induction of unresponsiveness to gamma interferon in macrophages infected with *Mycobacterium leprae.* Infect Immun 1988; 56: 1912–1919.
72. The International Chronic Granulomatous Disease Cooperative Study Group. A controlled trial of interferon gamma to prevent infection in chronic granulomatous disease. N Engl J Med 1991; 324:509–516.
73. Nathan CF, Kaplan G, Levis WR, et al. Local and systemic effects of intradermal recombinant interferon-γ in patients with lepromatous leprosy. N Engl J Med 1986; 315:6–15.
74. Badaro R, Falcoff E, Badaro FS, et al. Treatment of visceral leishmaniasis with pentavalent antimony and interferon gamma. N Engl J Med 1990; 322:16–21.
75. Holland SM, Eisenstein EM, Kuhns DB, et al. Treatment of refractory disseminated nontuberculous mycobacterial infection with interferon gamma. N Engl J Med 1994; 330:1348–1355.
76. Schnittman S, Lane HC, Witebsky FG, et al. Host defense against *Mycobacterium-avium* complex. J Clin Immunol 1988; 8:234–243.
77. Cheers C, Hill M, Haigh AM, Stanley ER. Stimulation of macrophage phagocytic but not bactericidal activity by colony-stimulating factor 1. Infect Immun 1989; 57:1512–1516.
78. Blanchard DK, Michelini-Norris MB, Pearson CA, et al. Production of granulocyte-macrophage colony-stimulating factor (GM-CSF) by monocytes and large granular lymphocytes stimulated with *Mycobacterium avium–M. intracellulare*: Activation of bactericidal activity by GM-CSF. Infect Immun 1991; 59:2396–2402.
79. Jeevan A, Asherson GL. Recombinant interleukin-2 limits the replication of *Mycobacterium lepraemurium* and *Mycobacterium bovis* BCG in mice. Infect Immun 1988; 56:660–664.
80. Chiu CP, Lee F. IL-6 is a differentiation factor for M1 and WEHI-3B myeloid leukemic cells. J Immunol 1989; 142:1909–1915.
81. Luger AT, Krutmann J, Kirnbauer R, et al. IFN-β_2/IL-6 augments the acitivity of human natural killer cells. J Immunol 1990; 143:1206–1209.
82. Bogdan C, Vodovotz Y, Nathan C. Macrophage deactivation by interleukin 10. J Exp Med 1991; 174:1549–1555.
83. Fiorentino DF, Zlotnik A, Mosmann TR, et al. IL-10 inhibits cytokine production by activated macrophages. J Immunol 1991; 147:3815–3822.
84. Bermudez LE, Champsi J. Infection with *Mycobacterium avium* induces production of interleukin 10 (IL-10), and administration of anti-IL-10 antibody is associated with enhanced resistance to infection in mice. Infect. Immun 1993; 61:3093–3097.
85. Porat R, Clark BD, Wolff SM, Dinarello CH. Enhancement of growth of virulent strains of *Escherichia coli* by interleukin-1. Science 1991; 254:430–432.
86. Denis M, Campbell D, Gregg EO. Interleukin-2 and granulocyte-macrophage colony-stimulating factor stimulate growth of a virulent strain of *Escherichia coli.* Infect Immun 1991; 59:1853–1856.

87. Luo G, Niesel DW, Shaban RA, et al. Tumor necrosis factor alpha binding to bacteria: Evidence for a high-affinity receptor and alteration of bacteria virulence properties. Infect Immun 1993; 61:830–835.

88. Bermudez L, Wu M, Petrofsky M, Young LS. Interleukin-6 antagonizes tumor necrosis factor-mediated mycobacteriostatic and mycobactericidal activities. Infect Immun 1992; 60:4245–4252.

89. Blanchard DK, Michelini-Norris MB, Pearson CA, et al. *Mycobacterium avium–intracellulare* induces interleukin-6 from human monocytes and large granular lymphocytes. Blood 1991; 77:2218–2224.

90. Shiratsuchi H, Toossi Z, Mettler MA, Ellner JJ. Colonial morphotype as a determinant of cytokine expression by human monocytes infected with *Mycobacterium avium*. J Immunol 1993; 150:2945–2954.

91. Michelini-Norris MB, Blanchard DK, Pearson CA, Djeu JY. Differential release of interleukin (IL)-1α, IL-1β, and IL-6 from normal human monocytes stimulated with a virulent and an avirulent isogeneic variant of *Mycobacterium avium-intracellulare* complex. J Infect Dis 1992; 165:702–709.

92. Johnson JL, Shiratsuchi H, Ellner JJ. Altered cytokine expression by monocytes from patients with AIDS stimulated with *Mycobacterium avium* (abstr). Clin Res 1993; 41:394A.

93. Furney SK, Skinner PS, Roberts A, et al. Capacity of *Mycobacterium avium* isolates to grow well or poorly in murine macrophages resides in their ability to induce secretion tumor necrosis factor. Infect Immun 1992; 60:4410–4413.

94. Chiu J, Nussbaum J, Bozzette S, et al. California Collaborative Treatment Group. Treatment of disseminated *Mycobacterium avium* complex infection in AIDS with amikacin, ethambutol, rifampin, and ciprofloxacin. Ann Inter Med 1990; 113:358–361.

95. Wong B, Edwards FF, Kiehn TE, et al. Continuous high-grade *Mycobacterium avium–intracellulare* bacteremia in patients with the acquired immune deficiency syndrome. Am J Med 1985; 78:35–40.

96. Washburn RG, Tuazon CU, Bennett JE. Phagocytic and fungicidal activity of monocytes from patients with acquired immunodeficiency syndrome. J Infect Dis 1985; 151:565.

97. Murray HW, Rubin BY, Masur H, Roberts RB. Impaired production of lymphokines and immune (gamma) interferon in the acquired immunodeficiency syndrome. N Engl J Med 1984; 310:883–889.

98. Bender BS, Davidson BL, Kline R, et al. Role of the mononuclear phagocyte system in the immunopathogenesis of human immunodeficiency virus infection and the acquired immunodeficiency syndrome. Rev Infect Dis 1988; 10:1142–1154.

99. Poli G, Bottazzi B, Acero R, et al. Monocyte function in intravenous drug abusers with lymphadenopathy syndrome and in patients with acquired immunodeficiency syndrome: selective impairment of chemotaxis. Clin Exp Immunol 1985; 62:136–142.

100. Müller F, Rollag H, Froland SS. Reduced oxidative burst responses in monocytes and monocyte-derived macrophages from HIV-infected subjects. Clin Exp Immunol 1990; 82:10–15.
101. Crowle AJ, Ross ER, Cohn DL, et al. Comparison of the abilities of *Mycobacterium avium* and *Mycobacterium intracellulare* to infect and multiply in cultured human macrophages from normal and human immunodeficiency virus-infected subjects. Infect Immun 1992; 60:3697–3703.
102. Sieraa-Madero JG, Toossi Z, Hom DL, et al. Relationship between load of virus in alveolar macrophages from human immunodeficiency virus–infected perosns, production of cytokines and clinical status. J Infect Dis 1994; 169: 18–27.
103. Schnittman SM, Psallidopoulos MC, Lane HC, et al. The reservoir for HIV-1 in human peripheral blood is a T cell that maintains expression of CD4. Science 1989; 245:305–308.
104. Massari FE, Poli G, Schnittman SM, et al. In vivo T lymphocyte origin of macrophage-trophic strains of HIV. J Immunol 1990; 144:4628–4632.
105. Gendelman HE, Orenstein JM, Baca LM, et al. The macrophage in the persistence and pathogenesis of HIV infection. AIDS 1989; 3:475–495.
106. Müller R, Rollag H, Gaudernack G, Froland SS. Impaired in vitro survival of monocytes from patients with HIV infection. Clin Exp Immunol 1990; 81:25–30.
107. Crowle AJ, Cohn DL, Poche P. Defects in sera from acquired immunodeficiency syndrome (AIDS) patients and from non-AIDS patients with *Mycobacterium avium* infection which decrease macrophage resistance to *M. avium.* Infect Immun 1989; 57:1445–1451.
108. Meylan PRA, Munis JR, Richman DD, Kornbluth RS. Concurrent human immunodeficiency virus and mycobacterial infection of macrophages in vitro does not reveal any reciprocal effect. J Infect Dis 1992; 165:80–86.
109. Newman GW, Kelley TG, Gan H, et al. Concurrent infection of human macrophages with HIV-1 and *Mycobacterium avium* results in decreased cell viability, increase *M. avium* multiplication and altered cytokine production. J Immunol 1993; 151:2261–2272.
110. Spear GT, Ou C, Kessler HA, et al. Analysis of lymphocytes, monocytes, and neutrophils from human immunodeficiency virus (HIV)-1 infected persons for HIV DNA. J Infect Dis 1990; 162:1239–1244.
111. Clouse KA, Cosentino CM, Weih KA, et al. The HIV-1 gp120 envelope protein has the intrinsic capacity to stimulate monokine secretion. J Immunol 1991; 147:2892–2901.
112. Merrill JE, Koyanagi Y, Chen ISY. Interleukin-1 and tumor necrosis factor α can be induced from mononuclear phagocytes by human immunodeficiency virus type 1 binding to the CD4 receptor. J Virol 1989; 63:4404–4408.
113. Nakajima K, Martinez-Maza O, Hirano T, et al. Induction of IL-6 (B cell stimulatory factor-2/IFN-β2) production by HIV. J Immunol 1989; 142:531–536.

114. Wahl LM, Corcoran ML, Pyle SW, et al. Human immunodeficiency virus glycoprotein (gp120) induction of monocyte arachidonic acid metabolites and interleukin-1. Proc Natl Acad Sci USA 1989; 86:621–625.

115. Molina JM, Scadden DT, Amirault C, et al. Human immunodeficiency virus does not induce interleukin-1, interleukin-6, or tumor necrosis factor in mononuclear cells. J Virol 1990; 64:2901–2906.

116. Shiratsuchi H, Johnson JL, Toossi Z, Ellner JJ. Modulation of the effector function of human monocytes for *Mycobacterium avium* by human immunodeficiency virus-1 envelope glycoprotein gp120. J Clin Invest 1994; 93:885–891.

117. Shiratsuchi H, Johnson JL, Ellner JJ. *M. avium*: Pathogenicity in HIV-1 infections. Res Microbiol 1994; 145:230–236.

118. Klatzmann D, Champagne E, Chamare S, et al. T-lymphocyte T4 molecule behaves as the receptor for human retrovirus LAV. Nature 1984; 312:767–768.

119. Melendez-Guerrero ML, Nicholson JKA, McDougal JS. In vitro infection of monocytes with HIV_{Ba-L}. Effect on cell surface expression of CD4, CD14, HLA-DR, and HLA-DQ. AIDS Res Hum Retroviruses 1990; 6:731–741.

120. Finbloom DS, Hoover DL, Meltzer MS. Binding of recombinant HIV coat protein gp120 to human monocytes. J Immunol 1991; 146:1316–1321.

121. Wagner RP, Levitz S, Bernardo J, et al. HIV envelope protein (gp120) decrease the anti-cryptococcal effect of human bronchoalveolar macrophages (abstr). 6th Int Conf AIDS 1990; 6:159.

122. Breen EC, Rezai AR, Nakajima K, et al. Infection with HIV is associated with elevated IL-6 levels and production. J Immunol 1990; 144:480–484.

123. Kalinkovich A, Engelmann H, Haopaz N, et al. Elevated levels of soluble tumor necrosis factor receptors (TNF-R) in patients with HIV infection. Clin Exp Immunol 1992; 89:351–355.

124. Seekinger P, Isaaz S, Dayer J. Purification and biologic characterization of a specific tumor necrosis factor α inhibitor. J Biol Chem 1989; 264:11966–11973.

125. Kruppa G, Thoma B, Machleidt T, et al. Inhibition of tumor necrosis factor (TNF)-mediated NF-κB activation by selective blockade of the human 55-kDa TNF receptor. J Immunol 1992; 148:3152–3157.

126. Wright SC, Jewett A, Mitsuyasu R, Bonavida B. Spontaneous cytotoxicity and tumor necrosis factor production by peripheral blood monocytes from AIDS patients. J Immunol 1998; 141:99–104.

127. Agostini C, Zambello R, Trentin L, et al. Alveolar macrophages from patients with AIDS and AIDS-related complex constitutively synthesize and release tumor necrosis factor alpha. Am Rev Respir Dis 1991; 144:195–201.

128. Trentin L, Garbisa S, Zambello R, et al. Spontaneous production of interleukin-6 by alveolar macrophages from human immunodeficiency virus type 1-infected patients. J Infect Dis 1992; 166:731–737.

129. Kekow J, Wachsman W, McCutchan JA, et al. Transforming growth factor β and noncytopathic mechanisms of immunodeficiency in human immunodeficiency virus infection. Proc Natl Acad Sci USA 1990; 87:8321–8325.

130. Zack JA, Arrigo SVC, Weitsman SR, et al. HIV-1 entry into quiescent primary lymphocytes: molecular analysis reveals a labile, latent viral source. Cell 1990; 61:213–222.

131. Osborn LO, Kunkel S, Nabel GJ. Tumor necrosis factor-α and interleukin 1 stimulate the human immunodeficiency virus enhancer by activation of the nuclear factor-κB. Proc Natl Acad Sci USA 1989; 89:2336–2346.

132. Mellors JW, Griffith BP, Oritz MA, et al. Tumor necrosis factor-α/cachectin enhances human immunodeficiency virus type 1 replication in primary macrophages. J Infect Dis 1991; 163:78–82.

133. Poli G, Bressler P, Kinter A, et al. Interleukin 6 induces human immunodeficiency virus expression in infected monocytic cells alone and in synergy with tumor necrosis factor α by transcriptional and posttranscriptional mechanisms. J Exp Med 1990; 172:151–158.

134. Clouse KA, Powell D, Washington I, et al. Monokine regulation of human immunodeficiency virus-1 expression in a chronically infected human T cell clone. J Immunol 1989; 142:431–438.

135. Estevez ME, Pittis G, Sternik G, Sen L. HIV-1 gp120 inhibits macrophage phagosome-lysosome fusion (abstr). 8th Int Conf AIDS 1992; 8:A64.

136. Bertram MA, Inderlied CB, Yadegar S, et al. Confirmation of the beige mouse model for study of disseminated infection with *Mycobacterium avium* complex. J Infect Dis 1986; 154:194–195.

137. Gangadharam PRJ, Perumal VK, Parikh K, et al. Susceptibility of beige mice to *Mycobacterium avium* complex infections by different routes of challenge. Am Rev Respir Dis 1989; 139:1098–1104.

138. Bermudez LE, Petrofsky M, Kolonosky P, Young LS. An animal model of *Mycobacterium avium* complex disseminated infection after colonization of the intestinal tract. J Infect Dis 1992; 165:75–79.

139. Poropatich CO, Labriola AM, Tuazon CU. Acid-fast smear and culture of respiratory secretions, bone marrow, and stools as predictors of disseminated *Mycobacterium avium* complex infection. J Clin Microbiol 1987; 25:929–930.

140. Orme IM, Furney SK, Roberts AD. Dissemination of enteric *Mycobacterium avium* infections in mice rendered immunodeficient by thymectomy and CD4 depletion or by prior infection with murine AIDS retroviruses. Infect Immun 1992; 60:4747–4753.

141. Brown ST, Edwards FF, Bewrnard EM, et al. Progressive disseminated infection with *Mycobacterium avium* complex after intravenous and oral challenge in cyclosporine-treated rats. J Infect Dis 1991; 164:922–927.

8

Pharmacokinetics of Drugs Used for the Therapy of *Mycobacterium avium*–Complex Infection

AARON D. KILLIAN
and THOMAS P. KANYOK

College of Pharmacy
University of Illinois at Chicago
Chicago, Illinois

G. L. DRUSANO

Albany Medical College
Albany, New York

I. Pharmacokinetic-assisted Drug Dosing

The utilization of pharmacokinetic data to assist clinicians in the design of appropriate dosing regimens for antibacterial agents is a familiar concept, particularly when applied to antimicrobials such as vancomycin or the aminoglycoside class of agents. Historically, the rationale behind monitoring bodily fluids for concentrations of these agents was related to minimizing toxicity while ensuring efficacy of antibiotic therapy. Today, hospital formularies contain many anti-infectives for which the ratio of toxic:therapeutic concentrations is relatively large and, thus, monitoring serum concentrations is less of a concern. The β-lactams are a classic example of antibiotics with large "therapeutic windows" which have allowed, in most cases, relatively standardized dosing methodologies to be employed without the need for serum concentration monitoring. However, the application of pharmacokinetics is just as important to the initial design of nonindividualized regimens as it is to individualized therapy in terms of effecting a clinical cure. This is espcially true for AIDS patients since many will, at one time or another, experience derangements in physiologic function(s) which may lead to alterations in antibiotic pharmacokinetics. In some patients, serum drug determinations may be required to ensure that therapeutic concentrations are achieved. Also, since mycobacteria reside predominantly within cells, it is necessary to understand the relationships between the extra- and intracellular pharmacokinetics of these antimicrobials.

II. Macrolides and Azalides

A. Clarithromycin

Clarithromycin is a 14-membered macrolide antibiotic which differs from erythromycin only by methylation of a hydroxyl group at position six. This simple substitution is likely responsible for clarithromycin's improved bio-availability, diminished gastrointestinal upset, broadened spectrum of activity, and increased intracellular activity (1,2). Some researchers have attributed these observations to the methyl group's ability to inhibit the decomposition of clarithromycin to inactive hemiketal and spiroketal by-products under acidic conditions in the gastrointestinal tract (3) and intracellular phagoly-sosomes (4,5). The adverse effects are related to hemiketal metabolite formation, but researchers are unsure of the mechanism behind the increased intracellular activity of clarithromycin. Recent investigations have refuted the theory that the increased intracellular activity is due to improved acid stability in the macrophage environment. Crowle and co-workers (6) have provided evidence suggesting that vesicles containing live *Mycobacterium avium* complex (MAC) from human macrophages are not acidic. Thus, the improved bioactivity may be a result of clarithromycin's lipophilicity and enhanced membrane penetrability or other unknown factors that are independent of cellular decomposition.

Certain in vitro environmental conditions such as pH (carbon dioxide), temperature, and incubation with serum may also influence the activity of clarithromycin (7–9). For example, it is difficult to compare clarithromycin susceptibility data from in vitro studies performed at varying pH, as it is known that clarithromycin is more active against MAC at a basic pH (10). Similarly, comparisons between in vitro and in vivo studies are fraught with hazard, since clarithromycin relies on the immune system for optimal drug delivery in the treatment of intracellular MAC infections. It is thought that clarithromycin is concentrated intracellularly within macrophages via an oxy-gen-dependent active transport mechanism which, in turn, relies on polymorphonuclear leukocytes (PMNLs), appropriate temperature, pH, and, of course, oxygen for activation (7).

Absorption

Following oral administrationn, clarithromycin is almost completely absorbed exhibiting an absolute bioavailability of 52–55% in healthy subjects (11,12). The absorption of clarithromycin and its metabolite 14-hydroxy-(R)-clarithromycin (14-OH-clarithromycin) is increased by about 25 and 9%, respectively, when given as a single 500-mg dose immediately after food (13). Since clarithromycin is a weak organic base, it is plausible that postprandial alterations in pH or gastric emptying time may alter its gastrointestinal dissolution or mucosal contact time suffiently to impact on its absorption. The modest increase in absorption as well as the disproportionate increase in parent to metabolite AUC (area under the serum concentration versus time curve) observed with ascending oral doses (14,15) lend further support to the theory that clarithromycin undergoes significant, capacity-limited first-pass metabolism (16). Suffice it to say, food is unlikely to impact on clarithromycin dosing regimens of ≤500 mg twice daily (13), but its effect on clarithromycin absorption may become more prominent with higher doses.

The drug also appears to be rapidly absorbed, as demonstrated in normal, healthy volunteers by an absorption rate constant (k_a) of 1.7 ± 0.9 hr^{-1} to 3.4 ± 6.4 hr^{-1} following single 500- and 250-mg doses, respectively (16). Also, after single 250- and 500-mg doses mean maximal plasma concentrations of clarithromycin were 0.78 and 2.1 mg/L, whereas those of 14-OH-clarithromycin were 0.61 and 0.83 mg/L, respectively. Steady-state, peak plasma concentrations are achieved after five doses with reported values for clarithromycin and 14-OH-clarithromycin of 1.0 and 0.62 mg/L (250 mg every 12 hr) and 2.7 and 0.88 mg/L (500 mg every 12 hr) (16).

Importantly, plasma concentrations of orally administered clarithromycin in human immunodeficiency virus (HIV)–infected adults and children appear similar to reported values in healthy individuals (17–19). In children, peak concentrations exceeded the minimal inhibitory concentration (MIC) of most pretherapy MAC isolates in the majority of patients receiving 7.5 mg/kg twice daily and in all patients at the 15 mg/kg twice daily dosage (19). However, diminished absorption of clarithromycin in HIV-infected adults and children with severe diarrheal disease is a concern and requires further investigation.

The relative contribution of 14-OH-clarithromycin to clarithromycin's antimycobacterial effect has not been extensively studied. Using the broth technique, Inderlied and co-workers (20) found that on a weight basis, clarithromycin was two- to six-fold more active than 14-OH-clarithromycin. The total activity of the metabolite, however, would depend on how well it distributes intracellularly. Both the parent and metabolite had MICs within one dilution of one another when tested by either agar or broth dilution methodology. At the present time, it is not known if the metabolite has any synergism when used in combination with other anti-MAC drugs.

Elderly volunteers show significant elevations in C_{max} (maximum serum concentration), C_{min} (minimum serum concentration), and AUC for both clarithromycin and 14-OH-clarithromycin when compared with young, healthy volunteers. These elevations are most pronounced for the active metabolite with mean values at least two-fold higher than in young adults (21). The investigators concluded that since the increases in circulating drug concentrations were small and well tolerated, elderly patients receiving 500 mg twice daily may not require dose adjustments solely on the basis of increased age. Similarly, Wallace and colleagues (22) found that 500 mg twice daily was tolerated in 9 of 10 elderly patients but 1000 mg twice daily resulted in discontinuation of high-dose therapy in 11 of 13 patients.

Distribution

As with other macrolide antibiotics, clarithromycin's lipid solubility allows extensive distribution outside of the vascular compartment into tissues. From limited data in volunteers receiving 250- and 500-mg doses of clarithromycin, the average apparent volumes of distribution (Vd/F with F being the bioavailability [fraction of drug reaching the systemic circulation after oral dosing]) for the parent compound after a single dose were 236 L (range 142–482 L) and 306 L (range 109–754 L), respectively (16). Although weight normalized volumes were not provided in this study, clarithromycin's distribution appears intermediate between that of erythromycin and the azalide azithromycin, which have reported values of 0.64 and 23.0 L/kg, respectively, following single, oral doses (2). Clarithromycin binds primarily to albumin, but it has a greater affinity for α_1-acid glycoprotein. Data from in vitro studies (23,24) suggest that clarithromycin is only 42–50% plasma protein bound; however, others maintain that binding is approximately 65–70% over a clinically achievable concentration range of 0.45 to 4.5 mg/L (unpublished data on file, Abbott Laboratories). Although not thought of as a highly protein bound drug, binding of clarithromycin is saturable at plasma concentrations above 1 mg/L leading to increased free plasma concentrations available for distribution and/or elimination within the body (24). Normally, increases in free fraction do not influence the free concentrations of drugs that undergo restrictive first-pass metabolism. However, clarithromycin exhibits a moderate degree of first-pass metabolism, and increases in free fraction could potentially reduce its bioavailability. Also, saturation of its metabolic processes may occur with higher doses. Thus, an increased free fraction can result in increased free concentrations which theoretically would mean greater availability of drug for distribution to sites of infection.

In humans, 4 hr after single or multiple doses of 500 mg, average concentrations of clarithromycin ranged from two- to seven-fold higher than concomitant plasma concentrations (25,26). At steady state, mean lung tissue concentrations of clarithromycin and 14-OH-clarithromycin were 54.0 and 5.1 μg/g, respectively, with mean parent:metabolite ratios of 11.3 for the lung and 2.4 for plasma (26). Concentrations of clarithromycin in other human tissues and blody fluids (nasal mucosa, middle ear fluid, saliva, skin, tonsils) have exceeded those in serum by 1.5 to 6-fold ratios. The serum concentrations of 14-OH-Clarithromycin have generally been about half of those observed for the parent compound (27).

Metabolism and Elimination

Clarithromycin is extensively metabolized in the liver by cytochrome P-450 enzymes through both oxidative and hydrolytic mechanisms. Animal studies have demonstrated the major metabolic route to be stereospecific hydroxylation at the 14 position of clarithromycin with the subsequent formation of the active R isomer (28). Minor metabolic pathways include N-demethylation and hydrolysis of the cladinose sugar to inactive metabolites (28–30). Clarithromycin's nonlinear pharmacokinetic profile is most likely attributable to saturation of the 14-hydroxylation and N-demethylation pathways. With a fivefold increase in the dose of clarithromycin, the AUC has been reported to increase approximately 13-fold (28). Further investigation into this nonlinearity revealed that saturation of the 14-(R)-OH metabolic pathway is most dramatic in healthy volunteers when doses equal or exceed 600 mg twice daily (16). Only small amounts of clarithromycin are excreted in the bile and feces. The drug is excreted into breast milk and is teratogenic in animals at doses producing serum concentrations 2–17 times normal therapeutic concentrations. Thus, it should be avoided in pregnancy unless no alternative agents are available (Package Insert Biaxin, 1994).

Renal excretion is also an important route of elimination for both the parent drug and its active metabolite. Urinary excretion accounts for up to 32% of the apparent total body clearance (CL/F) of both clarithromycin and its active hydroxy metabolite (27). Estimates of the metabolite's renal clearance were, for the most part, in excess of creatinine clearance, indicating a component of tubular secretion is likely involved in its elimination. In healthy volunteers, the steady-state terminal elimination half-life ($t1/2_\beta$) ranged from 3.5 to 4.8 hr with regimens of 250 and 500 mg twice daily (16). With mild reductions in creatinine clearance (reductions to $\geq$50 ml/min), the $t1/2_\beta$ of clarithromycin is only modestly increased, but the half-life for the hydroxy metabolite is significantly prolonged (21). In more severe renal disease, the reduction in clarithromycin elimination is more dramatic.

In the elderly, reductions in glomerular filtration and tubular secretion appear to be primarily responsible for decreases in the apparent clearance (CL/F) of clarithromycin and its renally eliminated metabolite, 14-OH-clarithromycin. Dosage adjustments may be considered in elderly patients, but they should be based on calculated creatinine clearance (CL_{cr}) rather than age alone (21). When the CL_{cr} falls below 30 mL/min, the dosing interval should be doubled.

The total body clearance of clarithromycin is not significantly altered with moderate to severe hepatic impairment, but the 14-hydroxylation of clarithromycin is reduced (3). An increase in the renal clearance (CL_R) observed in individuals with liver disease may partially explain why steady-state serum concentrations of clarithromycin do not deviate substantially from normal.

Drug Interactions

Clarithromycin has not been shown to impact on the pharmacokinetics of didanosine (ddI) or dideoxycytidine (ddC), but the AUC of zidovudine decreased by up to 34% when administered concurrently with clarithromycin 500 mg twice daily (data on file, Abbott Laboratories). Gustavson and coworkers found this interaction to be statistically significant at doses of 2 g twice daily (32). However, as previously suggested (33), it seems that the absorption of zidovudine is decreased when it is administered simultaneously with clarithromycin. If these agents are administered 2 hr apart, there is no significant effect of clarithromycin on zidovudine bioavailability (34). The pharmacokinetics of zidovudine were not altered in pediatric patients with MAC, but, in contrast to the previous study, drug administration times were not specifically recorded, and clarithromycin was administered as a suspension. It is not known if clarithromycin interacts with other nucleoside analogues (3-TC, D4T [stavudine]), nonnucleoside reverse transcriptase inhibitors (e.g., delavirdine, nevirapine), or protease inhibitors. However, interaction with the latter group of drugs is likely and requires further study.

Pharmacokinetic interactions with clarithromycin and the rifamycin derivatives are complex. First, clarithromycin serum concentrations are decreased significantly (>50%) during concomitant rifabutin therapy. Second, the AUCs of rifabutin and one of its metabolites, LM565, have been reported to increase 1.8- and 9.2-fold, respectively, when administered to HIV-infected patients receiving clarithromycin 500 mg twice daily (35). Anterior uveitis is a recognized ocular complication of rifabutin which is rare at doses of 300 mg daily but is more common when doses exceed 1 g per day (36,37). Thus, concurrent therapy with these two drugs may ultimately be limited due to the potential for both a decrease in clarithromycin activity and an increase in rifabutin toxicity. Rifampin is a much more potent enzyme inducer than rifabutin, and it is likely to be associated with more pronounced interactions (38).

Carbamazepine clearance is reduced by 17% with erythromycin and serum concentrations increase on the order of two- to four-fold (39). From limited data, it would appear that clarithromycin can also inhibit carbamazepine metabolism via the cytochrome P-450 IIIA4 pathway (4). Patients receiving concurrent carbamazepine therapy should be monitored clinically for signs of central nervous system (CNS) toxicity and may require serum carbamazepine concentration determinations. Honig and colleagues have found that both erythromycin and clarithromycin can inhibit the metabolism of terfenadine to a similar extent (41). With reduced carboxylate metabolite formation, terfenadine may accumulate and prolong the refractory period by delaying repolarization of cardiac muscle. Patients must avoid taking terfenadine (and astemizole) simultaneously with clarithromycin and should avoid these antihistamines within one week of cessation of clarithromycin therapy. (See Table 1 for complete clarithromycin Drug Interactions [39–44]).

B. Azithromycin

Azithromycin (AZI) is a 15-membered macrolide antibiotic with a methyl-substituted nitrogen atom rather than a carbonyl group at position 9a of the aglycone ring (45). Similar to the structural modifications involved with clarithromycin, this change results in increased bioavailability (46), decreased gastrointestinal toxicity (47), improved gram-negative activity (45), and increased intracellular activity (2). Also, cellular uptake is dependent on pH, cell viability, and the presence or absence of infection; the latter is likely due to cytokine and neutrophil activation which, in turn, regulate antibiotic uptake and transport in a manner analagous to that described for the macrolides (7). The major difference is that AZI concentrates intracellularly within phagolysosomes to a greater extent than any of the macrolides currently under

Table 1 A Summary of the Pharmacokinetic Parameters of Agents Used in the Prophylaxis and Treatment of MAC in Adults

Drug	Dose/route	Pharmacokinetic parameters						
		AUC (mg/L/hr)	C_{max} (mg/L)	F (%)	Cl_T (L/hr)	T_{max} (hr)	$T_{1/2}$ (hr)	Vd (L/kg)
Aminoglycoside								
amikacin	15 mg/kg/IV		30–40	100	varies with CrCl	0.5–1.5	2.0–4.0	0.22–0.3
streptomycin	15 mg/kg/IV		30–40	100		IM		
Fluoroquinolones								
ciprofloxacin	500 mg/PO	19.2 ± 1.1	1.6	63–85	23–43		3–5	2.6 ± 1.4
Macrolide/Azalide								
clarithromycin	500 mg/PO	20.8 ± 6.6	2.7	52–55	42–64	1.8–2.6	3.0–8.0	
azithromycin	500 mg/PO	3.39	0.41 (0.62)	37	6–11.4	2.5–3.0	11–14(α) 35–40(β)	23–31 L
Rifamycins								
rifabutin	300 mg/PO	9.2 ± 1.00	0.38 ± 0.27	53–85 (12–20)[a]	1.1	3.3 ± 0.9	45 ± 17 (38 ± 12)[a]	22.1 ± 0.7
	450 mg/dose			Varies			2–4	
rifampin	600 mg/PO	64	8–12	43–63	0.4 L/hr/kg		10 ± 4d(α) 70 d(β)	0.97 ± 0.4
	300 mg/PO		1.4					
Others								
clofazimine	5 mg/kg/PO	14.19 ± 4.19	4.0–5.0	80	20–30	2.8 ± 0.8	8.6 min(α) 2.5–3.6(β) 15 ± 1.7(δ)	0.36 1.65 (Vd_{ss})
ethambutol								

[a] HIV Infected individuals.

investigation (7,48). The intracellular/extracellular concentration ratio (IC: EC) for AZI in PMNLs is approximately three to six times greater than clarithromycin and erythromycin, respectively, after 1 hr of incubation. However, AZI continues to concentrate within the PMNLs for up to 24 hr, at which time the IC:EC exceeds that of erythromycin by about 26-fold (49).

Absorption

Although the absorption of AZI is not as complete as with clarithromycin, its acid stability improves the bioavailability to approximately 37% (compared with 25% for erythromycin). The AUCs of oral and intravenous (investigational) AZI increase over the first few days following a single 500-mg dose with AUC_{0-72} values of 3.39 and 9.08 mg/L, respectively (50). Maximal serum concentrations of orally administered drug are achieved within 2–3 hr of administration (5). Steady-state serum concentrations do not differ substantially from concentrations attained after single 250-mg doses (both approximately 0.2 mg/L) but increase slightly when the 500-mg dose is used (0.41 mg/L: single dose vs 0.62 mg/L: Cp_{ss}) (50). Thus, the slightly disproportionate increase in systemic availability suggests a minor component of saturable first-pass metabolism may occur with AZI.

A second serum peak has also been noted after both oral and intravenous administration of AZI approximately 2 hr after the initial peak. This phenomenon also occurs with intravenous AZI, which means discontinuous absorption of the oral formulation cannot explain this effect. Since the second peak is more noticeable after meals, it may represent biliary recycling of the drug (52–54). AZI and/or metabolic by-products are secreted into the hepatic parenchyma or gallbladder. The absorption of AZI can be decreased appreciably when it is given with food. Following a large meal, the C_{max} has been shown to decrease by 52%, whereas the AUC is reduced by approximately 43% (55). Thus, AZI should be administered 1 hr before or 2 hr following meals.

In contrast to clarithromycin, age and disease do not have a significant impact on the pharmacokinetics of AZI. According to one study in which HIV-infected patients were given weekly 1-g doses of AZI, peak serum concentrations normalized for dose were lower than in healthy volunteers (56). The investigators concluded that since the AUCs were similar between HIV-infected patients and healthy volunteers, the longer t_{max} (time to maximum serum concentration) in patients infected with HIV (3–4 hr vs 2–3 hr) was likely due to a slower rate of absorption (k_a). The data in HIV-infected patients is limited at the present time, and these conclusions should be interpreted tentatively until more information is available.

After a single 500-mg dose of AZI, patients with mild to moderate hepatic dysfunction did not demonstrate any consistent pharmacokinetic alterations in comparison to healthy volunteers (57). Total systemic clearance may be somewhat reduced with more severe liver disease, but this requires further study. Since most of AZI is excreted unchanged, alterations in its metabolism would not be expected to change the pharmacokinetic profile as dramatically as with the macrolide antimicrobials.

Similar to HIV-infected patients, elderly subjects exhibit a more prolonged absorption profile. In an open trial comparing 24 subjects (12 young and 12 elderly), the t_{max} on days 1 and 5 was significantly longer in elderly subjects (3.8 and 4.4 hr) compared with young volunteers (2.5 and 3.2 hr). Peak and trough serum concentrations were comparable between groups, but the AUC_{0-24} was significantly higher in the elderly (2.7 mg·hr/L) than in the younger age group (2.1 mg·hr/L (58). Changes in gastrointestinal pH induced by antacids or H_2-blocker therapy have little effect on AZI pharmacokinetics (59). Thus, although achlorhydria is a common finding in elderly and HIV-infected patients, it is unlikely to impact on the absorption of AZI. Reductions in first-pass metabolism or increases in absorption may be responsible for the increased extent of absorption (AUC) in the elderly. In HIV disease, the extent of absorption does not increase, which means changes in gastric motility or emptying time might be more likely explanations for the altered rate of absorption. It is plausible that altered gastrointestinal transit time may be a contributing factor to the prolonged absorption of AZI in both patient populations.

Limited data also support comparable pharmacokinetics in pediatric patients. Fourteen patients were given 10 mg/kg AZI suspension on day 1 and then 5 mg/kg on days 2 through 5 of the study. Pharmacokinetics estimated on day 5 using HPLC–mass spectrometry, showed an average C_{max}, t_{max}, and $AUC_{0-24} \pm$ SD of 0.38 $\pm$ 0.14 mg/L, 2.4 $\pm$ 1.1 hr, and 3.1 $\pm$ 1.0 mg·hr/L (60). The values reported for C_{max} and AUC are somewhat higher than in adults given a similar regimen (58) but are likely reflective of the higher milligram per kilogram doses received by the children in this study.

Distribution

As with the macrolide clarithromycin, AZI's low degree of ionization at physiological pH and moderately high degree of lipid solubility enable it to distribute extensively into various body fluids and tissues. Retsema and co-workers actually demonstrated preferential concentration of AZI in areas of infection. It is thought that AZI accumulates within PMNLs and macrophages and, during active inflammation, the drug can be transported via the host's cellular defenses to specific inflammatory sites (61).

In humans, the mean apparent Vd/F for AZI has been reported to be approximately 23–31 L/kg (62). Specific patient populations that might demonstrate significant alterations in distribution have yet to be identified. Concentrations of 1–100 μg/g have been observed in gastric (63), gynecological (64,65), (cervix, ovary, fallopian tube, uterus), pulmonary (66), prostatic (67), sinus (68) (acute sinusitis), and tonsillar tissue (69) following single 500-mg oral doses. The gastric tissue concentrations (2.3–4.6 mg/L) are 5- to 10-fold and 20-fold higher than those observed in gastric mucus and fluid, respectively (63). Favorable concentrations of AZI were retained in sputum, bronchial tissue, and alveolar macrophages for up to 96 hr after dosing (62).

In general, serum concentrations decline rapidly, whereas those in tissue peak at 48 hr after administration (70). This suggests that there is an initial rapid distribution phase followed by a second, much slower redistribution out of tissue (71). The redistribution of drug to the intravascular space is even slower than the initial tissue distribution phase. Tissue concentrations may persist for 72 hr or longer following single doses of AZI. AZI concentrations have been observed to decline biphasically, but a pattern of low tissue accumulation during the elimination of drug from serum, known as the gamma phase, occurs simultaneously (72).

The distribution of basic drugs such as AZI can be affected by the ''ion trapping'' phenomenon. Since AZI exists primarily in the unionized form, the drug may readily pass through epithelial or lipoidal barriers. The passage of drugs into breast milk is a classic example of how drugs such as AZI cross the breast epithelium and subsequently become ionized in acidic body fluids (73).

As in the case of tissue accumulation, there is also an antimicrobial hierarchy of penetrability into PMNLs (74). After 1 hr incubation with human PMNLs, the IC:EC for AZI is roughly 40:1 (48,49,74); the highest observed ratio among the currently available anti-MAC agents (see Table 2). This ratio increases to 79:1 and 336:1 after 2 and 24 hr of incubation, respectively. The corresponding concentration ratios in peritoneal macrophages are 62:1 (2 hr) and 110:1 (24 hr) (48,49,71). The ratio of IC:EC accumulation within alveolar macrophages is approximately 634 after 90 min of incubation with an efflux half-life of about 42 minutes in vitro (75).

Like clarithromycin, AZI also exhibits saturable plasma protein binding. Since saturation occurs with very small serum concentrations of the drug, the predominant serum protein involved is likely AAG (51). Using equilibrium dialysis, Foulds and colleagues demonstrated that the bound fraction

Table 2 Intracellular[a] and Extracellular Concentrations of Anti-MAC Drugs

Drug	Dose	Extracellular conc (mg/L)	Intracellular:extracellular ratio
Aminoglycosides			
amikacin	15 mg/kg/IV	30–40	
streptomycin	15 mg/kg/IV	30–40	1:10
Fluoroquinolones			
ciprofloxacin	500 mg/PO	1.6	12–20:1
Macrolide/Azalide	500 mg/PO	2.7	110:1 (24 hr)
azithromycin	500 mg/PO	0.41 (0.62)	17.3:1 (2 hr)
Rifamycins			
rifabutin	300 mg/PO	0.38 ± 0.27	7.0:1
Miscellaneous			
clofazimine	200 mg/PO	1	
ethambutol	300 mg/PO	4.0–5.0	2–6:1

[a]In macrophages.

increases from 7 to 37% as the serum concentration declines from 1 to 0.7 mg/L (50). With such a low degree of protein binding, the amount of drug that distributes to extracellular tissue sites is not expected to be altered appreciably by fluctuations in the serum concentration of AZI.

Metabolism and Elimination

More than 50% of AZI is eliminated unchanged in the feces largely through biliary excretion (75). It is thought that transintestinal excretion may be the primary route of elimination of unmetabolized drug (71). Urinary excretion of unchanged drug is a minor route of elimination responsible for only about 6–12% of orally ingested AZI (75). The renal clearance ranges from about 100–189 ml/min.

Hepatic metabolism of the drug also occurs with the primary pathway involving the N-demethylation at the 9A position of the azalide ring or of the desosamine sugar. Other minor pathways involve O-demethylation and hydrolytic reactions of the cladinose/desosamine sugars or the azalide ring (72). Despite the limited degree of hepatic metabolism, there may be as many as 10 metabolic by-products of AZI. None of the metabolites have been shown to have appreciable antibacterial activity (72).

The mean elimination half-life ($t1/2_\beta$) of AZI varies depending on the sampling interval. It has been reported to increase from 11 to 14 hr to 35 to

40 hr when studied for up to 1–3 days, respectively (50,56). The polyphasic elimination of drug from serum and tissues manifests as a rapid decay in serum drug concentration followed by fast tissue distribution and then a slow distribution and elimination phase (76). The dose of AZI does not have to be adjusted in the elderly, but Coates' group (58) found that a significant inverse relationship exists between creatinine clearance and AUC.

When compared with normal, healthy subjects, mild to moderate impairment of liver function leads to significant increases in t1/2_β (54 vs 68 hr) and mean residence time (60 vs 83 hr) (57). Thus, individuals with severe hepatic disease (especially if biliary secretory defects are present), hepatic and renal dysfunction, or mild to moderate liver disease on chronic MAC therapy will most likely require dosage adjustments. The manufacturer does not recommend its use in severe hepatic disease.

Drug Interactions

Macrolide antibiotics inhibit the cytochrome P-450 IIIA enzyme system by producing nitrosoalkanes which eventually complex and inactivate this isoenzyme (77). AZI, dirithromycin, and spiramycin, however, do not create nitrosoalkanes, which means drug interactions cannot occur via this mechanism (43). The C_{max} of AZI (500 mg/day for 3 day) is reduced by 24% with concomitant antacid administration, but the extent of absorption (AUC_{0-48}) is not affected (59). Although the extent of absorption is not altered, it is probably advisable to administer these drugs separately. With changes in the rate of absorption, the absorption of AZI may be altered if large doses are given or motility-altering drugs are used concomitantly. No pharmacokinetic interactions were detected with carbamazepine (78), cimetidine (59), methylprednisolone (79), theophylline (80,81), terfenadine (82), warfarin (79), or zidovudine (56).

III. Rifamycins

Rifabutin (RFB) is a semisynthetic ansamycin antibiotic derived from rifamycin S. The drug is bacteriostatic against MAC at normally achievable serum concentrations (83). It is thought that the mechanism of action of RFB against MAC is the same as rifampin for *Mycobacterium tuberculosis*. RFB acts to inhibit DNA-dependent RNA polymerase in mycobacteria that reside both outside and within macrophages (84). MAC isolates are more often resistant to rifamycin compounds than *M. tuberculosis*, which is likely due to alterations in cell wall architecture which limit entry of antimicrobial agents (85). The newer rifamycins, including RFB and rifapentine (cyclopentyl ansamycin), may have an advantage over rifampin in that they have better intracellular penetrability. This is probably an important feature for enhancing synergy with agents capable of altering the cell wall permeability of mycobacterial species (e.g., ethambutol) (86). RFB is currently indicated for the prevention of dMAC in advanced HIV disease, whereas RFP remains investigational at this time. Rather than devoting a special section to rifampin (RIF), the pharmacokinetics of this drug are summarized in Table 1.

A. Rifabutin

Absorption

RFB is incompletely absorbed following oral administration with a reported bioavailability of only 12 to 20% in early, symptomatic HIV-infected individuals (87). In normal volunteers, approximately 53% of the absorbed radiolabeled drug was recovered in the urine, which suggests that about half of the dose may be absorbed from the gastrointestinal tract (88). However, rifabutin metabolites likely account for a significant fraction of the recovered drug. In contrast to these two trials, another normal volunteer study demonstrated the relative bioavailability (F_{rel}) of the capsule dosage form to be 85% (89).

A high-fat meal causes a delay in the t_{max} from 3 to 5.4 hr but no significant change in $AUC_{0-\infty}$. Thus, RFB may be taken without regard to meals. In healthy volunteers, a single oral dose of 300 mg RFB was absorbed from the gastrointestinal tract with a mean ($\pm$SD) C_{max} of 375 $\pm$ 267 ng/ml (range 141–1033 ng/ml) and a mean t_{max} of 3.3 $\pm$ .9 hr (range 2 to 4 hr) (90). Interpatient variability is considerable with respect to the absorption of RFB; however, intrapatient fluctuations are much smaller. Also, steady-state serum pharmacokinetics of RFB appear to be more variable in the elderly (> 70 years) and symptomatic HIV-infected patients. Peak serum concentrations increase more or less proportionally as doses are increased over the range of 300–900 mg/day (125). The average steady-state trough concentrations (C_{min}^{ss}) achieved with standard doses of RFB range from 50–65 ng/ml in both normal volunteers and HIV-infected patients (91).

The AUC for RFB has been shown to decrease by about 28% from 5400 ng*hr/L to 3900 ng*hr/L after administration of 300 mg daily for 28 days (87). A similar phenomenon occurs with chronic RIF administration where the AUC may decrease by as much as 45% after 3 weeks of therapy (92,93). This is most likely a result of autoinduction. This has been shown to result in significantly lower AUC and C_{max} values. Benedetti and coworkers (94) demonstrated similar observed and theoretical plasma concentrations (mean ± SEM) after single doses of RFB (74 ± 4 ng*hr/ml vs 77 ± 7 ng*hr/ml) but markedly diminished observed values after 5 days of RFB (96 ± 16 ng/ml vs 187 ± ng/ml). After 450 mg daily for 10 days, the AUC on day 1 was 9287 ± 1001 ng/ml but only 5803 ± ng/ml by the end of the study. It appears that induction of presystemic extrahepatic metabolism is primarily responsible for the decrease in systemic availability of RFB, since its elimination half-life does not change appreciably following induction (94). That is, the decrease in AUC is due to a reduction in bioavailability rather than an increase in systemic clearance. Autoinduction is important to keep in mind when comparing various pharmacokinetic trials involving rifamycin compounds.

Distribution

RFB's enhanced lipophilicity enables widespread tissue and intracellular distribution. In general, the distribution volumes exceed total body water by about 15-fold. In a study involving seven HIV-infected subjects, the average (±SD) steady-state volume of distribution (Vd_{ss}) for intravenous RFB was estimated to be 8.2 ± 0.9 L/kg with a range of 8 to 11 L/kg. Plasma protein–binding studies indicate that RFB exhibits concentration-independent binding with a reported binding of 71–85% over the concentration range of 50–1000 ng/ml. The binding does not appear to be altered in the presence of renal or hepatic disease (87,90).

Peak tissue concentrations of RFB are generally achieved within 4 hr of oral dosing (88). The distribution half-life ($t1/2_\alpha$) of RFB is 1.2 ± 0.7 hr with daily regimens of 300 mg (87). Intracellular concentrations are significantly higher than concomitant plasma concentrations in both animals and humans. Studies are currently underway to assess the cerebrospinal fluid pharmacokinetics of RFB in humans (95). The manufacturer states that lung to plasma concentration ratios of 6.5 have been observed 12 hr after an oral dose of RFB in four surgical patients (data on file, Adria Laboratories). The uptake of RFB into mouse peritoneal macrophages was investigated by Dhillon and Mitchison (96). They were able to demonstrate that RFB had the best intracellular activity when compared with RIF, RFP, and FCE 22807. Intracellular penetration was assessed using a "double-titration" method which measured the ratio of the MIC in peritoneal macrophages to the in vitro MIC for *Mycobacterium macroti* and *M. tuberculosis*. These ratios were 2.0, 6.7, 26.0, and 20.0 for RFB, RIF, RFP, and FCE 22807, respectively. The lower ratio for RFB indicated that it had better activity despite previous reports of high intracellular concentration ratios of 61 and 3.5 for RFP (human peritoneal macrophages) (97) and RIF (human alveolar macrophages) (98), respectively.

Since RFB is structurally similar to RIF, one would expect it to cross the placenta and be excreted into breast milk (99–100). RIF may also cause CNS abnormalities and limb reduction (100–102). Thus, administration of rifamycin compounds during pregnancy should be avoided if at all possible.

Metabolism and Elimination

The elimination of RFB follows a biphasic pattern with a mean ($\pm$SD) terminal elimination half-life of 38 $\pm$ 12 hr in HIV-infected patients (87) and 45 $\pm$ 17 hr (range 16–69 hr) in healthy, adult subjects (90). RFB has a reported apparent clearance (CL/F) of 0.81 L/hr/kg in healthy, male volunteers indicating a moderately high rate of removal from plasma (89). Total body clearance (CL_T) ranged from 10 to 18 L/hr in symptomatic HIV-infected patients (87). Renal and biliary elimination account for about 5–10% of RFB's total apparent clearance. The renal clearance has been estimated to be approximately 18 $\pm$ 3 ml/min (87). As previously mentioned, about half of an oral dose is excreted in the urine, principally as metabolites (88). A total of five metabolites have been identified; two of which account for about 17% of the parent compound's plasma AUC. The principal breakdown product in humans is the 25-O-desacetyl metabolite (88). Based on the pharmacokinetic information, it has been estimated to account for approximately 10% of the total antimicrobial activity of RFB and is comparable in terms of antibacterial activity.

Drug Interactions

The majority of drug interactions with RIF occur as a result of induction of cytochromeP-450 IIIA, cytochromeP-450 IA, cytochromeP-450 IIC, and UDP-glucuronyltransferase hepatic enzymes (103,104). Since RFB is a structurally related compound, one would expect it to be capable of inducing the same metabolic pathways. One major difference between the two rifamycins, however, lies in the inherent inducing capabilities of each agent. For example, the clearance of delavirdine, a compound metabolized via the cytochromeP-450 IIIA4 system, is reduced approximately 27-fold by RIF, resulting in negligible serum concentrations of the antiretroviral. On the other hand, RFB reduces the clearance of delavirdine by about five-fold (105). Similarly, mean ($\pm$SD) steady-state serum concentrations of clarithromycin (500 mg bid) are reduced from 5.4 $\pm$ 2.1 mg/L to 0.7 $\pm$ 0.6 mg/L and 2.1 $\pm$ 1.5 mg/L in patients with MAC receiving equivalent daily doses of RIF or RFB, respectively (see Section II.A for complete interaction) (106). Theophylline is metabolized primarily through the cytochromeP-450 IA2 pathway, but it also undergoes oxidation through the IIIA4 route. As anticipated from the previous interactions, RFB did not alter the pharmacokinetics of theophylline, but RIF increased the oral clearance from 3.2 to 4.4 L/hr, whereas the AUC decreased from 140 mg·hr/L to 100 mg·hr/L (107). Thus far, it seems as though the cytochromeP-450 IA and IIIA systems are more likely to be induced with RIF than RFB. The induction potential of RFB on other isoenzymatic pathways known to be affected by RIF needs to be assessed in future investigations.

Initially, it was thought that RFB might increase the clearance of zidovudine. In one report, steady-state plasma concentrations (C_{max}^{ss}) and zidovudine AUC were decreased by 48 and 32% during concomitant RFB therapy (108). But a subsequent pharmacokinetic study was unable to confirm these findings (109).

Clinical reports on the ability of RIF to increase the clearance of dapsone, an antileprosy/pneumocystis drug, have been published previously (110,111). They have largely been dismissed because adequate serum dapsone concentrations are still achievable (112). However, increased formation of the metabolite of dapsone can result in clinically significant elevations of methemoglobin (113). This is a potentially dangerous pharmacodynamic interaction which deserves further study with RFB.

Owing to concerns of increased hepatotoxicity during isoniazid therapy, a study of the effects of RFB on isoniazid pharmacokinetics was performed in healthy volunteers (114). No alteration in the pharmacokinetics of isoniazid or acetylisoniazid were found.

Fluconazole has been shown to increase both the C_{max} and AUC of RFB and its metabolite LM-565 by at least 80% (115). In a posthoc analysis of the data from two double-blind, randomized, placebo-controlled trials (116,117), the prophylactic effect of RFB against MAC was found to be enhanced in patients receiving concurrent fluconazole therapy. It was suggested that higher systemic serum concentrations of RFB were responsible for this increased antimycobacterial effect. However, patients receiving the combination also had a higher incidence of neutropenia than those given RFB alone (17 vs 7%). Clinicians should be aware that ketocanazole has a greater in vitro inhibitory effect on microsomal enzymes than either fluconazole or itraconazole, and the potential exists for a drug interaction with other azole compounds. Furthermore, interactions with these antifungal agents are often unpredictable, patient specific, and dose dependent.

Table 3 Drug Interactions of the Agents Currently Used for the Prophylaxis and Treatment of MAC

Drug	Interacting drug(s)	Drug interaction	Action
Aminoglycosides amikacin streptomycin	Ototoxic or rental toxic agents General anesthetics Neuromuscular blocking agents	May potentiate the potential for ototoxicity, renal toxicity, or neurotoxicity when used in combination	Avoid concomitant use if possible.
Fluoroquinolones cipfloxacin	Antacids (Mg, Al, or Ca containing), Sucralfate Multivitamins (Fe, Zn containing)	↓ CIP conc. 14–50%	Avoid concomitant use or administer CIP 2 hr before or 4–6 hr after interacting drugs
	ddI	↓ ddI absorption by 90%	
	Probenecid	↑ CIP conc. up to 50% ↓ CIP CL_{renal} 50%	
	Theophylline	↑ Theo conc. 17–254% ↓ Theo CL by 20–35%	Avoid concomitant use or adjust dose of theo based on serum conc. monitoring.
Macrolide/Azalide clarithromycin	Zidovudine	↓ ZDV absorption ↓ AUC by up to 34%	Administer agents at least 2 hour apart.
	Rifabutin	↑ RFB conc. >50% ↓ Clarithromycin conc. >50%	Avoid concomitant use if possible.
	Carbamazepine	↓ CBZ clearance 17%	Monitor CBZ levels.
	Theophylline	↑ Theo conc. 20%	Monitor theo levels.
	Cyclosporine	Case report ↑ cyclosporine levels	Monitor cyclosprine levels

Rifamycins		
rifabutin	Delavirdine (U-90)	↓ clearance of U-90 five-fold
	Clarithromycin	See above
	Zidovudine	See text
	Dapsone	↓ CL dapsone. May ↑ conc of dapsone metabolite and ↑ methemoglobin conc.
	Fluconazole	↑ Conc. of **RFB** — ↑ Efficacy of **RFB** But ↑ neutropenia
Miscellaneous		
clofazimine	Isoniazid	↓ Tissue conc. of clof
ethambutol	Antacids (Al hydroxide)	↓ Conc. ethambutol — Separate doses by 2 hr

RFB has been shown to increase the clearance of cyclosporine in one patient 25 days after therapy was initiated. The clearance of cyclosporine increased from 0.26 L/hr/kg to 0.36 L/hr/kg. The interaction was not as severe as when the patient was previously treated with RIF (118). Table 3 provides a brief summary of some of the clinically significant interactions with RFB.

IV. Clofazimine

Absorption

Clofazimine (CFM) exhibits slow, dose-dependent absorption following oral administration (119). The biavailability decreases from 63% folowing a 100-mg dose to 43% after a 600-mg dose (120). The systemic availability is similar between the 300- and 600-mg doses, which suggests that saturable absorption occur at doses as low as 300 mg. Bioavailability is also dependent on the oral formulation. The early dosage forms contained CFM as coarse crystals which resulted in an average bioavailability of 20%. The commercially available preparation consists of a microcrystalline suspension of CFM in an oil-wax base which improves the drug's bioavailability to approximately 70% (121–123).

It is thought that absorption is improved if the drug is administered with fatty foods or high protein meals (122). When CFM was administered with food, the C_{max} and AUC increased by 28 and 62%, respectively. This resulted in a significant increase in serum concentrations. Normally, doses up to 200 mg daily do not produce serum concentrations much higher than 1 mg/L. In healthy volunteers, the mean C_{max} following a single dose of 200 mg has been reported to be about 0.5 mg/L (124). With repeated doses of 100, 200, or 300 mg, maximum serum concentrations were achieved within approximately 2 hr, resulting in values of 0.7, 1, and 1.4 mg/L, respectively (125).

Distribution

Accurate estimates of the volume of distribution (Vd) are not available, and plasma protein–binding studies have not been performed. Nonetheless, CFM has a tremendous volume of distribution with a predilection for the small intestine, reticuloendothelial system, fatty tissue, liver, adrenal glands, and gallbladder.

Tissue concentrations in these organs are often in excess of 2 mg/g. Variable concentrations, at times greater than 1 mg/g, have also been reported in the eye, heart, kidney, lung, lymph nodes, nerves, skin and spleen (126–

128). Large amounts of CFM crystals have been found in the intestine, liver, and mesenteric lymph nodes (119,126,129). A direct correlation exists between the number of macrophages present in a particular tissue and the magnitude of CFM accumulation (128). Crystals have recently been reported in alveolar macrophages in a patient with acquired immunodeficiency syndrome (AIDS) (127). CFM does not appear to be capable of crossing an intact blood-brain barrier (127,128).

CFM does cross the placenta and has been reported to discolor the skin of newborns (130). Since the drug is also excreted in breast milk, if a child is breastfed by a mother who continues to take CFM, the child will develop skin discoloration (131). In the absence of breastfeeding, the pigmentation generally fades and disappears after 1 year (119).

Metabolism and Elimination

Following oral administration of CFM, about 50% of the dose is excreted unchanged in the feces, which represents drug that has not been absorbed or has been excreted via the biliary system (125). Three urinary metabolites (I–III) have been recovered which account for less than 1% of the drug over a 24-hr period. Metabolites I, II, and III are produced via hydrolytic dehalogenation, hydrolytic deamination-glucuronidation, and hydration-glucuronidation, respectively. Feng and colleagues have hypothesized that metabolites I and II may be degraded by intestinal bacteria before drug is even absorbed. (132,133). It is plausible that the extensive distribution of the drug serves as a buffer to protect CFM from degradation and excretion.

CFM appears to be eliminated in two distinct phases. The first phase occurs with low-dose, short-term administration. This phase is characterized by a plasma half-life of 10.6 ± 4 days (122). The second phase occurs with high-dose, long-term administration and is represented by a plasma half-life of approximately 70 days (119). Computer simulations estimate that, in the absence of a loading dose, it would take 30 days to achieve steady state on a daily regimen of 50 mg. The reported R factor ($AUC_{ss}:AUC_1$), a measure of drug accumulation, is 4.85, which indicates a slow, gradual ascent to steady state (124). A small portion of drug is also eliminated from sebum and sweat (118).

Drug Interactions

In healthy volunteers, CFM delayed the t_{max} of RIF, but the C_{max} and AUC were unaltered (134). CFM may also reduce estrogen secretion in pregnant patients (135). In contrast to one report (113), three repeated-dose trials have found no influence of CFM on dapsone pharmacokinetics (136–138).

In patients receiving CFM 300 mg daily, isoniazid therapy was found to reduce CFM tissue concentrations. Also, serum and urine concentrations of CFM were increased. The investigators believed that isoniazid may mobilize CFM from tissue to produce elevations of drug in the central compartment (139).

V. Ethambutol

Absorption

Ethambutol (EMB) is rapidly and completely absorbed (140–143) with an estimated bioavailability of 80% (144). In normal volunteers, EMB doses of 4.0, 8.0, 12.5, 25.0, and 50.0 mg/kg produced proportional serum concentrations with an estimated t_{max} of 2–4 hr (141). Ameer and co-workers have dispelled previous notions that food can affect the absorption of EMB by demonstrating similar AUC values in fed and fasting states (145). Convolution methodology in animals suggest that the absorption of EMB comprises two, first-order processes, each with a half-life of approximately 30 min. This may be due to EMB's chemistry (ethylenediaminetetraacetic acid analogue) which permits enhanced chelation to various tissues, including the gastrointestinal tract (140).

An aqueous solution of EMB (15 mg/kg) produces a t_{max} and C_{max} of 1.9 ± 0.5 hr (range 1.5–2.5 hr) and 4.5 ± 0.9 mg/L (range 3.4–6.0 mg/L), respectively. This is in contrast to the tablet form (15 mg/kg) which yields a C_{max} of 4 ± 0.8 mg/L (range 3.3–5.6 mg/L) after 2.8 ± .8 hr (range 2.5–4.0 hr). Both the solution and tablet have similar bioavailability (140).

Maximal plasma concentrations may be affected by both renal and hepatic dysfunction. Of 100 subjects who received EMB at a dose of 25 mg/kg/day, 65, 22, and 13% had therapeutic (2–5 mg/L), elevated (5–12 mg/L), and depressed (<2 mg/L) values for C_{max} at 3 hr, respectively (146). In the group with elevated concentrations, 11 had renal disease, 3 had hepatic dysfunction, and 8 had body weights above 80 kg (doses > 2 g). The latter indicates that ideal body weight (IBW) is most appropriate for dosing.

Distribution

Using a two-compartment model, the volume of distribution of the central compartment (Vd_c) and at steady state (Vd_{ss}) in healthy volunteers was 0.36

and 1.65 L/kg, respectively. Noncompartmental analysis of the data over 72 hr gives a higher Vd of 3.85 L/kg (143). EMB has an estimated $t1/2_\alpha$ of 8.6 min, a $t1/2_\beta$ of 2.5–3.6 hr (mean 3.1), and a $t1/2_\gamma$ of 15.4 ± 1.7 hr when calculated over 72 hr (144). The latter phase ($t1/2_\gamma$) may represent elimination of EMB following its efflux out of erythrocytes. The Vd_c may be used as an approximation of the Vd_{ss}, since it is unlikely that the gamma ''accumulation'' phase would underpredict steady-state serum concentrations by much more than 10% (147).

A significant amount of EMB distributes into erythrocytes. EMB concentrates between two- and threefold at 1 hr but up to eightfold at 4.5 hr following dosing. Erythrocyte concentrations remain above 5 mg/L for approximately 24 hr. The IC:EC ratio within pulmonary alveolar macrophages was greater than RIF according to previous reports (IC:EC range of 2–6) (148,149). EMB is minimally bound to plasma proteins and, as with other basic drugs, it likely has an affinity for AAG. Equilibrium dialysis and ultrafiltration reported plasma protein binding of 20–30% over the concentration range of 0.5–2.0 mg/L (140). At concentrations of 4.8 mg/L, the binding is decreased to approximately 8% (123).

Metabolism and Elimination

About 80% of EMB is eliminated unchanged by the kidneys, and it is actively secreted in the renal tubules (mean renal clearance [CL_R] of 6.8 mL/min/kg; range 5.9–8.5 ml/min/kg) (144). The standard dose of EMB, in the absence of renal dysfunction, is 25 mg/kg. A dose of 15 mg/kg may be more appropriate for patients with a creatinine clearance (CrCL) between 70 and 100 ml/minute. Doses should be reduced further with more severe renal dysfunction. Some have recommended administering the drug every 24–36 hr or every 48 hr for patients with a CrCl of 10–50 ml/min and less than 10ml/min, respectively (123).

EMB was reported to be removed by hemodialysis (150), but the amount of EMB recovered in the dialysate was not given. A subsequent study of chronic dialysis patients found that the amount of EMB recovered in dialysate comprised only a small fraction of the total oral dose (151). The clearance increased from 0 to 3.1 L/hr in patients on hemodialysis receiving EMB (150). The beta (β) $t1/2_{on}$ dialysis has been reported to be about 2 hr, whereas the $t1/2_{off}$ is ≥ 7 hr (151). Thus, dosage supplementation in patients on hemodialysis is probably not necessary. In contrast, a significant amount of EMB is removed by peritoneal dialysis, and a dose of 18 mg/kg has been suggested as a supplement during peritoneal dialysis (152–154).

A dicarboxylic acid (metabolite I) and aldehyde intermediate (metabolite II) constitute the two main metabolites produced through oxidative reactions. About 10–20% of EMB is hepatically metabolized, although this figure may increase with significant renal disease (144). Using the noncompartmental techniques, the estimated nonrenal clearance is 6.2 L/hr or about 20% of the total clearance (30.2 L/hr) (144). Individuals with hepatic dysfunction likely do not require dosage adjustments unless there is coexistent renal disease (e.g., hepatorenal syndrome).

Drug Interactions

According to one report, the concomitant use of aluminum hydroxide may delay and lower peak serum concentrations of EMB. Thus, doses of EMB should be separated by about 2 hr from aluminum-containing antacids. Although no other significant interactions have been reported, other drugs which undergo tubular secretion may compete for elimination with EMB in the kidney and predispose patients to toxic serum concentrations of either agent.

VI. Quinolones
A. Ciprofloxacin

Ciprofloxacin (CIP) is a fluoroquinolone antimicrobial compound. As a class, the quinolone antimicrobial agents act as DNA gyrase inhibitors. This enzyme is required for induction of negative superhelical twists into double-stranded DNA (to unwind double strands) and for the catenation and decatenation of circular DNA linked in chains (155). CIP has excellent activity against most gram-negative aerobic bacilli, but also is effective against certain species of mycobacteria, including *M. tuberculosis* and *M. avium–intracellulare* (156–158). Unfortunately, the MICs for CIP against *M. avium* complex are much higher than for other mycobacteria. They are frequently in the 4 to >16 mg/L range, with only about 30% of *M. avium* strains retaining susceptibility to CIP ($\leq$2 mg/L) (158). Resistance develops rapidly (mutational frequency of 10^{-5}–10^{-7}) for rapidly growing mycobacterial pathogens if used as single drug therapy. Cross resistance is also a common feature shared among the quinolone antibiotics. Nonetheless, CIP has good intracellular penetration and has been used as a second-line agent in the treatment of dMAC (159,160).

Absorption

Following single oral doses of CIP, the mean C_{max} was reported to be 0.76, 1.6, 2.5, and 3.5 mg/L for the 250-, 500-, 750-, and 1000-mg doses, respectively (155). The C_{max} and AUC of both oral (161) and intravenous (162) CIP increase proportionally to the administered dose. In a comparative study of the pharmacokinetics of single-dose oral (750 mg) or intravenous (400 mg) CIP (162), the mean AUC (±SD) was 19.2 ± 1.1 mg/L·hr and 14.2 ± 1.1 mg/L·hr, respectively. Peak plasma concentrations were 6.7 ± 1.4 mg/L after intravenous and 3.9 ± 1.7 mg/L after oral administration.

The absolute bioavailabiity of CIP in normal volunteers ranged from about 63 to 85% (164,165). In addition to the effect of pH on the absorption of CIP (166), saturable intestinal secretion of the drug may also cause variability in estimates of systemic availability (167–170). Administration of CIP with food causes a delay in absorption resulting in prolonged values for t_{max} (approximately 2 hr with food and 1 hr with fasting), but the C_{max} and AUC are not affected (170–172). Thus, clinicians can recommend administration of CIP with food to avoid gastrointestinal upset.

The quinolones have not been used in pediatric patients until recently because of concerns over the potential for cartilage toxicity which occurs in animals. However, sophisticated monitoring techniques suggest that the quinolones do not cause arthropathy in humans (173). Nonetheless, CIP is only available on a compassionate use basis in prepubertal children. In one of the few pharmacokinetic studies performed in this age group, nine children were given a single oral dose of 15 mg/kg of CIP. The mean (±SD) C_{max} was 3.3 ± 1.3 mg/L and 2.1 ± 1.7 mg/L in infants (5–14 weeks) and children (1–5 years), respectively. Maximal absorption occurred at about 1 hr in both groups (173).

Distribution

The Vd_{ss} for CIP has recently been reported to be 2.6 ± 1.4 L/kg in patients with nosocomial pneumonia (174,175). According to ultrafiltration methodology, approximately 22% of CIP is bound to serum proteins (176). Estimated values were higher, averaging 40%, when ultracentrifugation techniques were used (177). Cosedimentation of free and bound drug, which occurs with higher molecular weight compounds (>300; CIP = 386), may have resulted in the sightly higher estimates with ultracentrifugation (178). Protein binding was independent of pH and concentration over the range of 0.25–1.0 mg/L.

The ratio of C_{max} in bronchial secretions:serum was about 33% after 4 days of intravenous CIP 200 mg every 12 hr. The overall penetration into bronchial secretions ranged from 50 to 66% as indicated by the AUC ratio in bronchial fluids:serum (179). CIP penetrates empyemic pleural fluid (100–200%) better than sterile fluid (30–90%) (180). Single intravenous doses of

200 mg produced CIP pulmonary tissue concentrations in excess of serum by three- to sevenfold: serum 0.6 mg/mL, bronchial mucosa 1.9 mg/g, lung parenchyma 3.4 mg/g, pleural tissue 1.7 mg/g (180). In contrast, steady-state values, using the same dose every 12 hr, yielded bronchial mucosa concentrations of 22 ± 5.6 mg/g 2 hr postadministration. The tissue:plasma ratios ranged from 10.1 to 26.3 (174). Bronchoalveolar lavage specimens have been found to contain extracellular lung fluid concentrations twice those in serum whereas alveolar macrophage concentrations were about 12- to 20-fold higher than serum concentrations (182). Metabolite concentrations are 10- to 100-fold lower than the parent compound in bronchial tissues, indicating they would not contribute to the drug's activity (183).

CIP concentrations in the cerebrospinal fluid (CSF) are approximately 6.5–39 and 9% of serum concentrations in bacterial and viral/tuberculous meningitis, respectively (184). However, concentrations of drug in the CSF are not predictive of those in the brain. Brain parenchymal tissue concentrations of single dose CIP or sparfloxacin exceed those in CSF by 1.8- to 19.4-fold (185).

CIP is secreted into human breast milk and breastfeeding should not be initiated within 48 hr of cessation of CIP therapy (186–188).

A good correlation exists between in vitro and in vivo distribution of CIP into PMNLs. Neutrophils recovered from healthy volunteers displayed IC:EC ratios ranging from 3.7 at 1.5 hr to 20 at 24 hr (189). Similarly, using a fluorometric assay, CIP was found to concentrate up to 12.7-fold in mouse peritoneal macrophages (190).

Metabolism and Elimination

Approximately 40–50% of CIP is eliminated as unchanged drug in the urine (191). Urinary excretion, following a single 250-mg oral dose, is nearly complete by 24 hr (165). The effect of dose on the serum pharmacokinetics of intravenous CIP was studied in nine healthy volunteers (19). The data were characterized best by a three-compartment model. Although values for CL_T and CL_R decreased with dose, these changes were not significant. The total mean (±SD) clearance was 0.53 L/hr/kg for intravenous doses of 100, 150, and 200 mg. The average CL_R was approximately threefold (range 2.9–3.4) larger than the measured CL_{cr}, indicating that the drug is actively secreted in the renal tubules. Renal clearance, on average, represents 60–70% of the total systemic clearance. The reported values for CL_T and CL_R in this paper are in good agreement with several other studies (191–194). The terminal elimination t1/2 ranged from 3 to 4.8 hr in these trials (192–194).

Hepatic metabolism of CIP produces four metabolites (I–IV). These metabolites account for 15% of an oral dose (165) and possess roughly one-quarter to one-half the activity of the parent compound (165). In general, metabolite II has the least antibacterial activity, whereas the minor metabolite (IV) is the most active (195). As indicated by the bioavailability, oral CIP has a relatively small first-pass effect and produces only slightly larger quantities of metabolic by-products than the intravenous dosage form (165). Approximately 15% of CIP is eliminated unchanged in the feces (165). Peak bile concentrations of 143 mg/L 3 hr after an oral dose of 750 mg were reported for one patient 3 hr after receiving CIP (196). In general, biliary secretion results in concentrations 8- to 10-fold higher than concomitant serum values (197). The bile is most likely an important route of elimination for CIP metabolites as well.

As mentioned in Section VI.A, transintestinal elimination may represent a second nonrenal mechanism of elimination for CIP. Transintestinal elimination may account for between 10 and 40% of the total clearance (167). This route of elimination may become more prominent in patients with impaired renal function where removal of excess drug is necessary to prevent significant accumulation. This may explain why a rather poor correlation exists between CL_{cr} and t1/2 and, in some patients, CL_{cr} and CL_T (167).

In renal dysfunction, the elimination of CIP and metabolites I–III are altered. Although the elimination t1/2 and AUC may double, the CL_T decreases to about half normal only in the presence of more severe renal disease (193). In these patients, it would seem prudent to reduce doses based on the degree of renal function *and* other factors such as age, coexistence of hepatic dysfunction, or signs and symptoms of toxicity. The dosing interval should be doubled when the CL_{cr} falls below 20 mL/min. CIP is moderately dialyzable and should be given after hemodialysis to avoid dose supplementation.

In children, oral doses of 10–15 mg/kg of cip tid produce plasma concentrations comparable to adult dosing regimens (6–10 mg/kg (198,199). A reduction in elimination t1/2 has been observed in children aged 1–5 years (t1/2 = 2.7 hr) and infants (t1/2 = 1.3 hr) compared with adults (t1/2 = 3–5 hr). Since data with prolonged administration of quinolones in children are limited, if CIP is required, it may be prudent to limit the duration of therapy.

Drug Interactions

CIP absorption is impaired when administered with antacids or other products containing aluminum, calcium, iron, magnesium, and zinc salts by a chelation with polyvalent ions (200,201). Aluminum-magnesium containing antacids (e.g., Maalox) can reduce CIP absorption by up to 90% (201–203). The interaction may be avoided completely by administering CIP 2 hr before or 6 hr after the antacid (203). Calcium carbonate can decrease the C_{max} 40%

and AUC 43% during concomitant administration (204). Administering calcium carbonate 2 hr before (205,206) or after (205) CIP administration prevents a reduction in bioavailability of this quinolone. Similarly, ferrous sulfate (100 mg elemental iron) reduces the AUC and C_{max} by 57 and 54%, respectively. Ferrous fumarate (200 mg) may decrease absorption by 70%, whereas the slow-release iron product FeroGradumet only reduces CIP by about 11% (201). Multivitamins with zinc reduce the absorption of CIP by up to 24% (207). Sucralfate contains aluminum cations and concomitant administration with CIP may result in almost complete unavailability of the antibiotic (208). Sucralfate should be administered 2–6 hr after CIP. Finally, didanosine has been shown to reduce the absorption of CIP by >90% (209). Since didanosine (ddl) chewable tablets contain aluminum and magnesium in the buffer, the interaction can be avoided if ddl is given 2–6 hours after the antibiotic.

The effect of enteral feeds on CIP absorption is controversial (210–212). Early reports suggested no interaction, but preliminary data suggest that CIP C_{max} and AUC can be reduced when given orally with Sustacal ($\downarrow C_{max}$ 48%; $\downarrow$ AUC 30%) or via G-tube with Jevity ($\downarrow C_{max}$ 37%; $\downarrow$ AUC 51%). Ironically, C_{max} and AUC values comparable to CIP administered without enteral feeds were achieved during the G-tube interaction. This interaction merits further study.

CIP interactions involving cytochromeP-450 enzyme inhibition can also occur. This results in decreases in the metabolic clearance of theophylline by 30% (212) and a doubling of the AUC of caffeine (P-450 IA2 mediated) (214).

CIP may inhibit gamma aminobutyric acid (GABA) binding to CNS receptors in a dose-dependent manner. Of the currently studied quinolones, CIP has one of the lowest affinities for GABA receptors (215). Thus far, nonsteroidal anti-inflammatory drugs have not been observed to potentiate CIP-induced CNS excitation, but clinicians should be aware of this potential interaction. Furthermore, patients with a history of seizures or structural CNS lesions and those receiving CIP with other drugs (216–218) capable of producing CNS excitatory effects or lowering the seizure threshold (e.g., foscarnet, imipenem, metronidazole, tricyclic antidepressants) should be carefully monitored for toxicity.

VII. Aminoglycosides

Although the drugs amikacin and gentamicin are different entities, they are often treated as a single drug with respect to their pharmacokinetics. A detailed description of the pharmacokinetics of the aminoglycosides (AMGs) is beyond the scope of this chapter, but a review of the salient features of these compounds is warranted.

Amikacin and gentamicin are usually administered intravenously over 30–60 min, although they can also be given intramuscularly. If given intravenously, it is best to use a volume of about 100 ml and infuse over 30 min to optimize the C_{max} (220). Peak serum concentrations are almost always achieved within 30–90 min after intramuscular injection, although the C_{max} may rarely be delayed out to 2 hr. The C_{max} following intramuscular injections are, on average, about 15–20% lower than the same dose given intravenously over 30 min (219).

The Vd for AMGs is generally quoted to be 0.25 L/kg, but there is tremendous inter- and intraindividual variation, which is most often due to changes in hydrational status (219) (see Table 1 for individual AMG pharmacokinetic parameters). The AMGs distribute primarily into extracellular body water, and thus the Vd fluctuates accordingly. The AMGs are distributed well into nearly all body fluids with the exceptions of the vitreous humor and cerebrospinal fluid.

Clinicians often estimate pharmacokinetic parameters using a one-compartment model, although the AMGs are best described by a three-compartment model (219). Despite the small Vd, the aminoglycosides do accumulate in so-called ''deep'' compartments. This accumulation phase is associated clinically with ototoxicity and nephrotoxicity (219,220). Clinicians should be aware that other medications (e.g., amphotericin B, pentamidine, foscarnet) may interact dynamically to increase nephrotoxicity.

The AMGs are nearly completely eliminated unchanged in the urine via glomerular filtration. A very small fraction of the AMGs is excreted into bile. Thus, the CL_T of these compounds is directly related to the CL_{cr} of the individual and, as a result, demonstrates significant interindividual variability (219). The serum elimination t1/2 is often between 2 and 4 hr in patients with normal renal function, but it increases in association with deteriorating renal function. The k_{21} (elimination rate of drug from deep, peripheral compartments) is the rate-limiting factor giving rise to a $t1/2_\gamma$ of 100 hr or longer, which allows for drug accumulation that may lead to toxicity. The AMGs are removed from the serum by hemodialysis, although the total amount of drug recovered in the urine during a dialysis session represents only a fraction of the total dose.

A. Liposomal AMGs

Liposomal encapsulated AMGs have been developed to provide a more optimal delivery technique for the treatment of MAC infections. The advantage of these preparations is that they are preferentially taken up by the reticuloendothelial system (RES) and macrophages, which allows drug to concentrate in tissues containing high amounts of mycobacteria (e.g., spleen, bone marrow). These agents have been under investigation for nearly a decade now. Early studies in beige mice with streptomycin (221,222), amikacin (223), and gentamicin (224) noted increased activity of the AMGs when incorporated into liposomes to treat experimental MAC infections.

More recently, the results of a phase I/II study of TLC G-65, or liposome-encapsulated gentamicin, were reported (225). TLC G-65 is a plurilamellar liposome made from egg phosphatidylcholine which contains 50 mg of phospholipid and 5 mg of gentamicin per milliliter. In a recent dose-escalation study, patients were given incremental dosage increases of 1.7 mg/kg/day if they did not experience a 99% reduction in MAC colony counts in blood and if no serious toxicity was observed. In each group (1.7, 3.4, and 5.1 mg/kg), the median colony count fell by more than 75% from baseline over a 6-week period. Although patients felt better subjectively, they continued to lose weight, and treatment failed to sterilize any of the subjects' blood. It was estimated that ≥ 8mg /kg of drug accumulated within subjects by the end of the study. The average C_{max} for liposome-bound drug at the 1.7, 3.4, and 5.1 mg/kg dose was 2, 8, and 29 mg/L, respectively. The average C_{max} of free drug was approximately 33% of the aforementioned values. One patient who experienced nephrotoxicity had liposome-bound C_{max} values of 15–42 mg/L and free C_{max} concentrations ranging from 6.5 to 12 mg/L. The patient's serum creatinine of 6.1 mg/dL returned to baseline 3 weeks later.

B. Aminosidine (Paromomycin)

Aminosidine is an older broad-spectrum aminoglycoside antibiotic first marketed worldwide in 1959 (226). It is available in both oral and intravenous formulations, although the latter is still investigational in the United States. It has been shown by Kanyok et al. (227,228) and Piersimoni, et al. (229) to have activity both in vitro and in vivo against *M. tuberculosis*, multi–drug-resistant *M. tuberculosis*, and MAC. After intravenous or intramuscular administration, aminosidine's pharmacokinetic parameters are similar to the other aminoglycosides (226). After oral administration, aminosidine is not absorbed to any significant degree. This makes it an ideal candidate for investigation as an oral prophylactic agent against dMAC infection (229). Additionally, its lack of cross resistance with SM (227,228) makes the parenteral form of the drug a candidate for the treatment of resistant disease when an aminoglycoside is indicated.

References

1. Sturgill MG, Rapp RF. Clarithromycin: review of a new macrolide antibiotic with improved microbiologic spectrum and favorable pharmacokinetic and adverse effect profiles. Ann Pharmacother 1992; 26:1099–108.
2. Piscitelli SC, Danziger LH, Rodvold KA. Clarithromycin and azithromycin: new macrolide antibiotics. Clin Pharm 1992; 11:137–52.
3. Kirst HA, Sides GD. New directions for macrolide antibiotics: structural modifications and in vitro activity. Antimicrob Agents Chemother 1989; 33:1413–18.
4. Anderson R, Joone G, van Rensburg EJ. An in vitro evaluation of the cellular uptake and intraphagocytic bioactivity of clarithromycin (A-56268, TE-031), a new macrolide antimicrobial agent. J Antimicrob Chemother 1988; 22:923–933.
5. Fernandes PB, Bailer R, Swanson R, et al. In vitro and in vivo evaluation of A-56268 (TE-031), a new macrolide. Antimicrob Agents Chemother 1986; 30:865–873.
6. Crowle AJ, Dahl R, Ross E, May MH. Evidence that vesicles containing live, virulent *Mycobacterium tuberculosis* or *Mycobacterium avium* in cultured human macrophages are not acidic. Infect Immun 1991; 59:1823–1831.
7. Ishiguro M, Koga H, Kohno S, et al. Penetration of macrolides into human polymorphonuclear leukocytes. J Antimicrob Chemother 1989; 24:719–729.
8. Hardy DJ, Hensey DM, Beyer JM, et al. Comparative in vitro activities of new 14-, 15-, and 16-membered macrolides. Antimicrob Agents Chemother 1988; 32:1710–1719.
9. Fernandes PB, Bailer R, Swanson R, et al. In vitro and in vivo evaluation of A-56268 (TE-031), a new macrolide. Antimicrob Agents Chemother 1986; 30:865–873.
10. Moinard D, Bourried Y, Bemer-Melchior P. Raffi F. Activity of clarithromycin against *Mycobacterium avium* complex determined with Bactec; pH effect. 2nd International Conference on the Macrolides, Azalides, and Streptogramins (ICMAS). Venice, Italy, January 1994.
11. Neu HC. The development of macrolides: clarithromycin in perspective. J Antimicrob Chemother 1991; 27(suppl A):1–9.
12. Chu S-Y, Deaton R, Cavanaugh J. Absolute bioavailability of clarithromycin after oral administration in humans. Antimicrob Agents Chemother 1992; 36:1147–50.
13. Chu S-Y, Park Y, Locke C, et al. Drug-food interaction potential of clarithromycin, a new macrolide antimicrobial. J Clin Pharmacol 1992; 32:32–36.
14. Chu S-Y, Sennello LT, Bunnell ST, et al. Pharmacokinetics of clarithromycin, a new macrolide, after single ascending oral doses. Antimicrob Agents Chemother 1992; 36:2447–2453.
15. Ferrero JL, Bopp BA, Marsh KC, et al. Metabolism and disposition of clarithromycin in man. Drug Metab Disp 1990; 18:441–446.

16. Chu S-Y, Wilson DS, Deaton RL, et al. Single- and multiple-dose pharmacokinetics of clarithromycin, a new macrolide antimicrobial. J Clin Pharmacol 1993; 33:719–726.

17. Gustavson LE, Chu S-Y, Fritz N, Gupta S. Pharmacokinetics of oral clarithromycin in adult and pediatric patients with HIV infection. 2nd International Conference on the Macrolides, Azalides, and Streptogramins (ICMAS). Venice, Italy, January 1994.

18. Gan VN, Chu S-Y, Kusmiesz HT, Craft JC. Pharmacokinetics of a clarithromycin suspension in infants and children. Antimicrob Agents Chemother 1992; 36:2478–2480.

19. Husson RN, Ross LA, Sandelli S, et al. Orally administered clarithromycin for the treatment of systemic *Mycobacterium avium* complex infection in children with acquired immunodeficiency syndrome. J. Pediatr 1994; 124:807–814.

20. Inderlied CB, Sandoval FG, Young LS. In vitro activity of Clarithromycin (CLARI) and 14-hydroxyclarithromycin against the *Mycobacterium avium* complex (MAC) alone and in combination with other agents. 31st Interscience Conference on Antimicrobial Agents and Chemotherapy. Chicago, September 29–October 2, 1991.

21. Chu S-Y, Wilson DS, Guay DRP, Craft C. Clarithromycin pharmacokinetics in healthy young and elderly volunteers. J Clin Pharmacol 1992; 32:1045–1049.

22. Wallace RJ, Brown BA, Griffith DE. Drug intolerance to high-dose clarithromycin among elderly patients. Diagn Microbiol Infect Dis 1993; 16:215–221.

23. Dette GA, Knothe H, Koulen G. Comparative in vitro activity, serum binding and binding activity interactions of the macrolides A-56268, RE-28965, erythromycin and josamycin. Drugs Exp Clin Res 1987; 13:567–576.

24. Suwa T,Yoshiida H, Kohno Y, et al. Metabolic fate of TE-031 (A-56268) III: absorption, distribution and excretion of 14C-TE-031 in rats, mice and dogs. Chemother 1988; 36:213–226.

25. Fraschini F, Scaglione F, Pintucci G., et al. The diffusion of clarithromycin and roxithromycin into nasal mucosa, tonsil and lung in humans. J. Antimicrob Chemother 1991; 27(suppl A):61–65.

26. Fish DN, Gotfried MH, Danziger LH, Rodvold KA, Penetration of clarithromycin into lung tissues from patients undergoing lung resection. Antimicrob Agents Chemother 1994; 38:876–878.

27. Peters DH, Clissold SP. Clarithromycin: a review of its antimicrobial activity, pharmacokinetic properties and therapeutic potential. 1992; 44:117–64.

28. Ferrero JL, Bopp BA, Marsh KC, et al. Metabolism and disposition of clarithromycin in man. Drug Metab Disp 1990; 18:441–446.

29. Adachi T, Sasaki J, Omura S. Hydroxylation and N-demethylation of clarithromycin (6-O-methylerythromycin A) by *Mucor circinelloides*. J Antibiot 1989; 17:1433–1437.

30. Adachi T. Morimoto S, Kondoh H, et al. Fourteen-hydroxy-6-O-methylerythromycins A, active metabolites of 6-O-methylerythromycin A in human. J Antibiot 1988; 16:966–975.

31. Chu S-Y, Granneman GR, Pichotta PJ. et al. Effect of moderate or severe hepatic impairment on clarithromycin pharmacokinetics. J Clin Pharmacol 1993; 33:480–485.
32. Gustavson LE, Chu S-Y, Mackenthum A, et al. Drug interaction between clarithromycin and oral zidovudine in HIV-1 infected patients (abstr). Clin Pharmacol Ther 1992; 165:577–580.
33. Petty B, Polis M, Haneiwich S, et al. Pharmacokinetic assessment of clarithromycin plus zidovudine in HIV patients. 32nd Interscience Conference on Antimicrobial Agents and Chemotherapy. Anaheim, CA, October 11–14, 1992.
34. Vance E, Guzman J, Kazanjian P. Clarithromycin and zidovudine pharmacokinetic study. 10th International Conference on SIDS: International Conference on STD. Yokohama, Japan, August 8–12, 1994.
35. DATRI 001 Study Group. Co-administration of clarithromycin (CL) alters the concentration-time profile of rifabutin (RFB). 34th Interscience Conference on Antimicrobial Agents and Chemotherapy. (A2) Orlando, FL, October 4–7, 1994.
36. Siegal FP, Eilbott D, Burger H, et al. Dose-limiting toxicity of rifabutin in AIDS-related complex: syndrome of arthralgia/arithritis. AIDS 1990; 433–441.
37. Havlir D, Torriani F, Dube M. Uveitis associated with rifabutin prophylaxis. Ann Intern Med 1994; 121:510–512.
38. Venkatesan K. Pharmacokinetic drug interactions with rifampicin. Clin Pharmacokin 1992; 22:47–65.
39. Wong YY, Ludden TM, Bell RD. Effect of erythromycin on carbamazepine kinetics. Clin Pharmacol Ther 1983; 33:460–464.
40. Albani F, Riva R, Baruzzi A. Clarithromycin-carbamazepine interaction: a case report. Epilepsia 1993; 34:161–162.
41. Honig P, Wortham D, Zamani K, et al. Effect of erythromycin, clarithromycin and azithromycin on the pharmacokinetics of terfenadine. 1993; 53:161(Pl-106).
42. Gillum JG, Israel DS, Polk RE. Pharmacokinetic drug interactions with antimicrobial agents. 1993; 25:450–482.
43. Periti P, Mazzei T, Mini E, Novelli A. Pharmacokinetic drug interactions of macrolides. 1992; 23:106–31.
44. Gersema LM. Porter CB, Russell EH. Suspected drug interaction between cyclosporine and clarithromycin. J Heart Lung Transplant 1994; 13:343–346.
45. Kirst HA, Sides GD. New directions for macrolide antibiotics: structure modifications and in vitro activity. Antimicrob Agents Chemother 1989; 33:1413–1418.
46. Fiese EF, Steffen SH. Comparison of the acid stability of azithromycin and erythromycin A. J Antimicrob Chemother 1990; 25(suppl A):39–47.
47. Omura S, Tsuzuki K, Sunazuka T, et al. Macrolides with gastrointestinal motor stimulating activity. J Med Chem 1987; 30:1941–1943.
48. Gladue RP, Bright GM, Isaacson RE, Newborg MF. In vitro and in vivo uptake of azithromycin (CP-62,933) by phagocytic cells: possible mechanism of de-

livery and release at sites of infection. Antimicrob Agents Chemother 1989; 33:277–282.

49. McDonald PJ, Pruul H. Phagocyte uptake and transport of azithromycin. Eur J Clin Microbiol Infect Dis 1991; 10:828–833.

50. Foulds G, Shepard RM, Johnson RB. The pharmacokinetics of azithromycin in human serum and tissues. J Antimicrob Chemother 1990; 25(suppl A):73–82.

51. Cooper MA, Nye K, Andrews JM, Wise R. The pharmacokinetics and inflammatory fluid penetration of orally administered azithromycin. J Antimicrob Chemother 1990; 26:533–538.

52. Pedersen V, Miller R. Pharmacokinetics and bioavailability of cimetidine in humane. J. Pharm Sci 1980; 69:394–398.

53. Colburn W. Pharmacokinetic analysis of cencentration-time data obtained following administration of drugs that are recycled in the bile. JP harm Sci 1984; 73:313–317.

54. Ziemniak JA, Welage LS, Schentag JJ. Cimetidine and ranitidine. In: Evand WG, Schentag JJ, Jusko WJ, eds. Applied Pharmacokinetics; Principles of Therapeutic Drug Monitoring, 2nd ed. Spokane: Applied Therapeutics, 1986; 24:182–246.

55. Zithromax product information. Pfizer Laboratories, New York, February 1992.

56. Chave J-P, Munafo A, Chatton J-Y, et al. Once-a-week azithromycin in AIDS patients: tolerability, kinetics, and effects on zidovudine disposition. Antimicrob Agents Chemother 1992; 36:1013–1018.

57. Mazzei T. Surrenti C, Novelli A, et al. P. Pharmacokinetics of azithromycin in patients with impaired hepatic function J Antimicrob Chemother 1993; 31(suppl E):57–63.

58. Coates P, Deniel R, Huston AC, et al. An open study to compare the pharmacokinetics, safety and tolerability of a multiple-dose regimen of azithromycin in young and elderly volunteers. Pharmacokinetics 1991; 10:850–852.

59. Foulds G, Hilligoss DM, Henry EB, Gerber N. The effects of an antacid or cimetidine on the serum concentrations of azithromycin. J Clin Pharmacol 1991; 31:164–67.

60. Nahata MC, Koranyi KI, Gadgil SD, et al. Pharmacokinetics of azithromycin in pediatric patients after oral administration of multiple doses of suspension Antimicrob Agents Chemother 1993; 37:314–316.

61. Retseema JA, Bergeron JM, Gerard D, et al. Preferential concentration of azithromycin in an infected mouse thigh model. J Antimicrob Chemother 1993; 31(Suppl E):5–16.

62. Baldwin DR, Wise R, Andrews JM, et al. Azithromycin concentrations at the sites of pulmonary infection. Eur Respir J 1990; 3:886–890.

63. Harrison JD, Jones JA. Morris DL. Azithromycin levels in plasma and gastric tissue, juice and mucus. Eur J Clin Microbiol Infect Dis 1991; 10:862–864.

64. Johnson RB. The role of azalide antibiotics in the treatment of chlamydia. Am J Obstet Gynecol 1991; 164:1794–1796.

65. Krohn K. Gynaecological tissue levels of azithromycin. Eur J Clin Microbiol Infect Dis 1991; 10:864–868.

66. Morris DL, De Souza A, Jones JA, Morgan WE. High and prolonged pulmonary tissue concentrations of azithromycin following a single oral dose. Eur J Clin Microbiol Infect Dis 1991; 10:859–861.

67. Foulds G, Madsen P, Cox C, et al. Concentration of azithromycin in human prostatic tissue. Eur J Clin Microbiol Infect Dis 1991; 10:868–871.

68. Karma P, Pukander J, Penttila M. Azithromycin concentrations in sinus fluid and mucosa after oral administration. Eur J Clin Microbiol Infect Dis 1991; 10:857–859.

69. Foulds G. Chan KH, Johnson JT, et al. Concentrations of azithromycin in human tonsillar tissue. Eur J Clin Microbiol Infect Dis 1991; 10:853–856.

70. Rodvold KA, Piscitelli SC. New oral macrolide and fluoroquinolone antibiotics: an overview of pharmacokinetics, interactions, and safety. Clin Infect Dis 1993; 17(suppl 1):S192–99.

71. Schentag JJ, Ballow CH. Tissue-directed pharmacokinetics. Am J Med 1991; 92(suppl 3A):5S–11S.

72. Peters DH, Friedel HA, McTavish D. Azithromycin: a review of its antimicrobial activity, pharmacokinetic properties and clinical efficacy. Drugs 1992; 44:750–799.

73. Kelsey JJ, Moser LR, Jennings JC, Munger MA. Presence of azithromycin breast milk concentrations: a case report. Am J Obstet Gynecol 1994; 170: 1375–1376.

74. Van der Auwera P. Matsumoto T, Husson M. Intraphagocyte penetration of antibiotics. J Antimicrob Chemother 1988; 22:185–192.

75. Wildfeuer A, Reisert I. Laufen H. Uptake and subcellular distribution of azithromycin in human phagocytic cells: demonstration of the antibiotic in neutrophil polymorphonuclear leucocytes and monocytes by autoradiography and electron microscopy. Arzneimittel Forschung 1993; 43:484–486.

76. Lalak NJ, Morris DL. Azithromycin clinical pharmacokinetics. Clin Pharmacokin 1993; 25:370–374.

77. Pessayre D, Larrey D, Funck-Brentano C, Benhamou JP. Drug interactions and hepatitis produced by some macrolide antibiotics. J Antimicrob Chemother 1985; 16(suppl A):181–194.

78. Raperport WG, Dewland PM, Muirhead DC, Forster PL. Lack of interaction between azithromycin and carbamazepine. Br J Clin Pharmacol 1992; 30:551P.

79. Hopkins S. Clinical toleration and safety of azithromycin. Am J Med 1991; 91(suppl 3A):40S–44S.

80. Gardner MJ, Coates PE, Hilligoss DM, Henry EB. Lack of effect of azithromycin on the pharmacokinetics of theophylline in man. Proceedings of the Mediterranean Congress of Chemotherapy. Athens, Greece, May 1992.

81. Clauzel AM, Visier S, Michel FB. Efficacy and safety of azithromycin in lower respiratory tract infections. Eur Respir J 1990; 3(suppl 10):89S.

82. Honig PK, Wortham DC, Zamani K, Cantilena L. Comparison of the effect of the macrolide antibiotics erythromycin, clarithromycin and azithromycin on

terfenadine steady-state pharmacokinetics and electrocardiographic parameters. Drug Invest 1994; 7:148–56.

83. Yajko D, Nassos PS, Hadley WK. Therapeutic implications of inhibition versus killing of *Mycobacterium avium* complex by antimicrobial agents. Antimicrob Agents Chemother 1987; 31:117–20.

84. Heifets LB, Lindholm-Levy PJ, Flory MA. Bactericidal activity in vitro of various rifamycins against *Mycobacterium avium* and *Mycobacterium tuberculosis*. Am Rev Respir Dis 1990; 141:626–630.

85. Rastogi N, Frehel C, Ryter A, et al. Multiple drug resistance in *Mycobacterium avium*: is the wall architecture responsible for exclusion of antimicrobial agents? Antimicrob Agents Chemother 1981; 20:666–677.

86. Hoffner SE, Svenson SB, Kallenius G. Synergistic effects of antimycobacterial drug combinations on *Mycobacterium avium* complex determined radiometrically in liquid medium. Eur J Clin Microbiol 1987; 6:530–535.

87. Skinner MH, Hsieh M. Torseth J, et al. Pharmacokinetics of rifabutin. Antimicrob Agents Chemother 1989; 33:1237–1241.

88. Battaglia R, Pianezzola E, Salgarollo G, et al. Absorption, disposition and preliminary metabolic pathway of ^{14}C-rifabutin in animals and man. J. Antimicrob Chemother 1990; 26:813–822.

89. Narang PK, Lewis RC, Bianchine JR. Rifabutin absorption in humans: relative bioavailability and food effect. Clin Pharmacol Ther 1992; 52:335–341.

90. Mycobutin product information. Adria Laboratories, Columbus, OH; December 23, 1992.

91. Colborn D, Lewis R, Narang P. HIV disease severity does not influence rifabutin absorption. 34th Interscience Conference on Antimicrobial Agents and Chemotherapy. (A42) Orlando, FL, October 4–7, 1994.

92. Loos U, Musch E, Jensen JC, et al. M. Pharmacokinetics of oral and intravenous rifampicin during chronic administration. Klin Wochenschr 1985; 63: 1205–1211.

93. Acocella G. Pagani V, Marchetti M, et al. Kinetic studies on rifampicin. 1971; 16:356–370.

94. Strolin Benedetti M, Efthymiopoulos C. Sassella D, et al. Autoinduction of rifabutin metabolism in man. Zenobiotica 1990; 20:1113–1119.

95. Strolin Benedetti M, Pianezzola E, Brughera M, et al. Concentrations of rifabutin in plasma and cerebrospinal fluid in Cynomolgus monkeys. J Antimicrob Chemother 1994; 34:600–603.

96. Dhillon J. Mitchison DA. Activity in vitro of rifabutin, FCE 22807, rifapentne, and rifampin against *Mycobacterium microti* and *M. tuberculosis* and their penetration into mouse peritoneal macrophages. Am Rev Respir Dis 1992; 145:212–214.

97. Pascual A, Tsukayama D. Kovarik J, et al. Uptake and activity of rifapentine in human peritoneal macrophages and polymorphonuclear leukocytes. Eur J Clin Microbiol 1987; 6:152–57.

98. Hand WL, Corwin RW, Steinberg TH, Grossman GD. Uptake of antibiotics by human alveolar macrophages. Am Rev Respir Dis 1984; 129:933–937.

99. Snider DE, Powell KE. Should women taking antituberculosis drugs breast-feed? Arch Intern Med 1984; 144:589.
100. Holdiness MR. Antituberculosis drugs and breast-feeding [letter]. Arch Intern Med 1984; 144:1888.
101. Chow AW, Jewesson PJ. Pharmacokinetics and safety of antimicrobial agents during pregnancy. Rev Infect Dis 1985; 7:287–313.
102. Peloquin CA. Antituberculosis drugs: pharmacokinetics. In: Heifets LB, ed. Drug Susceptibility in the Chemotherapy of Mycobacterial Infections. Boca Raton, FL, CRC Press, 1991:59–88.
103. Gillum JG, Israel DS, Polk RE. Pharmacokinetic drug interactions with antimicrobial agents. Clin Pharmacokin 1993; 25:450–482.
104. Bachmann K, Jauregui L. Use of single sample clearance estimates of cytochrome P450 substrates to characterize human hepatic CYP status in vivo. Xenobiotica 1993; 23:307–315.
105. Borin MT, Cox SR, Chambers JH, et al. Effect of rifampin on delavirdine pharmacokinetics in HIV+ patients. 34th Interscience Conference on Antimicrobial Agents and Chemotherapy. (A50) Orlando, FL, October 4–7, 1994.
106. Wallace RJ, Jr, Brown BA, Griffith DE, et al. Reduced serum levels of clarithromycin in patients on multidrug regimens including rifampin or rifabutin for treatment of *Mycobacterium avium-intercellulare* (MAI). 34th Interscience Conference on Antimicrobial Agents and Chemotherapy. (M59) Orlandi, FL, October 4–7, 1994.
107. Gillum JG, Sesler JM, Bruzzese VL, et al. Comparison of rifampin and rifabutin on the metabolism of theophylline in healthy volunteers. 34th Interscience Conference on Antimicrobial agents and Chemotherapy. (A1) Orlando, FL, October 4–7, 1994.
108. Narang P, Nightingale S, Manzone C, et al. Does rifabutin affect zidovudine disposition in HIV (+) patients? 8th International Conference on AIDS, (PO-B3888) 1992.
109. Narang PK, Sale M. Population based assessment of rifabutin effect on zidovudine disposition in AIDS patients. Clin Pharmacol Ther 1993; 53:219.
110. Balakrishnan S, Seshadri PS. Drug interactions: the influence of rifampicin and clofazimine on the urinary excretion of DDS. Lepr India 1981; 53:17–22.
111. Gelber RH, Gooi HC, Rees RFW. The effect of rifampicin on dapsone metabolism. Proc West Pharmacol Soc 1975; 18:330–334.
112. Venkatesan K, Bharadwaj VP, Ramu G, Desikan KV. A study of drug interactions in leprosy. Lepr India 1980; 52:229–235.
113. J Occhipinti DJ, Choi A, Danziger LH, Deyo K. Influence of rifampin and clofazimine on dapsone disposition and methbg concentrations. Clin Pharmacol Ther. In press.
114. Breda M, Pianezzola E, Strolin Benedetti M, et al. A study of the effects of rifabutin on isoniazid pharmacokinetics and metabolism in healthy volunteers. Drug Metabol Drug Interact 1992; 10:323–340.

115. Narang PK, Trapnell CB, Schoenfeder JR, et al. Fluconazole and enhanced effect of rifabutin prophylaxis (letter). N Engl J Med 1994; 330:1316–1317.

116. Nightingale SD, Cameron DW, Gordin FM, et al. Two controlled trials of rifabutin prophylaxis against *Mycobacterium avium* complex infection in AIDS. N Engl J Med 1993; 329:828–833.

117. Masur H, Public Health Service Task Force on Prophylaxis and Therapy for *Mycobacterium avium* Complex. Recommendations on prophylaxis and therapy for disseminated *Mycobacterium avium* complex disease in patients infected with the human immunodeficiency virus. N Engl J Med 1993; 329:898–904.

118. Vandevelde C. Chang A, Andrews, et al. Rifampin and ansamycin interactions with cyclosporine after renal transplantation. Pharmacotherapy 1991; 11:88–89.

119. Holdiness MR. Clinical pharmacokinetics of clofazimine. A review. Clin Pharmacokinet 1989; 16:74–85.

120. Mathur A, Venkatesan K, Bharadwaj VP, Ramu G. Evaluation of effectiveness of clofazimine therapy I. Monitoring of absorption of clofazimine from gastrointestinal tract. Indian J Lepr 1985; 57:146–49.

121. Yawalker SJ, Vischer W. Lamprene (clofazimine) in leprosy. Lepr Rev 1979; 50:135–44.

122. Venkatesan K. Clinical pharmacokinetic considerations in the treatment of patients with leproxy. Clin Pharmacokin 1989; 16:365.

123. Clofazimine, in American Hospital Formulary Service (AHFS). American Society of Hospital Pharmacists, 1992:455–459.

124. Schaad-Lanyi Z, Dieterle W, Dubois JP, et al. Pharmacokinetics of clofazimine in healthy volunteers. Int J Lepr 1987; 55:9–15.

125. Banerjee DK, Ellard GA, Gammon PT, Waters MRF. Some observations on the pharmacology of clofazimine (B663). Am J Trop Med Hyg 1974; 23:1110–1115.

126. Garrelts JC. Clofazimine: a review of its use in leprosy and *Mycobacterium avium* complex infection. Ann Pharmacother 1991; 25:525–531.

127. Mansfield RE. Tissue concentrations of clofazimine (B663) in man. Am J Trop Med Hyg 1974; 23:1116–1119.

128. Desikan KV, Balakrishnan S. Tissue levels of clofazimine in a case of leprosy. Lepr Rev 1976; 47:107–13.

129. Belaube P, Devaux J, Pizzi M, et al. Small bowel deposition of crystals associated with the use of clofazimine (Lamprene) in the treatment of prurigo nodularis. Int J Lep 1983; 51:328–330.

130. Holdiness MR. Teratology of the antituberculosis drugs: a review. Early Hum Devel 1987; 15:61–74.

131. Browne SG, Hogerzeil LM. B663 in the treatment of leprosy: preliminary report of a pilot trial. Lepr Rev 1962;33:6–16.

132. Feng PCC, Fenselau CC, Jacobson RR. A new urinary metabolite of clofazimine in leprosy patients. Drug Metab Disp 1982; 10:286–288.

133. Feng PCC, Fenselau CC, Jacobson RR. Metabolism of clofazimine in leprosy patients. Drug Metab Disp 1981; 9:521–524.

134. Mehta J, Ghandhi IS, Sane SB, Wamburkar MN. Effect of clofazimine and dapsone on rifampicin (Lositril) pharmacokinetics in multibacillary and paucibacillary leprosy cases. Indian J Lepr 1985; 57:297–310.
135. Duncan ME, Oakey RE. Reduced estrogen excretion due to clofazimine. Int J Lepr 1983; 51:112–113.
136. Grabosz JAJ, Wheate HW. Effect of clofazimine on the urinary excretion of dapsone. Int J Lepr 1975; 43:61–62.
137. George J, Balakrishnan S, Bhatia VN. Drug interaction during multidrug regimens for treatment of leprosy. Indian J Med Res 1988; 87:151–156.
138. Pieters FAJ, Woonink F, Zuidema J. Influence of once-monthly rifampicin and daily clofazimine on the pharmacokinetics of dapsone in leprosy patients in Nigeria. Eur J Clin Pharmacol 1988; 34:73–76.
139. Venkatesan K, Bharadwaj VP, Ramu G, Desikan KV. Study on drug interactions. Lepr India 1980; 52:229–235.
140. Lee CS, Gambertoglio JG, Brater DC, Benet LZ. Kinetics of oral ethambutol in the normal subject. Clin Pharmacol Ther 1977; 22:615–621.
141. Place VA, Thomas JP. Clinical pharmacology of ethambutol. Am Rev Respir Dis 1963; 87:901–904.
142. Peets EA, Sweeney WM, Place VA, Buyske DA. The absorption, excretion, and metabolic fate of ethambutol in man. Am Rev Respir Dis 1965; 91:51–58.
143. Place VA, Peets EA, Buyske DA. Metabolic and special studies of ethambutol in normal volunteers and tuberculous patients. Ann NY Acad Sci 1966; 135:775–795.
144. Lee CS, Brater DC, Gambertoglio JG, Benet LZ. Disposition kinetics of ethambutol in man. J Pharmacokin Biopharm 1980; 8:335–346.
145. Ameer B, Polk RE, Kline BJ, Grisafe JP. Effect of food on ethambutol absorption. Clin Pharm 1982; 1:156–158.
146. Strauss I, Erhardt F. Ethambutol absorption, excretion and dosage in patients with renal tuberculosis. Chemotherapy 1970; 15:148–157.
147. Benet LZ. Choice of appropriate predicting models in multiple dose chemotherapy. 10th International Congress of Chemotherapy. Zurich, 1977.
148. Johnson JD, Hand WL, Francis JB, et al. Antibiotic uptake by alveolar macrophages. J Lab Clin Med 1980; 95:429–439.
149. Hand WL, Corwin RW, Steinberg TH, Grossman GD. Uptake of antibiotics by human alveolar macrophages. Am Rev Respir Dis 1984; 129:933–937.
150. Christopher TG, Blair A, Forrey A, Cutler RE. Kinetics of ethambutol in renal disease. Proc Dialysis Transplant Forum 1973; 3:96–101.
151. Lee CS, Marbury TC, Benet LZ. Clearance calculations in hemodialysis: application to blood plasma and dialysate measurements for ethambutol. J Pharmacokin Biopharm 1980; 8:69–81.
152. Bennett WM, Aronoff GR, Morrison G, et al. I. Drug prescribing in renal failure: dosing guidelines for adults. Am J Kidney Dis 1983; 3:155–193.

153. Lee CS, Bambertoglio JG, Brater DC, et al. Kinetics of oral ethambutol in the normal subject. Clin Pharmacol Ther 1977; 22:615–621.
154. Dume T, Wagner C, Wetzels E. Zur pharmacokinetik von ethambutol bie gesunden und patienten mit terminaler niereninsuffizienz. Med Wochen 1971; 96:1430.
155. Wolfson JS. Hooper DC. The fluoroquinolones: structures, mechanisms of action and resistance, and spectra of activity in vitro. Antimicrob Agents Chemother 1985; 28:581–586.
156. Young LS, Berlin OGW, Inderlied CB. Activity of ciprofloxacin and other fluorinated quinolones against mycobacteria. Am J Med 1987; 82(suppl 4A): 23–26.
157. Salfinger M, Hohl P, Kafader FM. Comparative in-vitro activity of fleroxacin and other 6-fluroquinolones against mycobacteria. J Antimicrob Chemother 1988; 22(suppl D):55–63.
158. Leysen DC, Haemers A, Pattyn SR. Mycobacteria and the new quinolones. Antimicrob Agents Chemother 1989; 33:1–5.
159. Benson CA. Treatment of disseminated disease due to the *Mycobacterium avium* complex in patients with AIDS. Clin Infect Dis 1994; 18(suppl 3):S237–S242.
160. Recommendations on prophylaxis and therapy for disseminated *Mycobacterium avium* complex for adults and adolescents infected with human immunodeficiency virus: US Public Health Service Task Force on Prophylaxis and therapy for *Mycobacterium avium* Complex. MMWR 1993; 42(RR-9):14–20.
161. Tartaglione TA, Raffalovich AC, Poynor WJ, et al. Pharmacokinetics and tolerance of ciprofloxacin after sequential increasing oral doses. Antimicrob Agents Chemother 1986; 29:62–66.
162. Nix DE, Spivey JM, Norman A, Schentag JJ. Dose-ranging pharmacokinetic study of ciprofloxacin after 200-, 300-, and 400-mg intravenous doses. Ann Pharmacother 1992; 26:8–10.
163. Catchpole C, Andrews JM, Woodcock J, Wise R. The comparative pharmacokinetics and tissue penetration of single-dose ciprofloxacin 400 mg i.v. and 750 mg po. J Antimicrob Chemother 1994; 33:103–10.
164. Hoffken G, Lode H, Prinzing C, et al. Pharmacokinetics of ciprofloxacin after oral and parenteral administration. Antimicrob Agents Chemother 1985; 27: 375–379.
165. Campoli-Richards DM, Monk JP, Price A, et al.. Ciprofloxacin: a review of its antibacterial activity, pharmacokinetic properties and therapeutic use. Drugs 1988; 35:373–447.
166. Aronoff GE, Kenner CH, Sloan RN, Pottratz ST Multiple-dose ciprofloxacin kinetics in normal subjects. Clin Pharmacol Ther 1984; 3:384–388.
167. Griffiths NM, Hirst BH, Simmons NL. Active intestinal secretion of the fluoroquinolone antibacterials ciprofloxacin, norfloxacin and pefloxacin; a common secretory pathway? J Pharmacol Exp Ther 1994; 269:496–502.
168. Ramon J, Dautrey S, Farinoti R, et al. Intestinal elimination of ciprofloxacin in rabbits. Antimicrob Agents Chemother 1994; 38:757–760.

169. Griffiths NM, Hirst BH, Simmons NL. Active secretion of the fluoroquinolone ciprofloxacin by human intestinal epithelial Caco-2 cell layers. Br J Pharmacol 1993; 108:575–576.

170. Viell B, Krause B, Vestweber KH, et al. Transintestinal elimination of ciprofloxacin in humans—concomitant assessment of its metabolites in serum, ileum and colon. Infection 1992; 20:324–327.

171. Ledergerber B, Bettex J-D, Joos B, et al. Effect of standard breakfast on drug absorption and multiple-dose pharmacokinetics of ciprofloxacin. Antimicrob Agents Chemother 1985; 27:350–352.

172. Borner K, Hoffken G, Lode H, et al. Pharmacokinetics of ciprofloxacin in healthy volunteers after oral and intravenous administration. Eur J Clin Microbiol 1986; 5:179–186.

173. Schaad UB. Use of quinolones in paediatrics. Drugs 1993; 45(suppl 3):37–41.

174. Guay DRP, Auni WM, Peterson PK, et al. Pharmacokinetics of ciprofloxacin in acutely ill and convalescent elderly patients. Am J Med 1987; 82(suppl 4A): 124–129.

175. Fabre D, Bressolle F, Gomeni R, et al. Steady-state pharmacokinetics of ciprofloxacin in plasma from patients with nosocomial pneumonia; penetration of the bronchial mucosa. Antimicrob Agents Chemother 1991; 35:2521–2525.

176. Joos B, Ledergerber B, Flepp M, et al. Comparison of high-pressure liquid chromatography and bioassay for determination of ciprofloxacin in serum and urine. Antimicrob Agents Chemother 1985; 27:353–356.

177. Hoffken G, Lode H, Prinzing C, et al. Pharmacokinetics of ciprofloxacin after oral and parenteral administration. Antimicrob Agents Chemother 1985; 27: 375–379.

178. MacKichan JJ. Influence of protein binding and use of unbound (free) drug concentrations. In: Evans WE, Schentag JJ, Jusko WJ, eds. Applied Pharmacokinetics: Principles of Therapeutic Drug Monitoring. 3rd ed. Vancouver, WA: Applied Therapeutics, 1992:5.1–5.48.

179. Saux P. Martin C, Mallet M-N, et al. Penetration of ciprofloxacin into bronchial secretions from mechanically ventilated patients with nosocomial bronchopneumonia. Antimicrob Agents Chemother 1994; 38:901–904.

180. Joseph J. Vaughan LM, Basran GS. Penetration of intravenous and oral ciprofloxacin into sterile and empyemic human pleural fluid. Ann Pharmacother 1994; 28:313–315.

181. Dan M. Torossian K, Weissberg D, Kitzes R. The penetration of ciprofloxacin into bronchial mucosa, lung parenchyma, and pleural tissue after intravenous administration. Eur J Clin Pharmacol 1993; 44:101–102.

182. Baldwin DR, Wise R, Andrews JM, et al. Comparative bronchoalveolar concentrations of ciprofloxacin and lomefloxacin following oral administation. Respir Med 1993; 87:595–601.

183. Bacracheva N, Scholl H, Gerova Z, et al. The distribution of ciprofloxacin and its metabolites in human plasma, pulmonary and bronchial tissues. Int J Clin Pharmacol Ther Toxicol 1991; 29:352–356.

184. Barsic B, Himbele J, Beus I, et al. Entry of ciprofloxacin into cerebrospinal fluid during bacterial, viral and tuberculous meningitis. Neurol Croat 1991; 40: 111–116.

185. Davey PG, Charter M, Kelly S, Varma TR, et al. Ciprofloxacin and sparfloxacin penetration into human brain tissue and their activity as antagonists of GABAA receptor of rat vagus nerve. Antimicrob Agents Chemother 1994; 38:1356– 1362.

186. Briggs GG, Freeman RK, Yaffe SJ. Ciprofloxacin. In: Drugs in Pregnancy and Lactation (Update). 1990; 3:19–20.

187. Cover DL, Mueller BA. Ciprofloxacin penetration into human breast milk: a case report. Ann Pharmacother 1990; 24:703–704.

188. Gardner DK, Gabbe SG, Harter C. Simultaneous concentrations of ciprofloxacin in breast milk and in serum in mother and breast-fed infant. Clin Pharm 1992; 11:352–354.

189. Garraffo R, Jambou D, Chichmanian RM, et al. In vitro and in vivo ciprofloxacin pharmacokinetics in human neutrophils. Antimicrob Agents Chemother 1991; 35:2215–2218.

190. Chateau MT, Caravano R. Rapid fluorometric measurement of intra-cellular concentration of ciprofloxacin in mouse peritoneal macrophages. J Antimicrob Chemother 1993; 31:281–287.

191. Dudley MN, Ericson J, Zinner SH. Effect of dose on serum pharmacokinetics of intravenous ciprofloxacin with identification and characterization of extra-vascular compartments using noncompartmental and compartmental pharmacokinetic models. Antimicrob Agents Chemother 1987; 31:1782–1786.

192. Drusano GL, Plaisance KI, Forrest A, Standiford HC. Dose ranging study and constant infusion evaluation of ciprofloxacin. Amtimicrob Agents Chemother 1986; 30:440–443.

193. Drusano GL, Weir M, Forrest A, et al. Pharmacokinetics of intravenously administered ciprofloxacin in patients with various degrees of renal function. Antimicrob Agents Chemother 1987; 31:860–864.

194. Wise R, Lockley RM, Webberly M, Dent J. Pharmacokinetics of intravenously administered ciprofloxacin. Antimicrob Agents Chemother 1984; 26:208–210.

195. Zeiler H-J, Petersen U, Gau W, Ploschke HF. Antibacterial activity of the metabolites of ciprofloxacin and its significance in the bioassay. Arzneimittel Forschung 1987; 37:131–34.

196. Dan M, Verbin N, Gorea A, et al. Concentrations of ciprofloxacin in human liver, gallbladder and bile after oral administration. Eur J Clin Pharmacol 1987; 32:217–218.

197. Nix DE, Schentag JJ. The Quinolones: an overview and comparative appraisal of their pharmacokinetics and pharmacodynamics. J Clin Pharmacol 1988; 28: 169-xxx.

198. Lettieri JT, Rogge MC, Kaiser L, et al. Pharmacokinetic profiles of ciprofloxacin after single intravenous and oral doses. Antimicrob Agents Chemother 1992; 36:993–996.

199. Peltola H, Vaarala M, Renkonen O-V, Neuvonen PJ. Pharmacokinetics of single-dose oral ciprofloxacin in infants and small children. Antimicrob Agents Chemother 1992; 36:1086–1090.
200. Brouwers JR. Drug Interactions with quinolone antibacterials. Drug Safety 1992; 7:268–281.
201. Marchblanks CR. Drug-drug interactions with fluoroquinolones. Pharmacotherapy 1993; 13(2 Pt 2):23S–28S.
202. Nix DE. Drug-drug interactions with fluoroquinolone antimicrobial agents. 2nd ed. In Hopper DC, Wolfson JS, eds. Washington D.C.: American Society for Microbiology, 1993; 11:245–258.
203. Nix DE, Watson WA, Lener ME, et al. Effects of aluminum and magnesium antacids and ranitidine on the absorption of ciprofloxacin. Clin Pharmacol Ther 1989; 46:700–705.
204. Sahai J, Healy DP, Stotka J, Polk RE. The influence of chronic administration of calcium carbonate on the bioavailabiity of oral ciprofloxacin. Br J Clin Pharmacol 1993; 35:302–304.
205. Lomaestro BM, Bailie GR. Effect of staggered dose of calcium on the bioavailability of ciprofloxacin. Antimicrob Agents Chemoother 1991; 35:1004–1007.
206. Lomaestro BM, Bailie GR. Effect of multiple staggered doses of calcium on the bioavailabiity of ciprofloxacin. Ann Pharmacother 1993; 27:1325–1328.
207. Polk RE, Healy DP, Sahai J, et al. Effect of ferrous sulfate and multivitamins with zinc on absorption of ciprofloxacin in normal volunteers. Antimicrob Agents Chemother 1989; 33:1841–1844.
208. Nix DE, Watson WA, Handy L, et al. The effect of sucralfate pretreatment on the pharmacokinetics of ciprofloooxacin. Pharmacotherapy 1989; 9(suppl 6): 377-380.
209. Sahai J, Gallicano K, Oliveras L, et al. Cations in the didanosine tablet reduce ciprofloxacin bioavailability. Clin Pharmacol Ther 1993; 53:292–297.
210. Yuk JH, Nightingale CH, Sweeney KR, et al. Relative bioavailability in healthy volunteers of ciprofloxacin administered through a nasogastric tube with and without enteral feeding. Antimicrob Agents Chemother 1989; 33:1118–1120.
211. Yuk JH, Nightingale CH, Quintiliani R, et al. Absorption of ciprofloxacin administered through a nagogastric or a nasoduodenal tube in volunteers and patients receiving enteral nutrition. Diagn Microbiol Infect Dis 1990; 13:99–102.
212. Healy DP, Brodbeck M. Clendening C. Ciprofloxacin absorption impaired by enteral feedings given orally and via G-tube in patients. 34th Interscience Conference on Antimicrobial Agents and Chemotherapy. (A35) Orlando, FL, October 4–7, 1994.
213. Wijnands WJA, Vree TB, VanHerwaarden CL. The influence of quinolone derivatives on theophylline clearance. Br J Clin Pharmacol 1986; 22:677–683.
214. Mahr G, Sorgel F, Granneman GR, et al. Effects of temafloxacin and ciprofloxacin on the pharmacokinetics of caffeine. Clin Pharmacokinet 1992; 22(suppl 1):90–97.

215. Tsuji A, Sato H, Okezaki E, et al. Effect of the anti-inflammatory agent fenbufen on the quinolone-induced inhibition of g-aminobutyric acid receptor binding to rat brain membranes in-vitro. Biochem Pharmacol 1988; 37:4408–4411.

216. Fan-Havard P, Sanchorawala V, Oh J, et al. Concurrent use of foscarnet and ciprofloxacin may increase the propensity for seizures. Ann Pharmacother 1994; 28:869–872.

217. Semel JD, Allen N. Seizures in patients simultaneously receiving theophylline and imipenem or ciprofloxacin or metronidazole. South Med J 1991; 84:465–468.

218. Semel JD, Allen N. Combination effects of ciprofloxacin, clindamycin, and metronidazole intravenousy in volunteers. South Med J 1989; 84:465–468.

219. Zaske DE, Aminoglycosides. In: Evans WE, Schentag JJ, Jusko WJ, eds. Applied Pharmacokinetics: Principles of Therapeutic Drug Monitoring. 3rd ed. Vancouver, WA; Applied Therapeutics, 1992: 14.1–14.47.

220. Rotschafer JC, Zabinski RA, Walker KJ. Pharmacodynamic factors of antibiotic efficacy. Pharmacotherapy 1992; 12(6 Pt 2):64S–70S.

221. Duzgunes N, Perumal VK, Kesavalu, L, et al. Enhanced effect of liposome-encapsulated amikacin on *Mycobacterium aviium–M. intracellulare* complex infection in beige mice. Antimicrob Agents Chemother 1988; 32:1404–1411.

222. Gangadharam PRJ, Ashtekar DA, Ghori N, et al. Chemotherapeutic potential of free and liposome-encapsulated streptomycin against experimental *Mycobacterium avium* complex infections in beige mice. J Antimicrob Chemother 1991; 28:425–435.

223. Duzgunes N, Ashtekar DA, Flasher DL, et al. Treatment of *Mycobacterium avium–intracellulare* complex infection in beige mice with free and liposome-encapsulated streptomycin: role of kiposome type and duration of treatment. J Infect Dis 1991; 164:143–151.

224. Klemens SP, Cyamon MH, Swenson CE, Ginsberg RS. Liposome-encapsulated-gentamicin therapy of *Mycobacterium avium* complex infection in beige mice. Antimicrob Agents Chemother 1990; 34:967–970.

225. Nightingale SD, Saletan SL, Swenson CE, et al. Liposome-encapsulated gentamicin treatment of *Mycobacterium avium–intracellulare* complex bacteremia in AIDS patients. Antimicrob Agents Chemother 1993; 37:1869–1872.

226. Product Profile, Aminosidine. Farmitalia Carlo erba, 1979.

227. Kanyok TP, Reddy MV, Jagannath C, et al. In vivo activity of paromomycin against sensitive and multidrug-resistant *M. tuberculosis* and *Mycobacterium avium* complex. Antimicrob Agents Chemother 1994; 38(2):170–173.

228. Kanyok TP, Reddy MV, Jagannath C, et al. Activity of aminossidine (pharomomycin) for *Mycobacterium tuberculosis* and *Mycobacterium avium.* J Antimicrob Chemother 1994; 33:323–327.

229. Piersimoni C. Bornigia S, De Sio G, Scalise G. Bacteristatic and bactericidal activities of paromomycin against *Mycobacterium avium* complex isolates. 1994; 34:421–424.

9

Advances in the Treatment and Prophylaxis of *Mycobacterium avium* Complex in Individuals Infected with Human Immunodeficiency Virus

JOYCE A. KORVICK*

National Institute of Allergy
 and Infectious Disease
The National Institutes of Health,
Bethesda, Maryland

CONSTANCE A. BENSON

Rush Medical College/Rush-Presbyterian –
 St. Luke's Medical Center
Chicago, Illinois

I. Introduction

As disseminated *Mycobacterium avium*–complex disease (DMAC) was recognized with increasing frequency in patients with acquired immunodeficiency syndrome (AIDS), clinicians were faced with inadequate treatment options consisting of poorly tolerated and often ineffective multiple-drug regimens. Prior therapeutic efforts centered on pulmonary *Mycobacterium avium*–complex (MAC) infections in the patients without AIDS (Chapter 3). The Statement on Nontuberculous Mycobacteria of the American Thoracic Society recommended a standard three- or four-drug regimen for the initial treatment of pulmonary MAC to include isoniazid, rifampin, and ethambutol, with streptomycin to be added for 3–6 months for patients with extensive

---

*The comments contained herein are those of the author and do not reflect current policy of the National Institutes of Health or the Food and Drug Administration.

disease (1). In keeping with this recommendation, clinicians in the late 1980s treated patients with AIDS and DMAC with four- or five-drug regimens which included rifampin or rifabutin (ansamycin), ethambutol, clofazimine, ciprofloxacin, and amikacin. Continued work over the past 5 years has resulted in a number of advances in our ability to treat this opportunistic infection. The following chapter focuses on developments in treatment and prophylaxis of DMAC in individuals infected with the human immunodeficiency virus (HIV) (for further discussion of therapies for pulmonary MAC refer to Chapter 3).

II. Clinical Treatment Trials

A. Early Treatment Efforts

During the first decade of AIDS epidemic, cases of MAC bacteremia were noted with increasing frequency among patients with advanced HIV disease; whether DMAC was a preterminal event or treatable disease was highly debated (2,3). One of the earliest reported series described 29 cases of DMAC treated with two or more antimycobacterial drugs for a mean of 6 weeks (4). Most patients received rifabutin, clofazimine, and ethionamide or ethambutol. The microbiological and clinical results were disheartening: no clinical improvement or microbiological cure. Although MAC colony counts in the blood decreased in three patients, each patient with a premortem diagnosis of DMAC who underwent autopsy, whether treated or not, had DMAC present at postmortem examination. Masur et al. reported a series of 13 HIV-infected patients treated with rifabutin and clofazimine coupled with 1 or 2 additional agents, including amikacin, ciprofloxacin, cycloserine, or ethambutol (5). Only 6 of the 13 patients ultimately demonstrated two or more consecutive negative blood cultures; 2 of the 6 patients later relapsed with persistently positive cultures. In addition, only 1 of the 6 patients who became culture negative had clinical improvement in symptoms.

Despite these early failures, several investigators reported encouraging results (6–8). In one study, 7 of 10 patients were treated with isoniazid, 300 mg; ethambutol, 15 mg/kg; rifabutin, 150 mg; and clofazimine, 100 mg per day. In this same study, three patients refused treatment and were observed (6). Bacteremic clearing was observed in six of the seven treated patients. Cultures remained negative in one patient for 17 months and for 3–6 months preceding death in all other patients. Fever, night sweats, and weight loss resolved in patients who cleared the bacteremia. Bach et al. reported a series of four cases treated with three or four drug combinations of isoniazid, ethambutol, rifabutin, clofazimine, or ciprofloxacin (7). Each patient experienced symptomatic improvement, which lead the investigators to advocate treatment of DMAC in patients with AIDS. The first published prospective, nonrandomized study included 25 patients treated with a regimen of rifabutin (300–600 mg/day), clofazimine, isoniazid, and ethambutol (8). Twenty-two of these patients achieved ≥4 weeks of consecutive negative blood cultures, which remained negative in 16 patients for periods up to 72 weeks. Eighteen of these cases had complete resolution of symptoms. Doses of rifabutin used were higher in this study than those reported by Masur et al. (5). Ethambutol was also used more consistently in this study than in that reported by Masur (one patient only).

B. Activity of Single Agents

As clinical investigators converged around the question of whether and how to treat DMAC in patients with AIDS, several approaches were being initiated in clinical trials. These included (1) small pilot studies to evaluate the microbiological activity of single agents; (2) combination studies to evaluate agents shown to have preclinical efficacy in combination; and (3) strategies to deliver induction therapy with a maximum number of agents compared with using the minimal number of agents necessary to reduce symptoms and bacteremia. In vitro and in vivo (beige mouse or other animal models) studies suggested likely candidates for the treatment of DMAC based on the demonstrated activity of the agents in these settings (Chapter 5 and 6). Few combinations were shown to be consistently synergistic.

The need to demonstrate the contribution of single agents to the overall activity of multidrug regimens prompted short-duration pilot studies of the microbiological activity of single drugs (Table 1). Kemper et al. randomized patients with AIDS and DMAC to receive either clofazimine (200 mg/day), ethambutol (15 mg/kg/day), or rifampin (600 mg/day) alone for 4 weeks (9). Ethambutol produced the greatest quantitative reduction in colony counts of mycobacteria in blood (colony-forming units [CFU] per milliliter) followed by clofazimine and rifampin; the latter actually produced an increase of 0.2 $\log_{10}$ CFU/ml. The subsequent combination of ethambutol with rifampin or clofazimine did not appear to reduce MAC colony counts more than ethambutol alone.

Rifabutin, which appeared to be more active in vitro against *Mycobacterium avium* than rifampin (Chapter 5), was utilized by Sullam et al. in an active control trial design of combinations of clofazimine, 100 mg/day, and ethambutol, 15 mg/kg/day with or without rifabutin, 600 mg/day, in order to

Table 1   Clinical Studies of Single and Combination Antimycobacterial Agents

Ref.	Agent and dose	N	Change in $\log_{10}$ CFU/ml at week 4	% culture negative by week 12	% reduction in symptoms by week 12
14	Azithromycin, 500 mg/day	21	−1.2	28	−
15	Azithromycin				
	600 mg/day	65	−2.00	56	−
	1200 mg/day		−0.60	42	−
12	Clarithromycin	154			
	500 mg bid	(33)[a]	−1.5	41	60
	1000 mg bid	(31)[a]	−2.8	53	69
	2000 mg bid	(25)[a]	−2.7	41	75
9	Clofazimine, 200 mg/day	15	−0.2	−	−
	Ethambutol, 15 mg/kg/day	15	−0.6	−	−
	Rifampin, 600 mg/day	18	+0.2	−	−
17	Liposomal-gentamicin (variable 1.7–5.1 mg/kg/day)	21	−0.98[a]	−	−
16	Sparfloxacin				
	200 mg/day	10	*(4/10) −0.53		
	300 mg/day	12	†(3/12) −0.96		
	Sparfloxacin + ethambutol	22	‡(18/22) −0.95		
18	Ciprofloxacin, 750 mg bid† Ethambutol, 15 mg/kg/day† Rifampin, 600 mg/day† Amikacin, 7.5 mg/kg/day†	15	−1.5	18	60–70
19	Ciprofloxacin, 750 mg bid† Ethambutol, 15 mg/kg/day† Rifampin, 600 mg/day† Clofazimine, 100 mg/day†	31	−1.4	42	65–67
20	Rifampin, 600 mg/day† Ethambutol, 25 mg/kg/day† Ciprofloxacin, 750 mg bid† *or*	12	−0.2	−	−
	Placebo	12	+0.7	−	−

[a]Available cultures.
*Only 4 of 10 had a decline.
†Only 3 of 12 had a decline.
‡Only 18 of 22 had a decline.

determine the contribution of rifabutin to the regimen (10). Of the 11 patients randomized to the rifabutin-containing arm of the trial, 7 had either clearing of their bacteremia or $\geq 2 \log_{10}$ decrease in CFU/per milliliter of mycobacteria in blood compared with none of the 13 randomized to no rifabutin. This was a small study and conclusions could not be made regarding clinical benefit. Additional studies of the contribution of rifabutin to MAC treatment regimens are necessary to further elucidate the role of this drug.

Recognition of the in vitro antimycobacterial activity and enhanced intracellular penetration of the macrolide, clarithromycin, and the azalide, azithromycin, prompted further studies of the activity of these drugs as single agents in the treatment of DMAC. In a study by Dautzenberg et al., the microbiological activity of clarithromycin was determined by randomizing HIV-infected patients to 6 weeks of clarithromycin, 1000 mg bid, followed by placebo plus rifampin, isoniazid, ethambutol, and clofazimine for an additional 6 weeks or placebo alone for 6 weeks followed by clarithromycin plus the four other drugs (11). Of the eight patients initially randomized to clarithromycin alone, all had decreases in CFU per milliliter of mycobacteria in the blood by the end of 6 weeks; six of the patients had negative blood cultures. The five evaluable patients initially randomized to receive placebo had progressive increases in CFU per milliliter; when three patients were switched to clarithromycin plus the other four drugs, their quantitative colony counts decreased.

The activity of clarithromycin was further documented by two large-dose comparison studies (12,13). Chaisson et al. randomized 154 patients to one of three clarithromycin doses: 500 mg bid; 1000 mg bid; and 2000 mg bid (12). Overall, clarithromycin resulted in a decrease in mean CFU/per milliliter from 1.5 to 2.7 $\log_{10}$, depending on the dose. The most rapid clearing of the mycobacteremia occurred in patients randomized to 2000 mg bid (median of 54, 43, and 29 days, respectively, for 500, 1000, or 2000 mg bid). The 2000-mg bid dose was poorly tolerated owing mostly to gastrointestinal toxicity. Although the 1000-mg bid dose cleared the blood more rapidly than the 500-mg bid dose, the proportion of patients with negative cultures after 4 weeks of treatment was similar. During the first 12 weeks of double-blind treatment there was a survival advantage for those randomized to the 500-mg bid dose (3/53 [6%] vs 13/51 [25%] deaths, respectively, for the 500-mg bid and 1000-mg bid doses). This difference was statistically significant. Although there were minor differences among treatment groups, there were none of sufficient magnitude to explain the dose-related difference in acute survival. The second dose comparison study randomized 299 patients to either 500 mg bid or 1000 mg bid of clarithromycin (13). A bacteriological response, defined as a negative blood culture or a decline in colony counts by 1 $\log_{10}$ CFU/ml at the end of week 4, was reported for 72 and 82% of patients given the 500-mg bid or 1000-mg bid dose, respectively. A clinical response accompanied a bacteriological response in 75 and 82% of these cases, respectively. Based in part on these studies, the Food and Drug Administration (FDA) Advisory Committee recommended accelerated approval of clarithromycin, 500 mg bid, for the treatment of DMAC in HIV-infected patients in combination with at least one other agent having antimycobacterial activity (May 10, 1993, FDA, Antiviral Advisory Committee).

Despite the significant activity of clarithromycin in these studies, resistance to clarithromycin was demonstrated. Chaisson et al. reported 99% of the initial MAC isolates were susceptible to clarithromycin, with a minimum inhibitory concentration (MIC) of ≤ 4 μg/ml (12). Bacteriological relapses occurred during single-drug therapy in 21% of patients by week 12 and in another 26% thereafter. These were usually associated with recrudescence of symptoms and isolation of MAC with a clarithromycin MICs of >32 μg/ml. Although clarithromycin appeared very active in these studies, single-agent therapy is not recommended for the treatment of disseminated MAC because of the potential for the development of resistance.

Azithromycin in doses of 500, 600, and 1200 mg has also been shown to decrease the quantity of CFU/per milliliter of blood from 1.5 to 2.0 $\log_{10}$ compared with baseline after 30 days to 6 weeks of treatment (14,15). Among patients treated for either 20 or 30 days, fever and night sweats were alleviated (14). The most common adverse reaction was diarrhea.

Sparfloxacin has been evaluated in a pilot study in which doses of either 200 or 300 mg were administered for 4 weeks (16). Four of 10 patients and 3 of 12 patients assigned to 200 or 300 mg/day, respectively, had reductions in CFU/per milliliter of mycobacteremia at 4 weeks. The addition of ethambutol to either dose contributed to a further decline in CFU/per milliliter in 18 of 22 patients. The response of symptoms was difficult to assess. Although used in many multidrug regimens, single-agent studies of ciprofloxacin have not been performed; therefore, its singular antimycobacterial activity and its contribution to these regimens is unknown.

Liposome-encapsulated gentamicin has been evaluated as a single agent in a dose-escalating pilot study in patients with AIDS with MAC bacteremia in which the drug was administered for 4 weeks at doses ranging from 1.7 to 5.1 mg/kg/day (17). The median reduction in CFU was 0.98 $\log_{10}$. Symptoms were alleviated at the highest dose, but one of the patients given this dose developed nonoliguric renal failure.

C. Combination Therapy

Early studies of combinations of drugs included many of the conventional antimycobacterial agents (see Table 1). In a prospective study of a four-drug regimen, consisting of ciprofloxacin, ethambutol, rifampin, and amikacin, a 1.5 $\log_{10}$ decrease in blood MAC colony counts was demonstrated with a corresponding reduction in symptoms (18). However, the medical and logistical complications encountered during chronic intravenous therapy with amikacin made this a less attractive approach. In a prospective, nonrandomized trial, the California Collaborative Treatment Group evaluated the completely oral combination of ciprofloxacin, ethambutol, rifampin, and clofazimine (19). Similar reductions in MAC colony counts of 1.4 $\log_{10}$ were documented; however, 42% of the patients were culture negative by week 12 compared with 18% in the previous study. Improvement in associated symptoms was also observed. In a third study, Jacobson et al. randomized patients to receive either rifampin, 600 mg/day; clofazimine, 100 mg/day; and ethambutol, 15 mg/kg/day or placebo for 8 weeks (20). Patients randomized to the active treatment arm had a mean $\log_{10}$ decrease in CFU per milliliter of 0.2 versus an increase of 0.7 in the placebo group. The investigators concluded that this regimen had significant microbiological activity in the treatment of DMAC with some evidence of clinical activity; however, it was associated with a substantial rate of drug intolerance.

Few small studies have been reported with combinations of clarithromycin and other antimicrobial agents. One small combination study added ciprofloxacin and amikacin to clarithromycin (21). Mycobacteremia was cleared in all 12 patients after 2–8 weeks and symptoms resolved, although some patients had received treatment with other antimycobacterial drugs for up to 11 weeks prior to beginning clarithromycin therapy. In another small case series of 11 patients treated with clarithromycin plus clofazamine, all showed clinical improvement and cleared blood cultures by 12 weeks. Median survival from time of diagnosis of DMAC was estimated at 11.4 months (22).

AIDS Clinical Trials Group Protocol 135—a randomized, prospective, trial of ciprofloxacin, ethambutol, rifampin, and clofazimine with or without amikacin—enrolled 79 patients with AIDS and MAC bacteremia (23). Preliminary analyses showed that these combinations reduced geometrical mean quantitative MAC colony counts in the blood from 128 CFU/ml before treatment to 13 CFU/ml at the end of week 12; 49% of patients had negative cultures at week 4 (23,24). However, no significant differences in microbiological or clinical response were noted, suggesting no additional benefit to amikacin compared to 4-drug oral regimen for treatment of MAC bacteremia

(24). Patients subsequently received maintenance therapy with oral drug regimens containing azithromycin; follow-up studies are planned. Finally, in a retrospective review of 31 patients receiving ethambutol, 15 mg/kg; rifabutin, 6 mg/kg; and amikacin, 15 mg/kg (iv for 2–3 weeks), 22 of 31 patients showed a "response" after 14 days (25). Five patients relapsed but responded to additional treatment with amikacin.

Agents other than antibiotics may become part of the therapeutic approach to treatment of disseminated MAC in HIV-infected individuals. One recent report described seven HIV-seronegative patients with nontuberculous mycobacterial infections who were treated with interferon-γ as an adjunct to antimycobacterial therapy (26). Four of the patients had idiopathic CD4$^+$ T lymphocytopenia, and the other three patients were members of the same family with a common immune deficiency resulting in susceptibility to MAC infections. Six of the seven patients were infected with MAC and one patient was infected with *M. kansasii*. Subcutaneous interferon-γ, 25–50 g/M^2, was administered two or three times weekly. Marked clinical improvement was observed in all patients within 8 weeks of starting therapy. The use of interferon-γ is now being evaluated in preclinical studies as an adjunct for treatment of DMAC in HIV-infected individuals (Chapter 7). Recombinant granulocyte-macrophage colony-stimulating factor (Gm-CSF) has been shown to stimulate murine and human macrophages to inhibit growth and enhance intracellular killing of MAC. Bermudez et al. subsequently demonstrated significant reduction in the number of viable MAC in the liver, blood, and spleen of beige mice treated with combinations of either Gm-CSF and amikacin or azithromycin compared with control mice and those treated with Gm-CSF or antibiotics alone (27). A pilot study evaluating treatment of DMAC with the combination of azithromycin and Gm-CSF is in progress. Finally, low-dose dexamethasone (2 mg/day) was given to five patients who had DMAC and progressive weight loss and persistent fever despite multidrug antimycobacterial therapy (28): All patients had substantial weight gain, reduction of fever, and an improved sense of well-being. In addition, increases in serum albumin and decreases in alkaline phosphatase were documented. Future studies will determine what role these types of agents may have in the treatment of DMAC in HIV-infected individuals.

Many of the studies evaluating multidrug therapy for DMAC described above have been largely small nonrandomized, uncontrolled trials of short duration. Microbiological activity, measured by quantitative change in MAC CFU in the blood, were the primary endpoints of most studies. As a result of the aforementioned studies, our understanding of the potential activity of antimycobacterial drugs alone or in combination for treatment of MAC in

HIV-infected individuals has improved; however, larger, prospective, randomized controlled studies are needed to discern the overall clinical benefit of these regimens. Table 2 summarizes several currently ongoing prospective randomized treatment studies.

III. Prophylaxis of Disseminated MAC Infection

Because of the difficulty in treating MAC after tissue infection is established, prevention of disseminated infection has become a management goal. Presumably, there is a lower burden of organisms early in infection and the use of single-drug prophylaxis, modeled after the single-drug prophylaxis of tuberculosis with isoniazid, has been the most frequent approach. To date, three

Table 2 MAC Treatment Trials in Progress for Adult Patients with AIDS

Leading or sponsoring organization	Targeted enrollment	Treatment regimens
Abbott Laboratories (M93-069)	100	Clarithromycin + ethambutol
		Clarithromycin + ethambutol + clofazimine
California Collaborative Treatment Group (549)	200	Clarithromycin + ethambutol + clofazimine
		Clarithromycin + clofazimine
Pharmacia (087250)	312	Clarithromycin + ethambutol
		Clarithromycin + ethambutol + rifabutin (300 mg/day)
AIDS Community Research Consortium	40	Azithromycin
		Azithromycin + GM-CSF
Canadian HIV Trials Network	200	Clarithromycin + ethambutol + rifabutin (300 mg/day)
		Ciprofloxacin + ethambutol + clofazamine + rifampin
DATRI 001 (NIH)*	68	Clarithromycin + rifabutin
		Azithromycin + rifabutin
DATRI 007 (NIH)	24	Clarithromycin + ethambutol
US Veterans Administration Cooperative Group	100	Clarithromycin + ethambutol
		Azithromycin + ethambutol
Pfizer	108	Clarithromycin + ethambutol
		Azithromycin + ethambutol
AIDS Clinical Trials Group 223	246	Clarithromycin + ethambutol
		Clarithromycin + rifabutin
		Clarithromycin + ethambutol + rifabutin (450 mg/day)

*Pharmacokinetic interaction study.
(Adapted from AmFAR AIDS/HIV Treatment Directory)
Source: Ref. 50.

studies of single-agent prophylactic therapy, utilizing clofazimine, rifabutin, or clarithromycin have been completed; two of these studies are published (29,30).

The first controlled trial conducted for the prophylaxis of *Mycobacterium avium* complex in HIV-infected individuals utilized clofazimine, 50 mg/ day, versus no treatment (29). This open, randomized study was initiated in 1988 and enrolled 110 patients, of which 99 patients were evaluable. Patients were eligible if they had a prior episode of *Pneumocystis carinii* pneumonia, a CD4 cell count ≤ 100 cells/mm^3, and negative blood cultures for MAC prior to entry into the study. Patients were seen monthly, and a MAC blood culture was drawn only if symptoms of the clinical illness suggestive of MAC were reported. At the time of the first interim analysis, mean length of time on study was 299 days (median 283 days). MAC bacteremia was documented in 13 of 99 patients; 7 of 53 (13.2%) in the clofazimine treatment arm versus 6 of 46 patients receiving no prophylaxis (13.0%) (log rank test, $p = 0.76$). Kaplan-Meier estimates for probability of remaining free of MAC disease demonstrated no differences between the two groups (log rank test, $p = 0.6$). The evaluation of survival did not reveal any difference between the two treatment groups. Clofazimine was well tolerated during the study, with only three patients reporting gastrointestinal side effects, including nausea and diarrhea. Overall, the study was inconclusive regarding the utility of clofazimine for prophylaxis of *Mycobacterium avium*–complex bacteremia.

Rifabutin (Mycobutin*) was the first antibiotic approved as a single agent for prophylaxis of MAC disease in HIV-infected individuals. Two randomized, double-blind, multicenter clinical trials demonstrated the microbiological activity of rifabutin in this study population (30). Patients who were HIV seropositive with a prior AIDS-defining condition, had CD4 cell counts ≤ 200 cells/mm^3, and had two preentry cultures of both stool and blood negative for MAC were eligible. Both trials were initiated in 1990 and had identical study designs (study 023 and study 027). Blood cultures for MAC were obtained every month during the study. Study 023 enrolled 590 patients: 298 patients randomized to placebo and 292 patients to rifabutin. *Mycobacterium avium* bacteremia developed in 51 (17%) and 24 (8%) participants randomized to placebo or rifabutin, respectively. Study 027 enrolled 556 patients: 282 patients randomized to placebo and 274 patients to rifabutin. *Mycobacterium avium* bacteremia developed in 51 (18%) and 24 (9%) participants randomized to placebo or rifabutin, respectively. The relative risk of

---

*Mycobutin is a registered trademark.

M. avium–complex bacteremia in patients who received rifabutin as compared with placebo was 0.43 (95% confidence interval, 0.26 to 0.70; $p = 0.001$) for study 023, and 0.47 (95% confidence interval, 0.29 to 0.77; $p = 0.002$) for study 027. The time to development of MAC bacteremia while on study was significantly longer for patients receiving rifabutin ($p < 0.001$).

Although no statistically significant survival advantage was demonstrated between the two treatment groups, there were fewer deaths in the rifabutin group ($N = 33$) than the placebo group ($N = 47$) overall ($p = 0.086$). These studies were underpowered to detect a survival difference. Clinical benefit of rifabutin was detected in the analysis of signs, symptoms, and laboratory abnormalities associated with *Mycobacterium avium*–complex bacteremia. A significant reduction in the rifabutin treatment arm compared with the placebo was seen for the following: moderate, severe, or very severe fever and fatigue; a decrease of 20 or more points from baseline in the Karnofsky performance score; anemia, defined as a 10% decrease in the hemoglobin level from baseline; elevation of the alkaline phosphatase level, defined as a 50% increase from baseline, and hospitalization for any cause within 30 days of the last dose of study drug. Rifabutin was well tolerated during the study. Patients discontinued therapy for the following adverse events: rash (4%), gastrointestinal intolerance of the drug (3%), and neutropenia (2%). Myalgias, eructation, and dysgeusia ($\leq 3\%$) were more frequently reported in the rifabutin group. Uveitis was not reported in either study.

Since rifabutin has microbiological activity against *Mycobacterium tuberculosis*, concern regarding the potential development of drug-resistant pulmonary tuberculosis during prophylaxis was considered. In the two phase III trials for prophylaxis, tuberculosis was presumptively diagnosed in 7 of the 1146 patients enrolled. Three patients in the placebo arms of the trial subsequently had culture proven tuberculosis; susceptibility data were not available. *Mycobacterium tuberculosis* was never isolated from the four patients who were presumptively diagnosed in the rifabutin arm of the trial and little evidence was available to confirm the diagnosis.

The development of rifabutin-resistant *M. avium* complex was not detected among isolates studied. Studies of the MIC of rifabutin were performed for the first 59 of the 102 *M. avium*–complex isolates recovered from patients assigned to placebo and for the first 29 of the 48 isolates from patients receiving rifabutin. No differences were seen in the distribution of the MICs among the organisms tested.

Although clofazimine and rifabutin were the first agents studied for MAC prophylaxis, clarithromycin and azithromycin are likely to be effective given their in vitro and in vivo activity. Controlled clinical trials of these as single agents or in combination with rifabutin for prophylaxis are ongoing. Preliminary results of several studies have been reported (31–35). The largest and only prospective, randomized study, which was reported by Pierce et al., compared clarithromycin, 500 mg, bid twice daily (N = 343) to placebo (N = 341) in patients in AIDS with $CD4^+$ cell counts ≤100. Median time followed on study was 8.7 months (35). MAC bacteremia developed in 12.6% of placebo recipients compared with 4.5% of those receiving clarithromycin ($p < 0.001$). Seventy-four deaths occurred on the clarithromycin arm compared with 97 deaths in the placebo group ($p = 0.019$). Discontinuation of study drug due to adverse experiences occurred in 6% of the patients receiving clarithromycin and 4% on placebo. Resistance to clarithromycin was documented in 6 of 15 MAC isolates recovered from patients in the clarithromycin group and none of the 41 isolates in the placebo group. Currently, the safety and efficacy of long-term administration of these agents is unknown. In addition, the risk of the development of resistant mycobacteria or other bacteria (such as streptococci) is also of concern but unknown.

IV. Recommendations for Prophylaxis and Treatment of Disseminated *Mycobaterium avium* Complex Disease in HIV-Infected Individuals

The US Public Health Service Task Force on Prophylaxis and Therapy for MAC met in late 1992 to discuss the recent events in MAC therapy and prophylaxis (36). Although there were many unanswered questions, a substantial body of data had accumulated pointing to the potential usefulness of the macrolides and rifabutin. At the time the Task Force recommendations were made, azithromycin and clarithromycin were available to clinicians for the treatment of infections other than MAC but were not approved for treatment of MAC (Table 3). No definitive data were available on which to base a recommendation for the use of these agents in combination with other antimycobacterial drugs. However, clarithromycin was subsequently approved by the FDA for the treatment of MAC with the indication that it be used in combination with at least one other agent active against MAC (Table 4). The Task Force considered all of these data in making recommendations which provided several guiding principals to be used in the treatment and prophylaxis of DMAC in patients with AIDS. Subsequent to this, a second Task Force was convened in September 1994 by the US Public Health Service, the Infectious Diseases Society of America and the National Institute of Allergy and Infectious Diseases for the purpose of reviewing recommen-

Table 3 Task Force Recommendations for MAC Treatment and Prophylaxis

	MAC treatment	MAC prophylaxis
Indication	Blood culture positive for MAC	HIV-seropositive <100 CD4 cells/mm^3
Duration	Life long	Life long
Evaluations prior to therapy	Chest x-ray Skin test for TB	Chest x-ray Skin test for TB 1 or more blood cultures negative for MAC
Regimen	At least two agents active against MAC: one being a macrolide Clarithromycin 500, mg bid[a]	Rifabutin 300 mg/day[a]

[a]FDA approved indication.
Source: Ref. 36.

dations and establishing guidelines for the prevention of a broad range of opportunistic infections including MAC.

A. Prophylaxis Recommendations

The Task Force recommended that prophylaxis against MAC bacteremia should be initiated in patients with HIV infection whose CD4 cell count is fewer than 100 cells/mm^3. This recommendation was revised in 1994 stating that prophylaxis be considered when the CD4 cell count declined below 75 cells/mm^3 (36a) in those with a prior OI. Recommendations regarding other agents were deferred pending results of additional studies. The only drug currently approved for this indication is rifabutin in a dose of 300 mg/day. Because of the many unanswered questions regarding prophylaxis, as outlined above, both Task Forces suggested several considerations should be weighed prior to initiating prophylaxis with rifabutin: the potential for drug-drug interactions, the cost, and the potential to induce rifampin resistant tuberculosis in high risk groups.

Most patients eligible for prophylaxis are likely to be taking a number of concomitant medications. It is important to recognize that rifabutin can selectively induce enzymes of the cytochrome P-450 system and may decrease drug levels of agents metabolized through this pathway. Rifabutin has been shown to lower the area under the concentration curve (AUC) for zi-

Table 4   Antimycobacterial Agents Commonly Used in the Treatment of MAC Infections

Agent	Adult dose	Adverse effects
Amikacin	7.5–15 mg/kg qd iv[a]	Ototoxicity, nephrotoxicity
Azithromycin	500 mg/day	Nausea, diarrhea, vomiting, abdominal pain, headache, dizziness, elevations in hepatic enzymes
Ciprofloxacin	750 mg bid[b]	Anorexia, nausea, vomiting, abdominal pain, diarrhea, rash (rarely) mental status changes
Clarithromycin	500 mg bid[c]	Diarrhea, nausea, vomiting, elevations in hepatic enzymes, abdominal pain, renal insufficiency
Clofazimine	100–200 mg/day	Skin discoloration, ichthyosis, anorexia, nausea, vomiting, abdominal pain, peripheral neuropathy, (rarely) ocular changes
Ethambutol	15 mg/kg/day	Anorexia, nausea, vomiting, diarrhea, rash, elevations in hepatic enzymes, (rarely) ocular changes-retrobulbar neuritis.
Rifabutin	300 mg/day[3]	Anorexia, nausea, vomiting, diarrhea, rash, uveitis, myalgias, arthralgias, headache
Rifampin	10 mg/kg/day	Anorexia, nausea, vomiting, diarrhea, rash, elevations in hepatic enzymes

[a]OD iv; every day intravenously.
[b]BID; twice per day.
[c]FDA approved dose.
Source: Adapted from Ref. 51.

dovudine by about 30%; however, the clinical significance of this is unknown and no recommendations for the adjustment of zidovudine exist (37). Interaction studies with fluconazole and rifabutin showed that fluconazole levels were not affected by rifabutin; however, plasma levels of rifabutin were elevated by as much as 80% in some patients (38). Recently, an increased frequency of uveitis was observed in several trials of treatment or prophylaxis of MAC in which higher doses of rifabutin (450–900 mg/day) were administered alone or in combination with other agents, including clarithromycin and fluconazole. Uveitis has been reported in these settings in rates ranging from 3.5 to 45% of patients and is reversible with appropriate therapy and discontinuation of drug (39,40). The precise mechanism associated with this event is unknown, although a recent pharmacokinetic study reported a marked increase in rifabutin AUC (77% increase) when clarithromycin, 500 mg bid, and rifabutin, 300 mg daily, were coadministered (41). Finally, for those using low-dose oral contraceptive agents, breakthrough bleeding may occur due to increased metabolism of these agents induced by rifabutin.

Rifabutin does have activity against *M. tuberculosis*; however, in areas where the rate of tuberculosis is significant, there is a potential risk of treating undiagnosed tuberculosis infection with a single agent (rifabutin) when it is broadly used for MAC prophylaxis, thus inducing rifamycin-resistant tuberculosis. For this reason, all patients should be screened for the presence of active tuberculosis prior to starting rifabutin.

As additional studies of MAC prophylaxis are analyzed over the next 1–3 years, macrolide and/or combination therapies may be shown to be safe and effective for this indication. Faced with a patient today, the Task Force recommendations encompass the following courses of action (1) initiate rifabutin, 300 mg/day; and (2) no prophylaxis combined with close monitoring and expeditious initiation of therapy on diagnosis of disseminated MAC. At this time, recommendations regarding the safety and efficacy of macrolides for prophylaxis cannot be made.

B. Treatment Recommendations

The macrolide antibiotics have improved the armamentarium of agents available to treat MAC disease. Subsequent to the publication of the Task Force recommendations, clarithromycin was approved by the FDA for the treatment of MAC in combination with at least one other agent active against MAC supporting the Task Force recommendations. The approved dose of clarithromycin is 500 mg bid based on the higher mortality noted with larger doses. The Task Force clearly pointed out the danger of inducing resistance and subsequent failure of therapy as documented in the clinical trial by Chaisson et al. (12). Patients generally show a clinical response to treatment in 4–8 weeks, with cultures becoming negative by 12–16 weeks. At this point, the utility of susceptibility testing of isolates to guide the choice of initial therapy of disseminated MAC is unknown. If patients fail to respond clinically to initial treatment, or relapse with accompanying symptoms after having a negative culture or clinical response, the isolate should be tested for susceptibility to the macrolides. The Task Force suggested ethambutol as a useful second drug and listed a number of other drugs, including clofazimine, ciprofloxacin, rifampin or rifabutin, and amikacin, which might be added to a multidrug regimen. Ongoing studies of macrolides in combination with other agents should provide further information about the effect of various combinations on overall outcome.

V. Future Clinical Trials and Unanswered Questions

Clinical trials for treatment of disseminated MAC using two, three, or more agents in combination, as well as prophylaxis studies of the macrolides alone or in combination are ongoing (see Table 2). Future studies should address the following unanswered questions.

A. What is the Durability of Treatment Effect?

Longer duration of follow-up is needed to study the duration of effect. To date, studies have documented decreases in MAC CFU within 4–12 weeks of the initiation of therapy and have not focused on duration of clinical or bacteriological improvement with continuation of therapy.

B. When to Initiate MAC Prophylaxis?

Previous recommendations were to start prophylactic therapy when the $CD4^+$ T-lymphocyte count declines to below 100 cells/mm^3. However, patients who derived statistically significant benefit from rifabutin prophylaxis were those who entered the studies with fewer than 75 $CD4^+$ T lymphocytes prompting the recent changes in this recommendation. As understanding of the disease process improves, recommendations may depend on an as yet unidentified biological marker. Thus, a subset of patients may be identified who are at higher risk for MAC infection. Identifying those in need of prophylaxis will make it possible for others to avoid potential drug-drug interactions, toxicities, and costs.

C. What Is the Optimal Dose of Rifabutin for MAC Prophylaxis and/or Treatment?

The bioavailability of rifabutin is low, and attempts have been made to give patients higher doses (>300 mg/day). As a single agent rifabutin in doses of 1650–1800 mg/day has lead to cases of uveitis and an arthritis/arthralgia syndrome (42). The case has been made that patients with advanced AIDS have poor oral absorption of many drugs (43). Is the efficacy of rifabutin as a prophylactic agent at 450 or 600 mg/day better than 300 mg/day? The potential disadvantages of increasing the dosage of rifabutin include the induction of cytochrome P-450 microsomal enzymes, potential drug-drug interactions, and increased toxicities. The use of rifabutin and clarithromycin or rifabutin and fluconazole in combination may be problematic. In addition to the effect of clarithromycin on rifabutin kinetics, it has been demonstrated that rifabutin decreases the clarithromycin AUC as much as 50% when the two are coadministered (44). What effect this may have in a treatment regimen is unknown. No recommendations have been made for the dosage adjustment of clarithromycin; several experts have suggested that rifabutin should be used in a dose of 300 mg/day when combined with clarithromycin or fluconazole.

D. How Does One Evaluate the Clinical Benefit of Agents Based on Various Endpoints: Prevention of Bacteremia versus Survival?

To date, no large studies have demonstrated a survival benefit based on eradication or prevention of bacteremia. Recently, a prospectively followed cohort of 367 patients with AIDS and $CD4^+$ cell counts ≤ 50 has shown that DMAC was independently associated with an increased risk of death (45). Treatment (nonrandomized) increased duration of survival. Other reports support these findings (46).

Currently, culture techniques are used to detect and quantify MAC in the blood. Does the disappearance of MAC from the blood indicate eradication of the organism from tissues? It has been shown that patients with negative MAC cultures can have positive bone marrow or liver biopsy cultures (47–49). In prophylaxis studies, prevention of bacteremia is a useful endpoint; however, the rifabutin studies did not continue long enough to definitively show that prevention of bacteremia equated with an increase in MAC disease–free survival. Alternatively, in clinical trials evaluating various regimens for the treatment of disseminated MAC, sterilization of the blood and its relationship to prolongation of survival related to DMAC should be studied.

E. What Is the Potential for the Development of Drug Resistance During Therapy and What Impact Does Resistance Have on Outcome?

Resistance has been shown to occur with single-drug treatment of disseminated MAC. Does combination therapy prevent or reduce the development of resistant MAC isolates? Preliminary analysis of the clarithromycin prophylaxis trial has shown that this agent may induce resistant MAC isolates when used alone for prophylaxis. The relative and comparative risk of developing resistance during long-term prophylaxis remains to be determined.

F. What Are the Implications of Drug-Drug Interactions and of Polypharmacy in Patients with Advanced AIDS?

What effect does combination therapy have on the absorption of other agents, not only antimycobacterial but also antiretroviral and other opportunistic infection therapies? Few studies have been conducted to date to evaluate the drug interactions associated with many agents used in this patient population. As already mentioned, patients with advanced-stage HIV disease may have different absorption profiles than those in early stages or individuals who are not HIV infected. The number of pills and side effects of the agents used are important. As has been demonstrated in the management of tuberculosis, poor compliance leads to treatment failure. Patients with advanced AIDS are often taking numerous medications for various conditions, and the success of MAC treatment or prophylaxis may not only depend on the activity of the regimens used but also on the number of tablets and the timing of their administration. Studies of the pharmacodynamics (the clinical outcome affected by various drug doses/interactions) must be undertaken and can be nested in larger efficacy trials.

G. What Is the Optimal Treatment or Prophylaxis of Disseminated MAC?

Comparative trials with single and combination agents currently underway may further refine the dosing and efficacy and better define the population at risk for disseminated MAC.

VI. Conclusions

The single agents that have been most active in prospective clinical trials of therapy for DMAC are clarithromycin, azithromycin, and ethambutol. Rifabutin, rifampin, clofazimine, amikacin, and ciprofloxacin may contribute to the efficacy of multiple-drug regimens, but their individual contributions are unclear at this point. Trials to elucidate further the activity of various combination regimens are underway (see Table 2). In addition to these antimycobacterial drugs, the future effective treatment of DMAC may require adjunctive immune modulation, such as might be induced by the concomitant use of interferon-γ or Gm-CSF, with the latter being the first agent to be studied in an ongoing clinical trial in patients with AIDS. As data from ongoing trials become available in the next 3–4 years, treatment and prophylaxis of MAC disease will improve.

References

1. American Thoracic Society. Diagnosis and treatment of disease caused by nontuberculous mycobacteria. Am Rev Respir Dis 1990; 142:940–953.

2. Young LS. *Mycobacterium avium* complex infection. J Infect Dis 1988; 157: 863–867.

3. Horsburgh CR, Metchock B, Gordon SM, et al. Predictors of survival in patients with AIDS and disseminated *Mycobacterium avium* complex disease. J Infect Dis 1994; 170:573–577.

4. Hawkins CC, Gold JWM, Whimbey E, et al. *Mycobacterium avium* complex infections in patients with acquired immunodeficiency syndrome. Ann Intern Med 1986; 105:184–188.

5. Masur H, Tuazon C, Gill V, et al. Effect of combined clofazimine and ansamycin therapy on *Mycobacterium avium–Mycobacterium intracellulare* bacteremia in patients with AIDS. J Infect Dis 1987; 155:127–129.

6. Agins BD, Berman DS, Spicehandler D, et al. Effect of combined therapy with ansamycin, clofazimine, ethambutol and isoniazid for *Mycobacterium avium* infection in patients with AIDS. J Infect Dis 1989; 159:784–787.

7. Bach MC. Treating disseminated *Mycobacterium avium–intracellulare* infection [letter]. Ann Intern Med 1989; 110:169–170.

8. Hoy J, Mijch A, Sandland M, et al. Quadruple-drug therapy for *Mycobacterium avium–intracellulare* bacteremia in AIDS patients. J Infect Dis 1990; 161:801–805.

9. Kemper CA, Havlir D, Haghighat D, et al. The individual microbiologic effect of three antimycobacterial agents, clofazimine, ethambutol and rifampin on *Mycobacterium avium* complex bacteremia in patients with AIDS. J Infect Dis 1994; 170:157–164.

10. Sullam PM, Gordin FM, Wynne BA, Rifabutin Treatment Group. Efficacy of rifabutin in the treatment of disseminated *Mycobacterium avium* complex infection. Clin Infect Dis 1994; 19:84–86.

11. Dautzenberg B, Truffot C, Legris S, et al. Activity of clarithromycin against *Mycobacterium avium* infection in patients with acquired immune deficiency syndrome: A controlled clinical trial. Am Rev Respir Dis 1991; 144:564–569.

12. Chaisson RE, Benson CA, Dube MP, et al. Clarithromycin therapy for bacteremic *Mycobacterium avium* complex disease in patients with AIDS. Ann Intern Med 1994; 121:905–911.

13. Gupta S, Blahunka K, Dellerson M, et al. Interim results of safety and efficacy of clarithromycin in the treatment of disseminated *Mycobacterium avium* complex infection in patients with AIDS. In: Proceedings and Abstracts of the 32nd Interscience Conference on Antimicrobial Agents and Chemotherapy (abstr #892). Washington, DC: American Society for Microbiology; 1992.

14. Young LS, Wiviott L, Wu M, et al. Azithromycin for treatment of *Mycobacterium avium–intracellulare* complex infection in patients with AIDS. Lancet 1991; 388:1107–1109.

15. Berry A, Koletar S, Williams D. Azithromycin for disseminated *Mycobacterium avium–intracellulare* in AIDS patients. In: The First National Conference on Human Retroviruses and Related Infections (abstr #292). Washington DC: Centers for Disease Control and Prevention/National Institutes of Health, 1993.

16. Young LS, Wu M, Bender J for the Sparfloxacin Study Group. Pilot study of sparfloxacin for *Mycobacterium avium* complex (MAC) bacteremia complication AIDS. In: Program and Abstracts of the 32nd Interscience Conference on Antimicrobial Agents and Chemotherapy, (abstr #897). Anaheim, CA: American Society of Microbiology, 1992.

17. Nightingale SD, Saletan SL, Swenson CE, et al. Liposome-encapsulated gentamicin treatment of *Mycobacterium avium—Mycobacterium intracellulare* complex bacteremia in AIDS patients. Antimicrob Agents Chemother 2993; 37: 1869–1872.

18. Chiu J, Nussbaum J, Bozzette S, et al. Treatment of disseminated *Mycobacterium avium* complex infection in AIDS with amikacin, ehtambutol, rifampin and ciprofloxacin. Ann Intern Med 1990; 113:358–361.

19. Kemper CA, Meng RC, Nussbaum J, et al. Treatment of *Mycobacterium avium* complex bacteremia in AIDS with a four-drug oral regimen. Ann Intern Med 1992; 116:466–472.

20. Jacobson MA, Yajko D, Northfelt D, et al. Randomized, plkacebo controlled trial of rifampin, ethambutol and ciprofloxacin for AIDS patients with disseminated *Mycobacterium avium* complex infection. J Infect Dis 1993; 168:112–119.

21. deLalla F, Maserati G, Scarpellini P, et al. Clarithromycin-ciprofloxacin-amikacin for therapy of *Mycobacaterium avium—Mycobacterium intracellulare* bacteremia in patients with AIDS. Antimicrob Agents Chemother 1992; 36:1567–1569.

22. Saint-Marc T, Marneff E, Touraine JL. *Mycobacterium avium—intracellulare* infections. Treatment with clarithromycin-clofazimine. 18 observations. Press Med 1993; 22:1903–1907.

23. Jacobs MR, Morrissey AM, Bajaksouzian S. Changes in quantitative blood cultures. (colonial morphology and susceptibility of mycobacterium avium drug therapy (abst #1124). In: Program and Abstracts of the 33rd Interscience Conference on Antimicrobial Agents and Chemotherapy. Washington DC: American Society for Microbiology, 1993.

24. Parenti D, Ellner J, Hafner R, et al. A phase II/III trial of rifampin, ciprofloxacin, clofazimine, ethambutol, ± amikacin in the treatment of disseminated *Mycobacterium avium* infection in HIV-infected individuals. (August 6) Program and Abstracts of the 2nd National Conference on Human Retroviruses and related infections. Washington, DC: American Society for Microbiology, p. 56, 1995.

25. Jorup-Ronstrom C, Julander I, Petrini B. Efficacy of triple drug regimen of amikacin, ethambutol and rifabutin in AIDS patients with symptomatic *Mycobacterium avium* complex infection. J Infect 1993; 26:67–70.

26. Holland SM, Eisenstein DM, Kuhns DB, et al. Treatment of refractory disseminated nontuberculous mycobacterial infection with interferon gamma. A preliminary report. N Engl J Med 1994; 330:1348–1355.

27. Bermudez LE, Martinelli J, Petrofsky M, et al. Recombinant granulocyte-macrophage colony-stimulating factor enhances the effects of antibiotics against *My-*

cobacterium avium complex infection in the beige mouse model. J Infect Dis 1994; 169:175–180.

28. Wormser GP, Horowitz H, Dworkin B. Low-dose dexamethasone as adjuvant therapy for disseminated *Mycobacterium avium* complex infections in AIDS patients. Antimicrob Agents Chemother 1994; 38:2215–2217.

29. Abrams DI, Mitchell TG, Child CC, et al. Clofazimine as prophylaxis for disseminated *Mycobacterium avium* complex infection in AIDS. J Infect Dis 1993; 167:1459–1463.

30. Nightingale SD, Cameron DW, Gordin FM, et al. Two controlled trials of rifabutin prophylaxis against *Mycobacterium avium* complex infection in AIDS. N Engl J Med 1993; 329:828–833.

31. Sonnabend JA, Coulston DR, Payne DL. Clarithromycin for *Mycobacterium avium* complex prophylaxis in patients with AIDS (abst #I189). In: Proceedings and Abstracts of the 34th Interscience Conference on Antimicrobial Agents and Chemotherapy. Washington, DC: American Society for Microbiology, 1994.

32. Grossman HA, Greiger-Zanlungo P, Sonnabend J, Senior S. Clarithromycin 500 mg bid as primary prophylaxis for DMAC disease (Abst #I191). In: Proceedings and Abstracts of the 34th Interscience Conference on Antimicrobial Agents and Chemotherapy. Washington, DC: American Society for Microbiology, 1994.

33. Baker RL, Norris SA. Clarithromycin prophylaxis against MAC in AIDS. In: Proceedings and Abstracts of the 34th Interscience Conference on Antimicrobial Agents and Chemotherapy (abst #I193). Washington, DC: American Society for Microbiology, 1994.

34. Keith PE, Schiller TL. Clarithromycin as primary prophylaxis in patients with AIDS. In: Proceedings and Abstracts of the 34th Interscience Conference on Antimicrobial Agents and Chemotherapy (abstr #I193). Washington, DC: American Society for Microbiology, 1994.

35. Pierce M, Lamarca A, Jablonowski H, et al. A placebo controlled trial of clarithromycin prophylaxis against mycobacterium avium complex infection in AIDS patients. In: Proceedings and Abstracts of the 34 Interscience Conference on Antimicrobial Agents and Chemotherapy (abstr #A2). Washington, DC: American Society for Microbiology, 1994.

36. Masur H, Public Health Service Task Force on Prophylaxis and Therapy for Mycobacterium Complex. Recommendations on prophylaxis and therapy for disseminated mycobacterium avium complex disease in patients infected with the human immunodeficiency virus. N Engl J Med. 1993; 329:898–904.

36a. Centers for Disease Control and Prevention, National Institutes of Health, Infectious Disease Society of America. Recommendations for prevention of Opportunistic infections in HIV-infected persons. Clin Inf Dis 1995 (in press).

37. Nordic Medical Research Councils' HIV Therapy Group. Double blind dose-response study of zidovudine in AIDS and advanced HIV infection. Br Med J 1992; 304:13–17.

38. Trapnell CB, Narang PK, Li R, et al. Fluconazole increases rifabutin absorption in HIV positive patients on stable zidovudine therapy (abstr #PO B31-2212). In: IX Intl Conference on AIDS/HIV and the STD World Congress. Berlin, 1993.

39. Shafran S, Deschenes J, Miller M, et al. Uveitis and pseudojaundice during a regimen of clarithromycin, rifabutin and ethambutol. N Engl J Med 1994; 330: 438–439.

40. Uveitis associated with rifabutin therapy. Morb Mortal Week Rep 1994; 43:658.

41. DATRI 001 Study Group. Coadministration of clarithromycin alters the concentration-time profile of rifabutin. In: Proceedings and Abstracts of the 34th Interscience Conference on Antimicrobial Agents and Chemotherapy (abst #A2). Washington, DC: American Society for Microbiology, 1994.

42. Siegal F, Eilbott D, Burger H, et al. Dose-limiting toxicity of rifabutin in AIDS-related complex: Syndrome of arthralgia/arthritis AIDS 1990; 4:433–441.

43. Gordin SM, Horsburgh CR, Peloquin CA, et al. Low serum levels of oral antimycobacterial agents in patients with disseminated *Mycobacterium avium* complex disease. J Infect Dis 1993; 168:1559–1562.

44. The DATRi 001 Study Group. Clarithromycin plus rifabutin for MAC prophylaxis; evidence for a drug interaction. In: The First National Conference on Human Retroviruses and Related Infections (abstr #291). Washington, DC: Centers for Disease Control and Prevention/National Institutes of Health, 1993.

45. Chin DP, Reingold AL, Stone EN, et al. Impact of *Mycobacterium avium* complex bacteremia and its treatment on survival of AIDS patients; a prospective study. J Infect Dis 1994; 170:578–584.

46. Horsburgh CR, Metchock B, Gordin SM, et al. Predictors of survival in patients with AIDS and disseminated *Mycobacterium avium* complex disease. J Infect Dis 1994; 170: 573–577.

47. Wiley EL, Parry A, Nightingale SD, Lawerence J. Detection of *Mycobacterium avim* complex in bone marrow specimens of patients with acquired immunodeficiency syndrome. Am J Clin Pathol 1994; 101:446–451.

48. Lasseur C, Maugein J, Dupon M, et al. Usefulness of bone marrow aspiration culture for diagnosis of disseminated *Mycobacterium avium* complex infection (D-MAC) in patients with AIDS. In: Proceedings and Abstracts of the 34 Interscience Conference on Antimicrobial Agents and Chemotherapy (abstr #D57). Washington, DC: American Society for Microbiology, 1994.

49. Wong B, Edwards FF, Kiehn TE, et al. Continuous high-grade *Mycobacterium avium–intracellulare* bacteremia in patients with acquired immune deficiency syndrome. Am J Med 1985; 78:35–40.

50. AIDS/HIV Treatment Directory. Eds Abrams D, Cotton D, Mayer K. Compiled by the American Foundation for AIDS Research (AmFAR). June, 1994; 7:190–193.

51. Inderlied CB, Kemper CA, Bermudez LEM. The *Mycobacterium avium* complex. Clin Microbiol Rev 1993; 6:266–310.

10

Targeted Preclinical Drug Development for *Mycobacterium avium* Complex: A Biochemical Approach

MICHAEL McNEIL

Colorado State University
Fort Collins, Colorado

I. Introduction

The unique niche of mycobacteria among the prokaryotes follows directly from the well-known characteristic red acid-fast bacilli readily observed under the microscope. Although the exact mechanism of this acid fastness remains unknown (1), it undoubtedly results in some fashion from the lack of permeability of the unique cell wall of mycobacteria (1). Thus, the structure of the mycobacterial cell wall is different from classic gram-positive or gram-negative bacteria. It is this same structural difference that contributes to making treatment of mycobacterial infections generally difficult. Many drugs simply cannot make their way through the highly impermeable wall at a fast enough rate to be effective. Perhaps the most important example of this is the β-lactams. In a careful study of the permeability of these molecules and of mycobacterial β-lactamase activity, Nikaido and coworkers (2) showed that even relatively small amounts of β-lactamase activity were sufficient to render the drugs ineffective owing to the low permeability of the cell walls.

Thus, the β-lactamase activity in combination with the cell wall impermeability accounted for the observed very high minimum inhibitory concentration (MIC) values (512 to greater than 2048 μg/ml) of β-lactams, such as cefazolin, against the mycobacterial test organism, *Mycobacterium chelonae*. Without a doubt, this impermeability is the basic reason for the resistance of mycobacteria to a large number of other common chemotherapeutic agents as well.

Nevertheless, it is possible to effectively treat *M. tuberculosis, M. leprae,* and, to a lesser extent, *M. avium.* Active chemotherapeutic agents can be usefully divided into two types: compounds active against a broad range of bacteria, such as streptomycin and members of the rifamycin family; and compounds specific for mycobacteria, such as isoniazid (INH) and ethambutol. The first class of compounds clearly is able to penetrate the cell wall barrier and make it to their targets inside the cell. Thus, although the cell wall barrier is a formidable obstacle to effective chemotherapy, it can be penetrated, and some wide-spectrum antibiotics will work effectively against mycobacteria. The second class of drugs, in general, overcomes the protection of the cell wall permeability barrier by attacking the biosynthesis of the unique components of the mycobacterial cell wall itself. Not surprisingly, at least one of them, ethambutol, is strongly synergistic with the first class of drugs, particularly with rifabutin (3). The rationale is that ethambutol's action against the cell wall results in better uptake of the second antibiotic.

Testing mycobacteria with drugs that are effective against other bacteria remains a highly important *M. avium* drug development strategy. This is true even though a lack of permeability will likely result in many drug candidates being ineffective. An example of success in this area is the important new active compounds in the quinolone family that are being discovered (4–6). Interestingly, some of these drugs may work best in combination (5) with cell wall synthesis–inhibiting drugs. In addition, classic screening of natural products against whole mycobacteria remains important and viable. This is especially true since many compounds and cell supernatents have not been screened against mycobacteria because of the difficulty in using these organisms in a screen. This difficulty may now be largely overcome owing to the applications of powerful genetic techniques such as the firefly luciferase assay (7) to test for cell death.

In parallel with these methods, it is important to move toward the development of new drugs specifically targeted against the mycobacterial cell wall. Drugs of this sort, related with respect to their target to ethambutol and INH, have the potential to be effective agents alone and as agents combined with other drugs. However, the development of mycobacterial cell wall– active drugs requires a biochemical approach. The structure of the cell wall must be elucidated and the biosynthetic pathways must be determined. Then with this knowledge, enzyme assays can be devised and compounds screened. In addition, enzymes can be purified and crystallized and inhibitors then designed and synthesized.

This chapter discusses the biochemical approach to the generation of new antimycobacterials against the cell wall. The power of this basic science–oriented thrust to *M. avium* drug design has yet to be proven. As stressed above, it is seen as a complementary approach to other proven pharmaceutical development methods. It should be noted, however, that the synthesis of inhibitors based on detailed biochemical knowledge has recently yielded some spectacular innovations in antiviral drug development (8). Interestingly, this development involved carbohydrate metabolism (8).

This chapter proceeds with a discussion of the structure of the cell wall. A summary of what is known about cell wall biosynthesis will follow. The development of compounds based on this knowledge is in its infancy; nevertheless, targets will be discussed and some examples of classes of active compounds considered.

II. The Structure of the Mycobacterial Cell Wall

The basic biochemistry of the mycobacteria is a topic that received steady research attention from the 1930s through the early 1970s. These important research studies revealed the fact that the mycobacterial cell wall is composed of three covalently linked macromolecules. These components are peptidoglycan, a polysaccharide known as arabinogalactan, and the hallmark of mycobacteria, mycolic acids (9–11).

A. The Structure of Peptidoglycan

The peptidoglycan in mycobacteria is similar to that found in most eukaryotic bacteria; specifically it is very similar (1,11) to that found in the gram-negative organism *Escherichia coli* (12). Thus, mycobacterial peptidoglycan is relatively thin and highly cross-linked. Its structure is presented in Figure 1. One structural feature of mycobacterial peptidoglycan that is different from the peptidoglycan in other bacteria is the *N*-acyl substituent on the muramic acid. In the case of most bacteria, this is an acetyl group, but in mycobacteria, the acetyl group has been hydroxylated to make a glycolyl group. The effect of this change on the physiology of the mycobacteria is not known, although it is possible that the hydroxylation makes the peptidoglycan less susceptible to lysozyme. This is true because changes on the acylated amino groups have

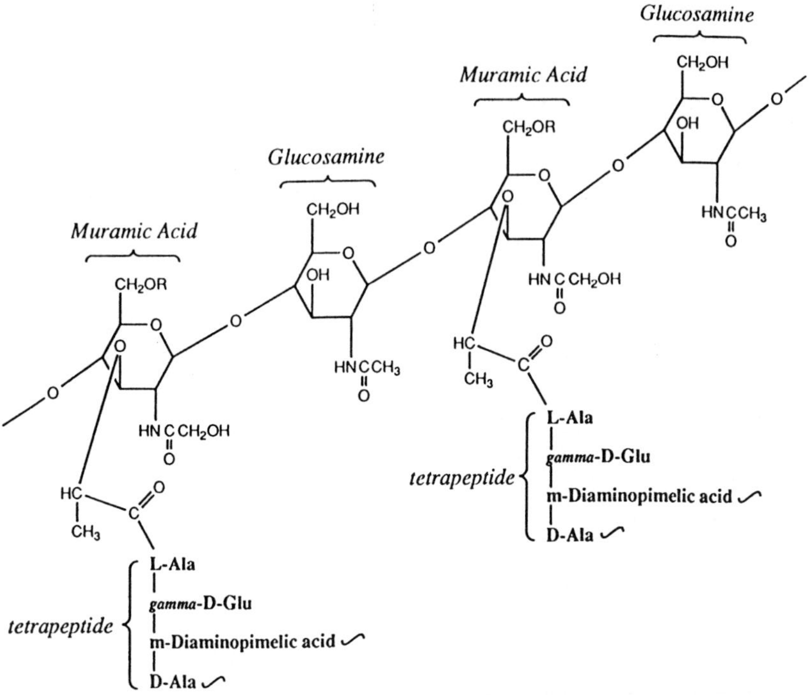

Figure 1 The structure of the peptidoglycan found in mycobacteria. The glycan and peptide regions are indicated, as are the positions of cross linking (~).

been shown in the past to inhibit lysozyme activity (13) where the *N*-acetyl group of the *N*-acetyl glucosamine was deacylated to make a free amine. Additionally, it has been found difficult to degrade mycobacterial peptidoglycan with lysozyme. A successful procedure has been to de-N-glycolylate followed by N-acetylation (14). Although the evidence is not conclusive, it appears that the N-glycolyl group on the muramic acid of mycobacterial peptidoglycan may result in protection of the organism from degradation.

B. The Linker Between Peptidoglycan and Arabinogalactan

The polymer arabinogalactan is attached to the peptidoglycan. This polymer is attached to *C*-6 of approximately every tenth muramic acid residue in the peptidoglycan by a structurally critical linker disaccharide phosphate (15). This arrangement is similar to that found in conventional gram-positive organisms for the attachment of polymers, such as teichoic acids, to the peptidoglycan (15–18). The disaccharide phosphate linker unit in the instance of mycobacteria is illustrated in Figure 2. It is composed of a L-rhamnosyl unit attached to a D-N-acetylglucosamine residue, which is in turn attached to the hydroxyl group at *C*-6 of every tenth muramic acid by a phosphodiester. The importance of this linker saccharide needs to be stressed. It could be considered somewhat analogous to a bolt holding two structural components of a steel framework together. Without the linker, the major components of the mycobacterial cell wall cannot be connected to each other.

C. Structure of the Arabinogalactan

The arabinogalactan is directly attached at its reducing galactofuranosyl end to the linker. It is a very complex polysaccharide, and only recently has its structure begun to be elucidated in detail. Early studies recognized that the arabinosyl residues were in the D absolute configuration (10). Although D-arabinose is a rather simple sugar, it is extremely rare in nature, and virtually all polysaccharides containing D-arabinosyl residues are found in mycobacteria and closely related genera. Thus, the arabinan polysaccharide is a particularly attractive drug target with regard to lack of toxicity in the human host. The early literature also suggested that the D-arabinose was in the furanose (five-membered ring) form (10,19) and recognized that at least some

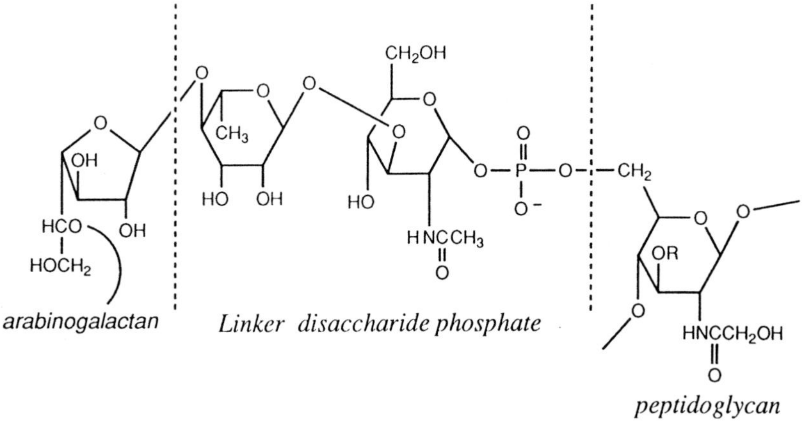

Figure 2   The structure of the linker disaccharide phosphate. The sugars of the arabinogalactan and peptidoglycan to which the linker is attached are also shown.

of the galactose was also in the furanose form (20). Later (21) it was shown that all of the D-arabinose and all of the D-galactose are in the furanose ring form. This fact has implications for drug development in that inhibitors of furanose galactose should not be toxic. This is true because galactose is always found in the pyranose or six-membered ring form in humans. Thus, the basic building blocks of mycobacterial cell wall arabinogalactan are known to be D-galactofuranose and D-arabinofuranose. The more difficult question is how are these building blocks put together to form the polymer?

Structure of the Cell Wall Galactan

Early studies (10) confirmed by recently published data (22) suggested that the arabinogalactan contained two major domains: an arabinan region and a galactan region. In a recent study (22), it was revealed that the galactan was attached directly to the linker disaccharide at its reducing end and that the galactan was essentially a linear polysaccharide (Fig. 3). This linear galactan contains about 30 galactofuranosyl residues and they are connected by alternating five and six linked residues as illustrated in Figure 3. Approximately two or three of the six-linked Gal*f* residues are branched at *C*-5. This branching point is where the arabinan is attached. Recent studies (23) have revealed that these branch points are very close to the nonreducing end of the galactan where it is attached to the linker disaccharide.

Structure of the Cell Wall Arabinan

The structure of the external regions of the arabinan, an important drug target (see below), is now precisely known. The structures of the first 24 arabinosyl residues at the nonreducing end are illustrated in Figure 4. It may be that the

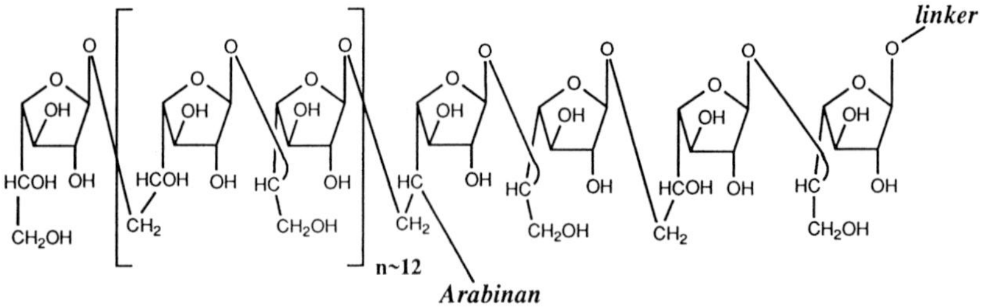

Figure 3   The structure of the cell wall galactan. The points of attachment to the linker and to arabinan are also shown.

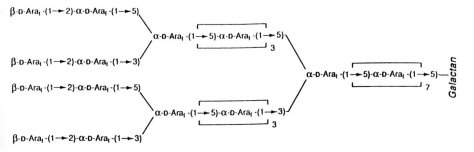

Figure 4 The structure of the cell wall arabinan. The structure of the individual D-Ara*f* units can be seen by examination of Figure 5.

reducing end of this "24'mer" is attached directly to the galactan at the five position of a six-linked D-Gal*f*, as discussed above. Contrarily, it may be that there are some additional D-Ara*f* residues between the 24'mer and the galactan. The arabinan is an incredible carbohydrate in that it is so large and yet has a precisely controlled structure.

Structure of the Mycolic Acids and Their Attachment to Arabinan

The mycolic acids are attached at the nonreducing terminal of the arabinan. Approximately two thirds of the nonreducing end pentasaccharides have four mycolic acids attached to them as illustrated in Figure 5 (24). Even though these units are at the nonreducing end of the arabinan, consideration of electron micrographs of mycobacterial cell walls (1,25) and of the complete structure of the arabinogalactan suggest that the "ester end" of the mycolic acids shown in Figure 5 is located quite close to the peptidoglycan. It is envisioned that the majority of the arabinan polysaccharide (see Figure 4) lies close to the peptidoglycan and then the mycolic acids form a dense lipophilic region extended outward in a perpendicular fashion (26,27).

The structure of the mycolic acids themselves is also illustrated in Figure 5. Their awesome lipid nature is evident. Note that they are α-branched β-hydroxy fatty acids. The α-branch is 22 carbon atoms long in *M. avium* and 24 carbon atoms long in *M. tuberculosis* (28–31). The main chain can contain up to 60 carbon atoms (28–31). They are driven to associate with each other through powerful hydrophobic, albeit noncovalent, interactions. Thus, the wall may be thought of as a two-layered affair. The innermost layer is the peptidoglycan component similar to that of many bacteria. The outer-

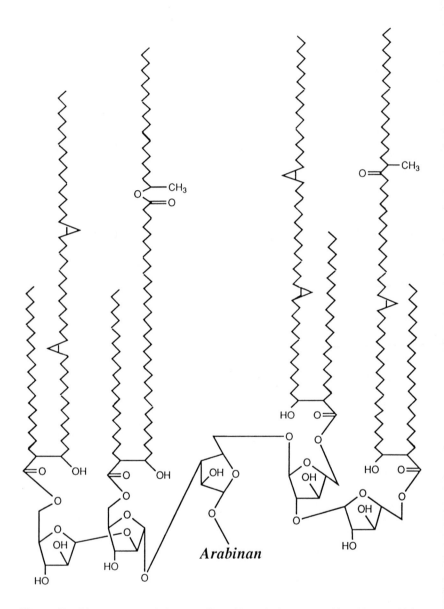

Figure 5   The structure of the mycolic acids and the pentaarabinoside to which they are attached.

most layer is the mycolic acid lipid "wall." The two layers are then held together by the arabinogalactan and linker region.

The theme of drug development focused on in this chapter is either inhibition of the synthesis of the outer layer of the wall directly (mycolic acids) or inhibition of the polysaccharide which connects it to the inner layer. These potentially new drugs are necessarily best designed with knowledge about how it is all put together.

III. Biosynthesis of the Mycobacterial Cell Wall

In this section, we describe what is known about the biosynthesis of the arabinogalactan. The key component of carbohydrate biosynthesis in general is an enzyme known as a glycosyl transferase (32). Inhibition of the mycobacterial cell wall glycosyl transferases, that is, the arabinosyl and/or galactosyl transferases, is an important drug development priority (see Sect. IV.B). Glycosyl transferases transfer a glycosyl unit from a glycosyl donor (see below) to the hydroxyl group of a growing oligosaccharide. The same glycosyl donor can be used by a number of glycosyl transferases. The specificity of the reaction results from any given glycosyl transferase recognizing only a specific sugar or group of sugars in the acceptor and then transferring the sugar from the donor to a specific hydroxyl group in a specific (α or β) anomeric configuration.

Glycosyl donors are generally found in nature in two forms. The more common form is known as a sugar nucleotide; for example, dTDP-Rha (Fig. 6). Here the sugar is glycosidically attached to the β-phosphate of a nucleotide diphosphate. Typically, many different glycosyl transferases will use the same sugar nucleotides as the specificity lies in the transferase molecule and the acceptor. Thus, dTDP-Rha is used by numerous gram-negative bacteria to insert rhamnosyl residues into a large number of lipopolysaccharide O-antigens. The second and less common glycosyl donor found in bacteria is a sugar phosphate polyprenol. In this case, the sugar is still glycosidically attached to a phosphate but the phosphate in turn is attached to a polyisoprene lipid. It generally contains 11 five-carbon units, but in mycobacteria it contains 10 five-carbon units at most (see Sect. III.C). These donors are membrane associated in contrast to sugar nucleotides, which are soluble. In the 1950s and 1960s, most of the common sugar nucleotides and sugar phosphate isoprenes were discovered and characterized (32). However, notably lacking were those involved in mycobacterial metabolism. These sugar nucleotides and sugar lipids are only now being isolated and identified. Inhibition of their formation as a strategy for designing new drugs is discussed in Section IV.A.

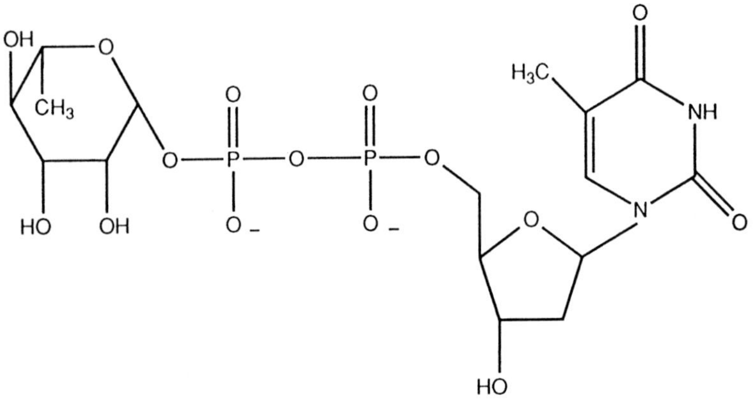

Figure 6   The structure of dTDP-Rha.

A. Mycobacteria Containing dTDP-Rha

Recent studies (33) have resulted in the recognition that the nucleotide donor of the rhamnosyl residue present in the linker region is likely to be dTDP-Rha (see Fig. 6). Mycobacteria are able to synthesize this sugar nucleotide from G1c-1-phosphate and TTP in the same fashion as gram-negative bacteria, which use L-rhamnose residues in their lipopolysaccharide (32). Since mammals do not use rhamnose, this is a good drug target.

B. UDP-Gal*p* Is a Mycobacterial Metabolite

The donor of the galactofuranosyl residues in the cell wall needs to be identified in order to begin to understand the biosynthesis of the cell wall and develop drugs against it. There is only one case of a previous biosynthesis study of a polymer composed of galactofuranosyl residues (34,35). In this case, a penicillin mold was found to synthesize a polysaccharide known as galactocarlose, which is composed of linear β-1, 5-galactofuranosyl residues (36). The investigators found that UDP-Gal*p* could in fact serve as a biosynthetic precursor of this polymer (34). Further investigations revealed that the UDP-Gal*p* was subsequently converted by an enzyme to UDP-Gal*f* (35) (Fig. 7) and that this sugar nucleotide was the donor of the galactofuranosyl residues. Studies (37) have commenced in various laboratories to ascertain whether a similar mechanism might occur in mycobacteria. Initial results have consistently shown that the UDP-Gal*p* is, in fact, a readily formed sugar nucleotide in mycobacteria. Since galactopyranosyl residues are not present

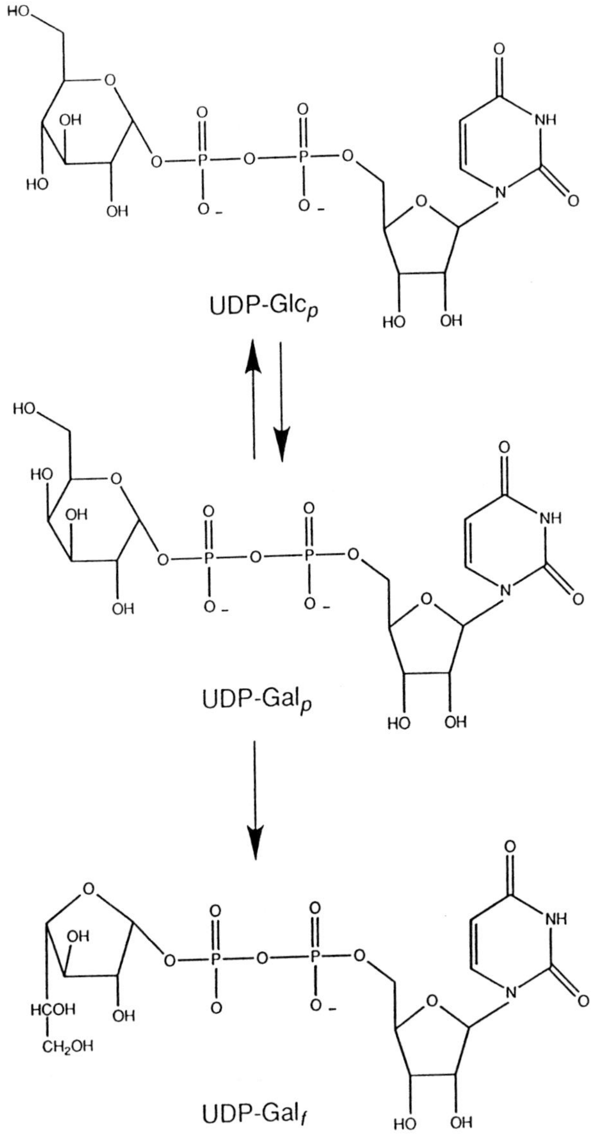

Figure 7 The formation of UDP-Gal*p* from UDP-Glc*p*, which has been shown to occur in mycobacteria. The formation of UDP-Gal*f* from UDP-Gal*p*, which has been postulated to occur in mycobacteria but remains to be definitively shown.

in mycobacteria, the logical explanation of the presence of UDP-Gal*p* is that, as in penicillin mold, this sugar nucleotide is a biosynthetic precursor of UDP-Gal*f*, the actual donor. Research to establish whether this is the case is still proceeding, but it appears likely that the donor of galactofuranosyl donors in mycobacteria is UDP-Gal*f*.

C. β-D-Ara*f*-Monophosphodecaprenol Is Found in Mycobacteria

Studies to look for a sugar nucleotide of Ara*f* residues in mycobacteria have been frustratingly slow and have not yet been successful to the author's knowledge. In fact, the biosynthetic origin of the carbon atoms of this relatively simple molecule (D-Ara) remains unknown. A bright spot in this gloomy picture is the isolation and characterization of β-D-Ara*f*-monophosphodecaprenol by Beata Wolucka and coworkers (38) (Fig. 8). This compound, by its structure, is expected to be a lipid-linked donor of arabinosyl residues. Preliminary experiments utilizing the compound in radioactive form (39) confirm this expectation, although more definitive studies need to be performed. How this compound is formed remains a mystery, but proof of its role as an arabinosyl donor will be highly beneficial to developing new drugs against the biosynthesis of the mycobacterial cell wall as described below.

D. Identification of the Donor of Mycolyl Residues Is an Important Undertaking

Although mycolic acids are obviously not carbohydrates, the concept of a mycolic donor is appropriate. The mycolic acids are not synthesized directly on the terminal arabinosyl residues but rather put together in a different context as an activated ester and eventually transferred to the arabinan. A possible donor of these mycolic acids has been suggested to be trehalose monomycolate (40). In this compound (40,41), a mycolic acid is attached to *C*-6 of trehalose 1,1'-α,α'-diglucose. Definitive studies confirming or disproving the role of this molecule as the donor of mycolic acids to the cell wall are

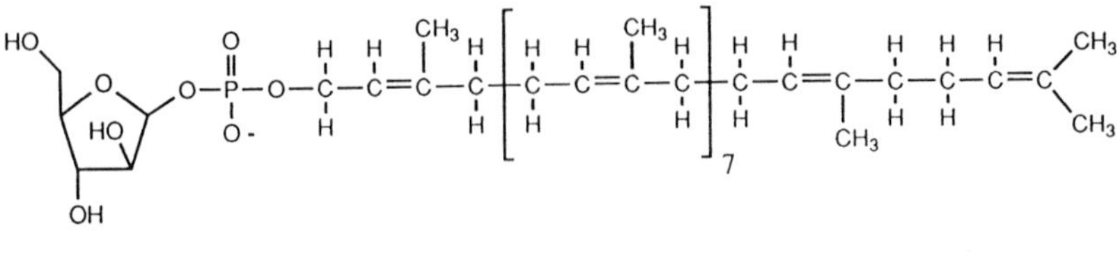

Figure 8   The structure of β-D-Ara*f*-monophosphodecaprenol.

urgently needed, as the attachment of mycolic acids to the cell wall arabinogalactan is an obvious drug target that cannot be developed without more fundamental information.

E. Sugar Acceptors

In the previous section, what was known about the sugar donors needed to synthesize the mycolylarabinogalactan was summarized, and it was seen that some progress has been made in this area. The identity of the acceptors in all cases remains a complete mystery in mycobacteria. Clearly, the acceptors are an oligosaccharide of arabinosyl or galactosyl residues, but the molecules they are attached to at their reducing end remains unknown. There is some precedence in other bacteria to suggest possibilities (42) but no evidence for the validity of extending these conclusions to mycobacteria. In parallel with other bacteria, it would be expected that the initial acceptor of arabinogalactan biosynthesis would be decaprenyl phosphate and N-acetylglucosamine phosphate would be transferred from UDP-GlcNAc to form α-D-GlcNAc-diphosphodecaprenol. This lipid sugar would then be the acceptor of a rhamnosyl residue donated from dTDP-Rha and the resulting disaccharide diphosphate lipid the acceptor for the galactosyl residues of the galactan. In theory, the whole arabinogalactan could be built upon this lipid acceptor and transferred after complete synthesis to the six position of a peptidoglycan muramic acid in the same fashion as teichoic acids in gram-positive bacteria (42).

F. Glycosyl Transferases

No glycosyl transferase activity has been well defined in mycobacterial cell wall arabinogalactan biogenesis. In contrast, the transfer of mannosyl residues to mycobacterial glycolipids from GDP-Man has been demonstrated (43,44), as has the transfer of mannosyl residues to exogenously supplied oligomannosides from β-D-Man$p$-monophosphodecaprenol (45). Hopefully, now that the sugar donors involved in cell wall biosynthesis are now beginning to be identified, reactions catalyzed by specific cell wall glycosyl transferases will also be carried out soon.

IV. Designing Inhibitors

It should be clear to the reader that although the cell wall arabinogalactan offers a superb target for rationally designed chemotherapy, capitalization of this potential remains extremely difficult because of the lack of basic biochemical information on its synthesis. Thus, the most important priority in developing drug targets based on the cell wall of arabinogalactan lies in gaining a basic understanding of this organelle is biosynthesized. Nevertheless, it is possible at this time to point out some of the more promising targets that are emerging.

A. Inhibition of Donor Formation

As discussed above, evidence that dTDP-Rha is synthesized by mycobacteria coupled with the key role of rhamnose in the linker region (see Fig. 6) suggests inhibition of the formation of this sugar nucleotide to be an area ripe for exploitation. This idea is furthered by the fact that the four enzymes known for its formation are well characterized in other bacteria (Fig. 9), and there is preliminary evidence that the same enzymes are utilized in mycobacteria as well (33). In addition, the enzymes involved have been cloned and sequenced from many bacteria (46–48). An approach to developing drugs against the formation of dTDP-Rha in mycobacteria involves cloning the relevant four enzymes and developing inhibitors against the reactions they catalyze. The development of such inhibitors can proceed based on published mechanisms (49) or most powerfully by crystallizing the proteins in question. Obtaining x-ray diffraction structures and designing inhibitors based on the active site environments has been done most dramatically for an antiviral (8) drug. The job is not complete once good inhibitors of the enzymes have been identified. The next step is to get an inhibitor that will be capable of entering the mycobacteria and getting to the target. Actually, of the two jobs, the second task is probably the more challenging.

Inhibitors of the formation of the other two donors, UDP-Gal$f$ and β-D-Ara$f$-monophosphodecaprenol, are also attractive drug targets. Realistically, realization of this goal will first require definition of the enzymatic routes by which these compounds are formed and development of the assays of enzymes involved in their synthesis. Once such assays are in place, compounds can be tested for activity and enzymes can be purified to yield further basic information needed to enhance the possibility of successful new drug production along similar lines to those described above for dTDP-Rha.

B. Designing Inhibitors of Glycosyl Transferases

Although the structures of the acceptors are not known in detail (see Section III.F), the structure of the arabinogalactan allows some information about the donor to be deduced. For example, it is clear in Figure 4 that an arabinosyl transferase must exist which recognizes the disaccharide α-D-Ara$f$(1→5)α-D-Ara$f$ and transfers a third arabinosyl residue to it. This is true even though it is not clear what the disaccharide is attached to in the mycobacteria as

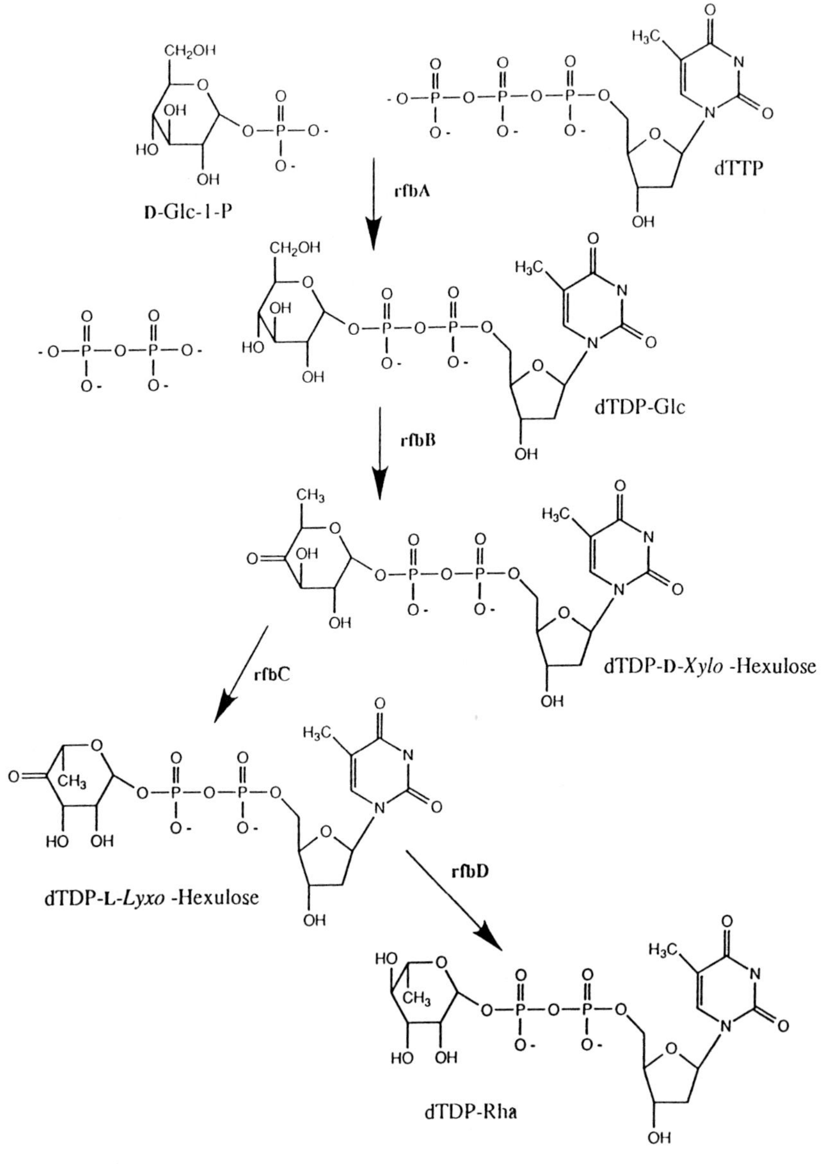

Figure 9 The formation of dTDP-Rha from TTP and glucose-1-phosphate.

arabinan biosynthesis proceeds. Thus, the enzyme must recognize and bind to the above disaccharide. Inhibitors based on the structure of the acceptor saccharide have been designed in other systems (50) and similar strategies should be applicable to mycobacteria. This is not only the case for the arabinosyl transferase described above but also applies to galactosyl transferases.

C. Designing Inhibitors of Mycolic Acid Biosynthesis

An exciting report (51) has recently appeared on the design of an inhibitor of mycolic acid biosynthesis. Even though the entire biosynthetic pathway of mycolic acid formation is not known, an important step has been recognized and a compound designed to inhibit this transformation prepared. As illustrated in Figure 10, the saturated unbranched C-24 fatty acid is desaturated at the five position. These types of unsaturations were known from other systems to be inhibited by cyclopropene rings and the investigators thus prepared a cyclopropene C-24 derivative. The compound was shown to inhibit the formation of mycolic acids by a cell-free system (51). Therefore, the next step in this encouraging development is further to test the compound against whole bacteria for activity.

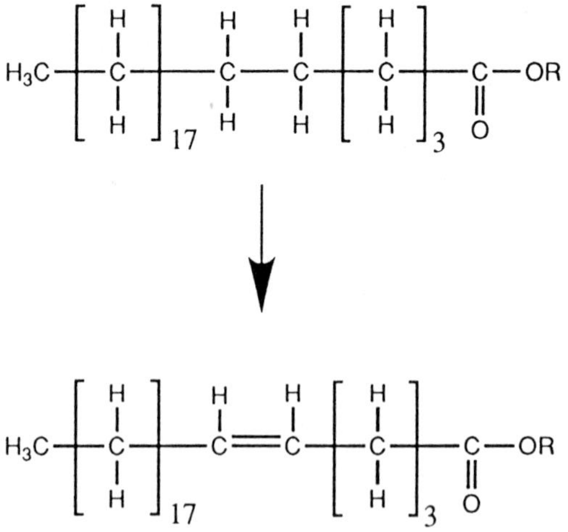

Figure 10 The desaturation of C-24 fatty acid to form a double bond between carbons five and six. The reaction is on the pathway to mycolic acid biosynthesis and inhibitors against it have been prepared (51). The identity of R is unknown.

D. Designing Inhibitors of Cell Walls Utilizing Known Cell Wall Drugs

Although the detailed mechanism of action of isoniazid (INH) has resisted many attempts at elucidation, it is known to act against cell wall mycolic acid biosynthesis. An important development in this field is the recognition of how mycobacteria develop resistance to this drug. In one study, a mutation in the *kat*G gene was shown to result in resistance to this drug. Interestingly, this gene encodes for an enzyme showing both catalase and peroxidase activity (52,53). A mutation in the gene resulted in INH resistance. Conversely, introduction of the gene restores sensitivity to INH (53). The reason why the catalase peroxidase is necessary for INH activity remains unclear, and, unfortunately, since the loss of the activity of this gene results in resistance, it is not immediately clear how this finding can be exploited to develop new novel inhibitors of mycolic acid synthesis. However, in another study, a second gene, *inh*A (which has nothing to do with the role of catalase-peroxidase) (54) was identified. Sequencing of this gene showed homology to an *E. coli* enzyme *env*M, a gene coding for a protein thought to be involved in fatty acid biosynthesis. Furthermore, cell-free assays suggested that the gene product of *inh*A is involved in mycolic acid biosynthesis. The investigators suggest that the gene product of *inh*A may be the primary target of action of INH and the related drug ethionamide. Therefore, this research can be moved toward new drug development. The protein can be expressed, perhaps crystallized, and new inhibitors of its actions developed. It will be important to define exactly what reactions it catalyzes.*

A final example of using known drugs to develop new targets against the cell wall concerns ethambutol. Genes confirming resistance to ethambutol have been recently cloned (55). Although not yet demonstrated biochemically, these gene products could be proteins necessary for cell wall biosynthesis, as numerous studies have shown that ethambutol inhibits cell wall biosynthesis probably by inhibiting arabinan biosynthesis. In this approach, an enzyme critical to cell wall biosynthesis may have been isolated. As has been the running commentary of this review, exploitation of these results will

---

*Note added in proof: This work has developed in an almost unbelievable fashion [Dessen, A., A. Quemard, W. R. Jacobs, Jr., and J. C. Sacchettini. 1995. J. of Cellular Biochemistry Abs. Sup. 19B:B3-109:67(Abstract)]. The *inh*A protein has been expressed and shown to catalyze the reduction of a double bond in mycolic acid biosynthesis. The enzyme was crystallized allowing inhibitors to be designed. These inhibitors were then shown to inhibit the growth of mycobacteria.

first require understanding of the basic biochemistry catalyzed by the enzymes that have been cloned.

References

1. Draper P. The anatomy of mycobacteria. In: Ratledge C, Sanford J, eds. The Biology of Mycobacteria, Vol. I. London: Academic Press, 1982:9–52.
2. Jarlier V, Gutmann L, Nikaido H. Interplay of cell wall barrier and beta-lactamase activity determines high resistance to beta-lactam antibiotics in *Mycobacterium chelonae*. Antimicrob Agents Chemother 1991; 35:1937–1939.
3. Hoffner SE, Svenson SB, Kallenius G. Synergistic effects of anti-mycobacterial drug combinations on *Mycobacterium avium* complex determined radiometrically in liquid medium. Eur J Clin Microbiol 1987; 6:530–535.
4. Tomioka H, Saito H, Sato K. Comparative antimycobacterial activities of the newly synthesized quinolone AM-1155, sparfloxacin, and ofloxacin. Antimicrob Agents Chemother 1993; 37:1259–1263.
5. Hoffner SE, Kratz M, Olsson Liljequist B, et al. In-vitro synergistic activity between ethambutol and fluorinated quinolones against *Mycobacterium avium* complex. J Antimicrob Chemother 1989; 24:317–324.
6. Young LS, Berlin OGW, Inderlied CB. Activity of ciprofloxacin and other fluorinated quinolones against mycobacteria. Am J Med 1987; 82:23–26.
7. Cooksey RC, Crawford JT, Jacobs WR, Shinnick TM. A Rapid method for screening antimicrobial agents for activities against a strain of *Mycobacterium-tuberculosis* expressing firefly luciferase. Antimicrob Agents Chemother 1993; 37:1348–1352.
8. von Itzstein M, Wu WY, Kok GB, et al. Rational design of potent sialidase-based inhibitors of influenza virus replication. Nature 1993; 363:418–423.
9. Melancon-Kaplan J, Hunter SW, McNeil M, et al. Immunological significance of *Mycobacterium leprae* cell walls. Proc Natl Acad Sci USA 1988; 85:1917–1921.
10. Misaki A, Seto N, Azuma I. Structure and immunological properties of D-arabino-D-galactan isolated from cell walls of Mycobacterium species. J Biochem 1974; 76:15–22.
11. Petit JF, Lederer E. The structure of the mycobacterial cell wall. In: Kubica GP, Wayne LG, eds. The Mycobacteria, a Sourcebook. New York: Marcel Dekker, 1984:301–322.
12. Ghuysen J-M. Use of bacteriolytic enzymes in determination of wall structure and their role in cell metabolism. Bacteriol Rev 1968; 32:425–464.
13. Araki Y, Nakatani T, Nakayama K, Ito E. Occurrence of N-nonsubstituted glucosamine residues in peptidoglycan of lysozyme-resistant cell walls from *Bacillus cereus*. J Biol Chem 1972; 247:6312–6322.

14. Kanetsuna F, San Blas G. Chemical analysis of a mycolic acid-arabinogalactan-mucopeptide complex of mycobacterial cell wall. Biochim Biophys Acta 1970; 208:434–443.

15. Kaya S, Yokoyama K, Ito E. N-Acetylmannosaminyl (1-4) N-acetylglucosamine, a linkage unit between glycerol teichoic acid and peptidoglycan in cell walls of several Bacillus strains. J Bacteriol 1984; 158:990–996.

16. Heptinstall J, Coley J, Ward PJ, et al. The linkage of sugar phosphate polymer to peptidoglycan in walls of *Micrococcus sp.* 2102. Biochem J 1978; 169:329–336.

17. Coley J, Tarelli E, Archibald AR, Baddiley J. The linkage between teichoic acid and peptidoglycan in bacterial cell walls. FEBS Lett 1978; 88:1–9.

18. Ward JB, Curtis CAM. The biosynthesis and linkage of teichuronic acid to peptidoglycan in *Bacillus licheniformis.* Eur J Biochem 1982; 122:125–132.

19. Misaki A, Ikawa N, Kato T, Kotani S. Cell wall arabinogalactan of *Mycobacterium phlei.* Biochim Biophys Acta 1970; 215:405–408.

20. Vilkas E, Amar C, Markovits J, et al. Occurrence of a galactofuranose disaccharide in immunoadjuvant fractions of *Mycobacterium tuberculosis* (cell walls and wax D). Biochim Biophys Acta 1973; 297:423–435.

21. McNeil M, Wallner SJ, Hunter SW, Brennan PJ. Demonstration that the galactosyl and arabinosyl residues in the cell wall arabinogalactan of *Mycobacterium leprae* and *Mycobacterium tuberculosis* are furanoid. Carbohydr Res 1987; 169: 299–308.

22. Daffe M, Brennan PJ, McNeil M. Predominant structural features of the cell wall arabinogalactan of *Mycobacterium tuberculosis*–specific as revealed through characterization of oligoglycosyl alditol fragments by gas chromatography/mass spectrometry and by ^{1}H and ^{13}C-NMR analyses. J Biol Chem 1990; 265:6734–6743.

23. Besra GS, Khoo K-H, McNeil M, et al. A Multiply branched tricosaarabinoside and non-branched linear tricosgalactoside are present in mycobacterial cell wall arabinogalactan. Unpublished data 1994.

24. McNeil M, Daffe M, Brennan PJ. Location of the mycolyl ester substituent in the cell walls of mycobacteria. J Biol Chem 1991; 266:13217–13223.

25. Barksdale L, Kim K-S. Mycobacterium. Bacteriol Rev 1977; 41:217–372.

26. Nikaido H, Kim SH, Rosenberg EY. Physical organization of lipids in the cell wall of *Mycobacterium chelonae.* Mol Microbiol 1993; 8:1025–1030.

27. Minnikin DE. Chemical principles in the organization of lipid components in the mycobacterial cell envelope. Res Microbiol 1991; 142:423–427.

28. Minnikin DE, Goodfellow M. Lipid composition in the classification and identification of acid-fast bacteria. In: Goodfellow M, Board RG, eds. Microbiological Classification and Identification. London: Academic Press, 1980:189–256.

29. Minnikin DE, Minnikin SM, Parlett JH, et al. Mycolic acid patterns of some species of Mycobacterium. Arch Microbiol 1984; 139:225–231.

30. Minnikin DE, Polgar N. The mycolic acids from human and avian tubercle bacilli. Chem Comm 1967; 18:916–918.

31. Minnikin DE, Polgar N. The methoxymycolic and ketomycolic acids from human tubercle bacilli. Chem Comm 1967; 22:1172–1174.

32. Shibaev VN. Biosynthesis of bacterial polysaccharide chains composed of repeating units. In: Anonymous. Advances in Carbohydrate Chemistry and Biochemistry. Academic Press, 1986:277–339.

33. Scherman M, Brown R, McNeil M. Formation of dTDP-Rha in mycobacteria. Unpublished data, 1994.

34. Trejo AG, Haddock JW, Chittenden GJF, Baddiley J. The biosynthesis of galactofuranosyl residues in galactocarolose. Biochem J 1971; 122:49–57.

35. Trejo AG, Chittenden GJF, Buchanan JG, Baddiley J. Uridine diphosphate α-*D*-galactofuranose, an intermediate in the biosynthesis of galactofuranosyl residues. Biochem J 1970; 117:637–639.

36. Gander JE, Jentoft NH, Drewes LR, Rick PD. The 5-O-β-D-galactofuranosyl–containing exocellular glycopeptide of Penicillin charlesii. J Biol Chem 1974; 249:2063–2072.

37. Brown R, Bournonville LK, Wolucka BA, et al. Formation of UDP-Gal*p* from UDP-Glc in mycobacteria. Unpublished data, 1994.

38. Wolucka BA, McNeil MR, Hoffmann E, et al. Recognition of the likely carrier lipid for arabinan biosynthesis and its relation to the mode of action of ethambutol in mycobacteria. Unpublished data, 1994.

39. Brennan PJ, Mikusova K, Besra GS. Transfer of arabinose into arabinan containing polymers using β-D-Ara*f*-decaprenyl phosphate as a donor. Unpublished data, 1994.

40. Kilburn JO, Takayama K, Armstrong EL. Synthesis of trehalose dimycolate (cord factor) by a cell-free system of *Mycobacterium smegmatis*. Biochem Biophys Res Commun 1982; 108:132–139.

41. Strain SM, Toubiana R, Ribi E, Parker R. Separation of the mixture of trehalose 6,6′-dimycolates comprising the mycobacterial glycolipid fraction. Biochem Biophys Res Commun 1977; 77:449–456.

42. Ward JB. Teichoic and teichuronic Acids: Biosynthesis, assembly, and location. Microbiol Rev 1981; 45:211–243.

43. Brennan PJ, Ballou CE. Biosynthesis of mannophosphoinositides by *Mycobacterium phlei*. J Biol Chem 1968; 243:2975–2984.

44. Brennan PJ, Ballou CE. Biosynthesis of mannophosphoinositides by *Mycobacterium phlei*. J Biol Chem 1967; 242:3046–3056.

45. Yokoyama K, Ballou CE. Synthesis of alpha 1-6 mannooligosaccharides in *Mycobacterium smegmatis*. Function of beta-mannosylphosphoryldecaprenol as the mannosyl donor. J Biol Chem 1989; 264:21621–21628.

46. Xiang SH, Haase AM, Reeves PR. Variation of the rfb gene clusters in *Salmonella enterica*. J Bacteriol 1993; 175:4877–4884.

47. Jiang XM, Neal B, Santiago F, et al. Structure and sequence of the rfb (o antigen) gene cluster of *Salmonella serovar typhimurium* (strain LT2). Mol Microbiol 1991; 5:695–713.

48. Rajakumar K, Jost HB, Sasakawa C, et al. Nucleotide sequence of the rhamnose biosynthetic operon of *Shigella flexneri* 2a and role of lipopolysaccharide in virulence. J Bacteriol 1994; 176:2362–2373.

49. Yu Y, Russell RN, Thorson JS, Liu L, Liu H. Mechanistic studies of the biosynthesis of 3,6-dideoxyhexoses in *Yersinia pseudotuberculosis.* J Biol Chem 1992; 267:5868–5875.

50. Hindsgaul O, Kaur KJ, Srivastava G, et al. Evaluation of deoxygenated oligosaccharide acceptor analogs as specific inhibitors of glycosyltransferases. J Biol Chem 1991; 266:17858–17862.

51. Wheeler PR, Besra GS, Minnikin DE, Ratledge C. Inhibition of mycolic acid biosynthesis in a cell wall preparation from *Mycobacterium smegmatis* by methyl 4-(2-octadecylcyclopropen-1-yl) butanoate, a structure analogue of a key precursor. Lett Appl Microbiol 1993; 17:33–36.

52. Zhang Y, Garbe T, Young D. Transformation wit katG restores isoniazid-sensitivity in *Mycobacterium tuberculosis* isolates resistant to a range of drug concentrations. Mol Microbiol 1993; 8:521–524.

53. Zhang Y, Heym B, Allen B, et al. The catalase-peroxidase gene and isoniazid resistance of *Mycobacterium tuberculosis.* Nature 1992; 358:591–593.

54. Banerjee A, Dubnau E, Quemard A, et al. inhA, A gene encoding a target for isoniazid and ethionamide in *Mycobacterium tuberculosis.* Science 1994; 263: 227–230.

55. Suzuki A, Inamine J. An operon responsible for resistance to ethambutol. Unpublished data, 1994.

AUTHOR INDEX

Italic numbers give the page on which the complete reference is listed.

SUBJECT INDEX

A

Absorption (*see* specific drugs)
Acquired resistance, 116
Agar:
  Löwenstein-Jensen medium, 120–121
  Middlebrook 7H10, 120–121
Agar dilution method, liquid medium and, 125
AIDS patients (*see* dMAC)
Alkaline phosphatase, dMAC and, 89–90
Alternative complement pathway, 165
  antibodies and, 167
  glycopeptidolipid, 165
  phagocytosis, 165–168

American Thoracic Society, recommendations, 241–242
Amikacin:
  animal models and, 151
  combination studies, 247–248
  pharmacokinetics, 224–226
Aminoglycosides, 224–226
  liposomes and, 225–226
Aminosidine (Paromomycin), 226
Anemia, dMAC and, 88–89
Animal models, 141–158
  active agents in, 145
  amikacin and, 151
  azithromcyin, 153–154
  BAY 3118 and, 154
  beige mouse, 144
  characteristics of, 142